Between Anthropology and Psychiatry

Between Anthropology and Psychiatry

Roland Littlewood and Simon Dein

berghahn
NEW YORK • OXFORD
www.berghahnbooks.com

First published in 2026 by
Berghahn Books
www.berghahnbooks.com

Library of Congress Cataloging-in-Publication Data
A C.I.P. cataloging record is available from the Library of Congress
Library of Congress Cataloging in Publication Control Number: 2026000158

British Library Cataloguing in Publication Data
A catalogue record for this book is available from the British Library

EU GPSR Authorized Representative
LOGOS EUROPE, 9 rue Nicolas Poussin, 17000, LA ROCHELLE, France Email: Contact@logoseurope.eu

ISBN 978-1-83695-461-3 hardback
ISBN 978-1-83695-462-0 epub
ISBN 978-1-83695-463-7 web pdf

https://doi.org/10.3167/9781836954613

In loving memory of Professor Roland Littlewood, a pioneer in the study of Anthropology and Psychiatry (d. 22nd November 2025).

Contents

ACKNOWLEDGEMENTS

We are grateful to our co-authors and to the journal editors for permission to reprint these papers.

1. Roland Littlewood and Simon Dein (1995), 'The Effectiveness of Words', *Culture, Medicine and Psychiatry* 19: 359–83.
2. Simon Dein (2010), 'A Messiah from the Dead: Cultural Performance in Lubavitcher Messianism', *Social Compass* 57: 537–54.
3. Roland Littlewood and Simon Dein (2013), 'Did Christianity Lead to Schizophrenia? Psychosis, Psychology and Self-Reference', *Transcultural Psychiatry* 50: 397–420.
4. Roland Littlewood and Goffredo Bartocci (2005), 'Religious Stigmata, Magnetic Fluids and Conversion Hysteria: One Survival of "Virtual Force" Theories in Scientific Medicine?', *Transcultural Psychiatry* 42: 596–609.
5. Simon Dein, Malcolm Alexander and David Napier (2008), 'Jinn, Psychiatry and Contested Notions of Misfortune among East London Bangladeshis', *Transcultural Psychiatry* 45: 31–55.
6. Simon Dein and Satoi Sermbhi (2001), 'The Use of Traditional Healing in South Asian Psychiatric Patients in the U.K.: Interactions between Professional and Folk Psychiatries', *Transcultural Psychiatry* 38(2): 243–57.
7. Roland Littlewood (2002), 'Trauma and the Kanun: Two Responses to Loss in Albania and Kosova', *International Journal of Social Psychiatry* 48(2): 86–96.
8. Roland Littlewood (2001), 'Social Institutions and Psychological Explanations: Druze Reincarnation as a Therapeutic Resource', *British Journal of Medical Psychology* 74: 213–22.

9. Simon Dein and Roland Littlewood (2005), 'Apocalyptic Suicide: From a Pathological to an Eschatological Interpretation', *International Journal of Social Psychiatry* 51: 198–210.

10. Roland Littlewood (2021), 'The Advent of the Adversary: Negative Power in Certain Religio-Therapeutic Systems', *Anthropolitan*, 20 October, N.P.

11. Simon Dein and Roland Littlewood (2011), 'Religion and Psychosis: A Common Evolutionary Trajectory?', *Transcultural Psychiatry* 48: 318–25.

12. Roland Littlewood (2009), 'Neglect as Project: How Two Societies Forget', *Journal of the Royal Anthropological Institute* 15(1): 113–30.

13. Simon Dein (2003), 'Against Belief: The Usefulness of Explanatory Model Research In Medical Anthropology', *Social Theory and Health* 1: 149–62.

Introduction

Monotheism and Mental Order

So, mental order, not mental disorder.

Ever since the three disciplines of anthropology, psychology and psychiatry differentiated themselves out of a more general nineteenth-century 'human science', many have argued about the question of normality or pathology accorded to certain novel patterns once observed by colonial officials, missionaries and travellers in non-European societies. Such patterns as *amok, latah, koro, kuru, witigo* or various spirit possession states were often picked up and observed by the European because they seemed bizarre and exotic, maybe even insane. They were initially simply observed and described, but then Western psychiatrists wondered if they might be included in the pattern of mental illness then described in European and American mental hospitals. Most notable among these was *amok*, a Malay word which has passed into English for indiscriminate and unmotivated violence by a person against others.

In one of the first discussions of the problems of comparing psychiatric illness across societies, the German hospital psychiatrist Emile Kraepelin, after a brief trip to Java during which he collected accounts of amok and observed hospitalized patients, noted that 'reliable comparison is of course only possible if we are able to draw clear distinctions between identifiable illnesses' (Kraepelin 1902). This proved difficult given the wide variety of local patterns together with the intention, which Kraepelin enthusiastically shared, to fit them into the restricted number of categories identified in European hospitals. He happily included various local patterns into this clinical nosology, arguing that whilst their 'content' may differ from Western illness, their essential 'form' remained the same. As Kraepelin's pupil Karl Birnbaum put it, the pathoplastic envelopes of culture just gave 'content, colouring and contour to individual illness whose both form and character have already been biologically established' (Birnbaum 1923). Wittgenstein critically likened this sort of approach in the psychological sciences to our picking away the leaves of an artichoke, in a hopeless attempt to uncover some real artichoke, on the assumption that (to use the anthropologist Clifford Geertz's sarcastic aphorism) 'culture is icing, biology cake. . . difference is shallow, likeness deep'. Even our later, statistical attempt to develop an international nomenclature favoured by epidemiologists in the 1970s and 1980s resulted in circular and quite varied arguments about categorization and universality.

Multitudes of colonial doctors, journalists and other commentators described local patterns of ritual, distress and therapy as if they were Western illnesses: shamans and prophets were regarded as severely disordered, even mentally ill. Possession cults and revitalist movements were considered hysteria, bodily transformations as self-mutilation, gender-based ceremonies as perverse sexuality, metaphysical speculations as delusion. Local treatments were useless superstition and dumb acceptance. This all ignored the possibility that certain reactions such as eating disorders, parasuicide, depression, obsessions or multiple personality disorder might be understood in (Euro-American) social or cultural terms. In other words, 'psychopathology' was considered devoid of any meaning and could only be explained as a biological contingency.

Anthropologists however continued to debate possession states and so on in non-pathological language until the pervasive influence of psychoanalysis in the United States academic world resulted in the Culture and Personality school of the 1930s to 1950s. This presumed that variant patterns could be understood on the basis of individual psychological development as presumed by Western psychodynamic theory. A generation of American cultural anthropologists became dominated by psychoanalysis. In the most extreme case, whole societies came to be identified with psychological patterns which were characteristic of severe mental illness in Western societies (e.g. Benedict 1935). The occasional social anthropologist objected that whole cultures could not be identified through individual psychological norms and that patterns of infant weaning – a favourite idiom of the C&P School – could not be said to determine the adult personality expected in a particular community, although they might exemplify it (Harris 1957).

By the late 1950s American psychiatry and anthropology had gradually found psychoanalysis less persuasive and the newly dominant McGill school of transcultural psychiatry in Canada, with its influential journal, was founded on a more descriptive and less normalizing basis. This was exemplified by the World Health Organisation's purely empirical studies as to whether schizophrenia was a universal disease or whether it could be explained by certain patterns of Western family life, as some argued. Those 'exotic' reactions which had appeared as possibly pathological were now classified as 'culture-bound syndromes' (Yap 1967) which were variously regarded as exaggerations of local culture or specific reflections of local culture, or as psychological conflict between the two. Patterns which could be more easily fitted into international universal classification or which seemed 'organic' (biological in origin) were generally excluded from this new category and from the developing area of cultural psychiatry.

Social anthropologists generally continued purely descriptive studies of diverse social roles and institutions or religion, based on eclectic sociological theory rather than on clinical or psychoanalytical presumptions, though they occasionally referenced an appropriate psychological theory. By the 1980s the American Arthur Kleinman had announced a new cross-cultural psychiatry which would emphasize the full exploration of local patterns and local explanations before one attempted to fit them into a medical framework. It was in this period that we both trained in social anthropology (before the separate speciality of medical anthropology developed) in a pattern earlier advocated by W.H.R. Rivers, the English anthropologist and psychiatrist in 1916. (He is now more generally remembered for his work on 'shell shock'.)

The area between anthropology and psychiatry remains a murky area. Social anthropology and psychiatry are two different modes of thought, each with their particular paradigms and methods. They often deal with the same phenomenon from their different starting points, but we cannot reduce one to the other, any more than we can reduce interpretation to explanation – or the reverse. Both remain necessary in what we once called an 'ironic simultaneity' (Littlewood 1993). In some of the chapters here we have generally emphasized the descriptive social anthropological side; in others we have offered a more pathological and medical explanation.

Why psychiatry at all? We have revisited some of those traditional patterns and motifs which are of interest to cultural psychiatry without presuming an explanation necessarily rooted in pathology – patterns such as messianism, bereavement, local categorizations of illness and cure, the history of syndromes, bodily stigmata, sorcery and suicide. Indeed, we have previously argued against the very utility of the pathological idiom at all in psychiatry (Littlewood 1991). These interests just come under a general rubric of medicine because they are often undesirable and painful, whether we consider them abnormal psychologically or statistically, but to announce them prematurely as a disease entirely (as pathology) is not helpful. In some cases, such as in our Druze chapter, we argue that a pattern which strikes the

European rationalist as bizarre may be considered as having some therapeutic value, i.e. in reducing suffering. We bear in mind the (hypothetical) Proto-Indo European term *tarpen ali*, or 'ritual substitute', the conjectured root of our term 'therapy', to derive some equivalence between the social and the medical. We tried to hold both in play.

Given the salience of religion in those societies studied by social anthropologists, the background of cultural psychiatry frequently indicates 'religious' cognitions and actions. Contemporary research into religion and psychiatry largely focuses on healing psychological troubles (e.g. Koenig 2015).

And on the prevalence and outcomes of mental illness in those who are religious, we build upon the work of James (1902) and note that the overlaps between normative religious experience and psychopathology have attracted recent academic attention (Dein 2010). Both psychiatry and religion focus on the understanding and amelioration of suffering, providing different epistemological frameworks in which redemption and healing can occur. Both attempt to deal with the nature of human agency and its displacement in religious experience and mental illness, and thus with questions of self-harm and its boundaries. Beyond these lie certain moral issues and their possible resolution. In forensic psychiatry, evil and illness run perilously close together.

The papers we have chosen here for reprinting for a wider audience are limited to those from the so-called 'Abrahamic tradition' – from Western monotheism, whether Judaism, Christianity and Islam – or at least from cultures strongly influenced by these. Our use of the term 'monotheism' is not to suggest theology or high doctrine. Perhaps 'vernacular monotheism' might be a better if rather clumsy term. We are dealing with the everyday perceptions of ordinary people, not the esoteric deliberation of churchmen or clerics. While there are many similarities between the Abrahamic religions in terms of notions of the Divine, salvation, afterlife and understandings of suffering, our choice of papers reflects our ethnographic interests rather than any overarching theological or psychological framework.

We have selected these papers out of our various interests and have not proposed here to reprint our earlier work on racism and mental health, pathomimesis, the dramaturgical model of neuroses and spirit possession, on the Albanian 'third sex', euhemerism, Haitian zombification, or recent work on Hindu conversion to Christianity. The papers included nevertheless employ a variety of different approaches apart from general descriptive psychiatry and anthropology: interpretive semiotics, phenomenology, psychodynamics, the history of psychiatry, evolutionary psychology, even – in one case – patristic theology. We strongly adhere to an exploration of the psychiatry/anthropology domain which uses a diversity of methods and theories. We employ here both the naturalistic and the personalistic in a complementary antinomy. Neither is true, nor false.

The first section is dedicated to healing and redemption in Judaism – more specifically to practices among one ultra-orthodox Hasidic group in Brooklyn and east London. Chapter 1 looks at how they deal with sickness and their recourse to biomedicine and religious healing. According to their key text – Tanya – there is an intrinsic link between religious words and the physical body. At times of sickness Lubavitchers communicate with their leader, the Rebbe, whose manipulation of religious words results in bodily healing. This conforms with the anthropologist Malinowski's suggestion that the symbolic comes into play when the pragmatic fails. Mediated through the person of the Rebbe, testimonials offered by sufferers evoke images of exile and restitution which derive from Kabbalistic texts. Both Kabbalah and medical anthropology attempt to transcend not dissimilar epistemological dualisms: here those characteristic of monotheism and of contemporary science. Yet the 'lower root' of Kabbalah affirms a material reality known through immediate sensory experience which recalls the rationale of biomedicine.

The second chapter considers the local situation after the death of the Rebbe, the spiritual leader who was frequently identified as the Jewish Messiah, and who would supposedly reveal himself as such, ushering in the redemption. When he died in 1994, he had not fulfilled his followers' messianic expectations. We look at the role of phenomenological experience and embodiment, the prophetic milieu, and modern communication media in maintaining a sense of the Rebbe's continuing presence. This ritualized reaffirmation of belief seems to provide the bereaved followers with social and psychological meaning in the wake of 'failed' prophecy and thus render their experiences less distressing.

The next chapter deals with popular Christianity. 'Does Christianity Lead to Schizophrenia?' argues that our most devastating psychiatric illness, schizophrenia, has not been a constant over history, nor is it universal across contemporary societies. Using some phenomenological arguments, we suggest that a more affectively-laden psychosis, probably close to manic depression (bipolar disorder), which we term here proto-schizophrenia, is modified under the self-reflection and self-directed scrutiny of Christianity and modernity into an illness now recognized in the west as clinical schizophrenia.

The next chapter in this section describes our encounter with a southern Italian religious stigmatic and visionary, who at Easter time physically demonstrates in her body the signs of Jesus' crucifixion. We review the psychiatric concept of 'hysterical conversion' and consider Natuzza's experience in the light of her personal history. Since we wrote the original paper, she has died and there is now a more detailed account of her life and fame published in Italy (Turi 2009).

Two chapters come from the Islamic tradition. 'Jinn, Psychiatry and Contested Notions of Misfortune' records a project among the east London

Bangladeshi population as to their understanding of *Jinn* spirits; whilst all Muslims are presumed to accept the idea of *Jinn,* our informants showed a variety of opinions concerning them. 'The Use of Traditional Healing in South Asian Psychiatric Patients in the UK: Interactions between Professional and Folk Psychiatries' explores the use of traditional healing among psychiatric patients from India, Bangladesh, Pakistan or Sri Lanka living in London. Individuals with a range of psychiatric problems deployed both Western psychiatry and traditional healing concurrently, with little understanding of (nor interest in) how these treatment modalities worked.

Chapter 7 examines 'Two Responses to Loss in Albania and Kosova'. Social anthropology has proposed that social institutions and psychological reactions may at times be alternative ways of dealing with similar situations; and that at a high level of generality, they may be conceived of as variants of similar (psycho-social) phenomena. Response to sudden bereavement in Albanian Kosova may follow two routes: the customary law arguing stoicism but retribution, and the psychological idiom of 'trauma' recently introduced by Western European aid agencies. Similarities and differences between what at first appear two quite distinct responses are outlined.

The chapter on Druze reincarnation in Lebanon concerns a community which derives from Islam but should now be considered as a separate religion. The Druze adhere to a very non-Islamic idea of reincarnation which we argue attenuates the grief the family experienced about the members who died in the Lebanese civil war. We might compare this to responses to the death of the Rebbe in Chapter 2, both denying the finality of death.

The next three chapters deal with more general themes. 'Apocalyptic Suicide' criticizes purely psychological explanations of mass suicide, charisma and millennialism, to emphasize eschatological dualism in monotheistic and post-monotheistic communities. Chapter 10 considers the introduction into certain religious therapeutic systems of a second and contrary principle which has implications for our understanding of complementary opposition. 'Religion and Psychosis' uses ideas from evolutionary psychology, anthropology and the Cognitive Science of Religion – taking 'religion' in a more general sense than we have used it so far – as the recognition of something like human sensibility and agency in ultrahuman entities. We emphasize theory of mind and agent hyper-identification as significant in normal cognition, and hence in religious and psychotic cognitions.

The last two chapters reflect a number of concerns in medical anthropology relating to explanatory models, trauma, forgetting and medical pluralism. Chapter 12 considers how two societies deal with forgetting the recent past. A millennial community in the Caribbean have a centrally directed policy of ignoring the modern industrial world. By contrast a post-Communist village in Albania gradually let the Hoxha period just slide away, allowing buildings and institutions of that time to decay without referring to them, with no rancour or recriminations. The final chapter discusses the limitations of the explanatory model paradigm, most importantly the neglect of the socio-political context of health seeking and the often observed discrepancy in ethnographic fieldwork between what informants say and what they actually do in practice.

These chapters thus take a wide variety of traditional motifs, with theoretical positions emphasizing a plurality of methodologies, the naturalistic and the personalistic each encroaching on the other in recursion not in essence.

We do not attempt to produce new definitions of this area of 'cultural psychiatry', but rather we presume forays into the area from each side until they disintegrate, sometimes emphasizing the individual and psychological, sometimes the social anthropological and cultural, in a way that recalls George Devereux' somewhat different notion of complementarity (Devereux 1978). In either case we hope to provide new insights into a fascinating area: fascinating and confused.

We owe an enormous debt to our own patients and critics, and to our fieldwork and informant hosts: there are far too many to list here, but we would like to pay an especial tribute to Dr Maurice Lipsedge of Guy's Hospital, our former clinical teacher, who many years ago did so much to encourage us to venture into the contested but fertile ground between anthropology and psychiatry.

References

Benedict, R. 1935. *Patterns of Culture.* London: Routledge and Kegan Paul.

Birnbaum, K. 1923. 'Des Aufbau der Psychoses', trans. as 'The Making of a Psychosis', in S.R. Hirsch and M. Shepherd (eds), *Themes and Variations in European Psychiatry.* Bristol: Wright.

Dein S.J. 2010. 'Judeo-Christian Religious Experience and Psychopathology: The Legacy of William James', *Transcultural Psychiatry* 47: 523–47.

Devereux, G. 1978. *Ethnopsychoanalysis: Psychoanalysis and Anthropology as Complementary Frames of Reference.* Berkeley: California University Press.

Geertz, C. 1968. 'The Impact of the Concept of Culture on the Concept of Man', in Y.A. Cohen (ed.), *Man in Adaptation.* Chicago: Archive.

Harris, C. 1957. 'Possession "Hysteria" in a Kenyan Tribe', *American Anthropologist* 59: 1046–68.

James, W. 1902. *The Varieties of Religious Experience.* New York: Simon & Schuster.

Kleinman, A. 1987. 'Anthropology and Psychiatry: The Role of Culture in Cross-Cultural Research on Illness', *British Journal of Psychiatry* 151: 447–54.

Koening, H.G. 2015. 'Religion, Spirituality and Health: A Review and an Update', *Advances in Mind-Body Medicine* 29: 19–26.

Kraepelin, E. 1904. 'Vergleichende Psychiatrie', trans. As 'Comparative Psychiatry', in S.R. Hirsch and M. Shepherd (eds), *Themes and Variations in European Psychiatry.* Bristol: Wright.

Littlewood, R. 1991. 'Against Pathology', *British Journal of Psychiatry* 159: 696–702.

______. 1993. *Pathology and Identity.* Cambridge: Cambridge University Press.

______. 1996. 'Psychiatry's Culture', *International Journal of Social Psychiatry* 42: 245–68.

Rivers, W.H.R. 1924. *Medicine, Magic and Religion.* London: Keegan Paul, Trench and Trubner.

Turi, A.M. 2009. *Netuzza Evolo La Mystica Di Paravati.* Rome: Edizioni Mediterranee.

Yap, P.M. 1967. 'Classification of the Culture-Bound Reactive Syndromes', *Australian and New Zealand Journal of Psychiatry* 1: 172–79.

Chapter 1

The Effectiveness of Words

Letters to the Rebbe

And I shall behold God through my flesh.

—Job 19:26

The Lubavitch Hasidim of Stamford Hill in London are members of a world-wide Jewish movement, whose leader, the seventh Lubavitcher Rebbe, lives in New York.[1] Every year he receives hundreds of petitions (*kvitlekh*) about episodes of sickness and misfortune. He responds to many with reassurance and advice, sometimes suggesting that the household's religious objects are impure and should be checked. A 60-year-old rabbi living in the community recalls how he became dangerously ill following a heart attack: after discharge from hospital, he continued to experience chest pains, so his concerned wife wrote to the Rebbe in Brooklyn asking why this had happened and what could be done. The Rebbe replied simply that 'one should check one's *mezuzot*.' (The mezuzah is a parchment scroll inscribed with the *shema*, the affirmation of faith in God, enclosed in a metal case and placed upon the door frames of the observant Jewish home.) After a thorough examination of the family's *mezuzot* by a scribe, it was found that in one, in the ordinance 'thou shalt love thy God with all thy heart' (Deuteronomy 6:5), the word for heart was wrongly spelt. A new, kosher, mezuzah was obtained and subsequently the man experienced no more chest pains. Both husband and wife maintain that the error in transcription was the ultimate cause of the illness, and its correction was essential to his recovery. The Rebbe's knowledge was, in their words, 'truly miraculous'.

The 'Double Register' Efficacy and Meaning in the Anthropology of Healing

The incident certainly recalls the conventional understanding of a 'miracle'. Cause and effect are recognized in the material world through our everyday sensory experience, but also on occasion through direct knowledge of (or actual intercession by) a transcendent other worldly register which ultimately justifies suffering, one which is generally opaque to full human awareness but which we can supplicate if not sometimes actually constrain.

The anthropology of what has been termed 'symbolic' or 'mythic' healing explained such *efficacité symbollique* (Lévi-Strauss 1949) as a close coupling of embodied experience to a society's received cognitions (ibid.; Rivers 1924; Dow 1986). Since Mauss (1950) and Moerman (1979), few social scientists would now claim any intrinsic association between the body as biological fact and such language-based representations. Where a formal isomorphism has been recognized between the body and the social order (e.g. Durkheim and Mauss 1903; Douglas 1966, 1973), transformations in either are no longer explained as somehow participating in or casually influencing the other. Indeed, when challenged as to the relationship between the body understood naturalistically and its symbolizations, many – whilst admitting some Kantian antinomy yet discreetly avoiding any apology for 'magic' – evoke the local moral rhetoric of the body to interpret what it is to be healed (Scheper-Hughes and Lock 1987; Good 1994). Phenomenological anthropology argues similarly that the experiencing self must be understood without recourse to any objectifications of the material world (Csordas 1994a, 1994b). If any psychological consequences of 'symbolic therapies', systematized or folk, are still recognized by medical anthropologists, then these are assumed to be through non-specific mechanisms such as alleviating anxiety or somehow promoting the body's immunological response (McGuire 1983; Laderman 1987). With contemporary interest in the political context of biomedicine, the naturalistic body has itself become theoretically redundant, as just another social representation of an external reality whose ontological status is no concern of anthropology.

This shift from empirical explanation to cultural interpretation and thence phenomenology parallels certain developments in Western psychotherapy whose nineteenth-century origins lay in explanations of hysteria which presumed a direct homology between the psychological body and its representation, akin to the homunculus inscribed in figures of the cerebral cortex to illustrate cortical localization: an isomorphism generally accessible to awareness but not in the 'dissociated' patient who in treatment was returned to this awareness (Grunbaum 1984). Similarly, 'hypertension' not only stood for but physically expressed 'emotional tension' (Alexander 1939). Psychotherapy, like anthropology and complementary medicine (Beckford 1985), has only with reluctance abandoned this powerful idea of a 'double-register' with its direct and intrinsic correspondence between physiology and its social cognition, between two rather difficult states of being – or, as we might now say, different maps of reality. Rather, psychotherapy too is now concerned not with efficacy but with 'meaning', 'self-actualization' and 'awareness': as Frazer might have argued, with those problems still resistant to immediate biophysical intervention.

Western monotheisms, the 'revealed religions', had expressly distinguished material experience from some type of ultimate, here divine, meaning (Tambiah 1990). Christianity's explicitly paradoxical elision of nature and divinity in the Incarnation enhances a tendency in the Jewish scriptures to mark a sharp distinction between the two (with theological problems of them establishing the relations between them [Brown 1989]),[2] a distinction which was developed later into the increasingly secular dualism of Renaissance science, thence to the epistemologies of Sydenham, Locke and Kant, and to contemporary scientific empiricism (Foucault 1966; Rorty 1980; Tambiah 1990; Gellner 1992; Littlewood 1993; Good 1994). Whether simply appropriating Jewish and Christian dualism which identified ultimate reality with the divine meaning, or reversing it to privilege the material, one level or other was taken as outside human agency and thus as somehow more 'real' (Berger and Luckman 1966) and determining of human interests.[3] Such an attempt might be termed 'structuralist' or even 'foundationalist' (Piaget 1968; Ardener 1978; McMullin 1978; Hage and Harary 1983; Lawson and McCauley 1993): one which is exemplified by the Comptean hierarchy of explanation which still underpins biomedicine, and by those expressly 'structuralist' approaches in the human sciences which place some generative power (and thus for the theorist the formal analytical key) in social relations (Durkheim), practical instrumentality (Marx), psychology (Tylor, Freud, Malinowski) or neuro-psychology (Chomsky, Lévi-Strauss). And these carry with them certain assumptions about 'representation' and 'symbolization': less an arbitrary correspondence between fairly autonomous registers than the necessary enactment of the one 'real' level as individual agency and thus as historical event. In Lévi-Strauss' words (1970: 10) there is an attempt 'to reduce apparently arbitrary data to some kind of order, and to attain a level at which a kind of necessity becomes apparent, underlying the illusions of liberty.'

Medical anthropology's shift from an empirical and sociological perspective to the discursive is characteristic of recent tendencies in the social sciences, away from the idea of such privileged analytical access to the 'real' level (whether biological or social) which determines subjective agency and implicit knowledge at another, to a single understanding in which both local experience and our analysis are taken as culturally and historically intended (e.g. Clifford 1988; Crapanzano 1992). It is not surprising that the discipline which has been central in the move away from structuralism is anthropology, with its concern with alternative epistemologies in non-Western societies where things may quite variously hang together in local knowledge even if one or another mode of reality was identified by ethnographers as primary. In this sense then, the varieties of post-structuralism all signal an apparent rupture with a Western mode of understanding which goes back to the Jewish scriptures with their privileging of some determining reality. As Hegel predicted, our distinction between form and function has perhaps finally broken down.

Some sort of 'congruence' (Torrey 1971) between bodily illness as experienced and the systematized social representation of it is still recognized (Kleinman and Sung 1979; Dow 1986; Good and Good 1986; Bilu et al. 1990; Kirmayer 1993). Indeed, it seems difficult to characterize any social action as 'healing' without assuming some agreement on a shared representation of the immediate problem. And it is this agreement which itself now constitutes what Tambiah (1977) terms 'performative efficacy', successful healing being justified not through some objective criterion of health external to the understanding of healing – as biomedicine still argues – but rather in the acceptance by patient and others that a transformation of bodily state or sensibility has been effected (McGuire 1983; Csordas 1988; Good 1994), 'Ritual' in general is now taken as an action intended in some way by participants to aesthetically evoke or modify their consensual experience, as well as (or indeed instead of) instrumentally effecting events in the material world (Tambiah 1968, 1990; Young 1976; Ahern 1979; Kapferer 1993; Csordas 1994a), together with a more subtle distinction between instrumental and representational models (Caws 1974; Holy and Stuchlik 1981). If for some anthropologists there remain a number of paths from psychical experience to representation which are not mediated by agency and language (Sperber 1980), the observer cannot claim to fully elucidate the 'meaning' of healing symbols but merely record what they evoke in a particular situation. 'Symbolic meanings' are now not only naturalistically arbitrary, polysemous and manifest creatively in immediate situations (Good 1994) but are to be demonstrated as the participants' own understanding and intentions, through description rather than explanation (Parkin 1982; cf. Lawson and McCauley 1993). As such they may be quite diverse (Sperber 1985), circumscribed (Caws 1974), of variable 'depth' (Feinberg 1990; Barrett and Lucas 1993), unrelated to actual experience (Jackson 1983), ambiguous (Bourdieu 1977; Hobart 1982) or of little general concern (Sperber 1975; Schieffelin 1985). Healing idioms may be considerably less systematized than anthropologists recognize (Young 1976; Laderman 1987; Kirmayer 1993) and indeed may gain their very efficacy through some meta-communicative unintelligibility (Last 1981; McGuire 1983; Csordas 1988) – Malinowski's 'coefficient of weirdness.'

The so-called 'interpretive turn' in medical anthropology, like its phenomenological successors, claims a greater closeness to individual agency and intention than that achieved through an objective and context-free criterion of efficacy derived from biophysical medicine: for biomedicine is now recognized as a map not a mirror. Whilst we have criticized elsewhere anthropology's complete abandonment of the objectified naturalistic body as one valid commentary on human experience (Littlewood 1991, 1995; *pace* Csordas 1994c), our concern here is rather different. Does the emphasis on 'meaning' do justice to the explicit concerns of those involved situationally as sick individuals?[4] Medical anthropologists still imply some greater validity to their own 'holistic' methodologies in, typically, suggesting that the flux of experiencing should not be reified into entities and that a dualist epistemology is in some way misconceived (Lock and Scheper-Hughes 1990; Good 1994; Csordas 1994b). The generality of bodily afflictions is however experienced as real, as immediate and arbitrary (Ellen 1977; Feinberg 1990; Littlewood 1993); neither 'symbolic' nor demanding rhetorical transformation, they have a compelling physical urgency which demands instrumental redress in the same register (Last 1981; Gellner 1992). While we may sometimes, particularly with chronic afflictions (Kleinman and Sung 1979; Good 1994), be driven to a search for significance and justification, we are generally concerned with immediate practical amelioration: with countering the 'first spear' as best we can before worrying about the second, to use Evans-Pritchard's Zande idioms.

The structuralist schema had required what Ardener (1980) terms 'P-structures', paradigms or blueprints which had some primary instrumental or formal relationship to the secondary registrar, whether as base and superstructure, myth and experience, or simply template and artefact. Structuralist models of healing such as that of Lévi-Strauss (1949) seemed to correspond closely with local exegesis in societies where body and its sickness were indeed already highly 'mythologized': where upper and lower register, mythic reality and bodily experiences (and, as in this chapter, social group) were understood as already reflecting and recreating each other in a ubiquitous and closed narrative, where psychology was a cosmology, a mythic reality being experienced by individuals as in accordance with events and actions which were not seen as situationally specific, nor generally justified as personal agency.[5] In increasingly less 'tight' societies ('low grid, low group' in Douglas' [1973] terminology), such as the pluralistic postmodern world where biomedicine, whilst arguably evoking core notions of self and agency (Lock and Gordon 1988), has considerably less representational coherence and certainly no obvious formal homology with some ultimate reality, we may expect the notion of 'mythic healing' to become more extraordinary both for the observer and participants.[6] The greater the gap between divinity and experience, the more miracles are indeed 'miracles'.

The Besht

While Western monotheisms radically distinguished the sensible world from its ultrahuman reality, an explicit image of 'healing' has been common to both the restoration of the body to health and safety and to the deliverance of a 'wounded spirit' or indeed the redemption of a whole community (cf. GK. *soteria*, Lat. *salvus*). Prophets and the founders of new religious dispensations commonly engage in, or are recorded by later hagiographers as having employed, miracles of healing. They assert a double register, usually enhancing the very separation, yet at the same time they show that it may be mediated by certain individuals; indeed, their very authority appears to be justified through their tapping into higher realities to heal sickness and insanity, as well as to predict or avert other misfortunes, evil forces or disasters to the community. The expectations for a prophet to reconcile the two worlds through healing – and his occasional resistance to these – are well demonstrated for Jesus in the Christian Gospels (Mathew 4:23, 8:16, 9:32, 12:22; Mark 5:25), together with his use of the idiom of 'healing' for an increased turning to the spiritual, through confession and absolution, with conversion of the sick soul to a fundamentally new perspective.

In this chapter we are not concerned with whether the conversion of individuals to the new religious perspective can be usefully termed 'therapeutic' (Heelas and Haglund-Heelas 1988; Witztum and Greenberg 1990; Littlewood 1993), so much as with the public apologies for physical illness offered by its members. However, such testimonials, and those offered by their Rebbe, come back to the moment of awakening to the moment's ideals, an experience which is frequently couched in a therapeutic idiom.

Hasidism developed as a popular movement in Eastern Europe in the eighteenth century.[7] Its immediate founder was the Master of Good Name, the Baal Shem Tov, popularly known by the acronym Besht. Epstein (1959) argues that two events were instrumental in its emergence: the Cossack insurrections of 1648–1649, which killed tens of thousands of Jews in Poland and the Ukraine, and the subsequent Sabbathian crisis. Buber (1984) and Sharot (1982) both emphasize the increasing gap between the urban rabbinate and the rural Jewish population after the death of Sabbatai Svi (1626–1676) whose messianic claims and antinomian acts had swept the Jewish diaspora with promises of immediate redemption and speedy release from all their trials (Scholem 1973). When Sabbatai converted suddenly to Islam, some followers returned to rabbinical Judaism or converted to Islam or Christianity. Other maintained Sabbatian ideas under the guise of orthodoxy, citing the Kabbalah to explain how Sabbatai had committed the ultimate transgression of apostasy; for the Messiah had to descend to the lower levels to redeem the divine sparks exiled there since the beginning of time (Scholem 1971; Littlewood 1995).

The relationship of Hasidism to the Sabbatian movement remains controversial and some scholars deny any direct continuity.[8] The Besht, a clay-digger and itinerant healer of humble origin, taught that every present moment contained the possibility of redemption for each individual and for the community. Every person, whatever his status, wealth or learning, could participate in this cosmic process. Between the scholarly elitism of the rabbis and the apocalyptic messianism of the Sabbatians, the Besht's followers put forward an egalitarian interpretation of the Kabbalistic teachings which we consider below. They taught that God was to be known immediately in all aspects of life, since the physical world existed with Him and within Him, and He could be reached through everyday activities (Jacobs 1973). People were encouraged to 'cleave to God' and experience Him though ecstatic song, prayer, and dance and even, initially, by the use of tobacco and alcohol. Any act – eating, work, sexual relations – was a religious act if the intention was to attach oneself to God.

The Besht was apparently well known in his hometown as a healer, 'a master of practical Kabbalah, a magician' (Scholem 1954). It has been suggested that he employed the existing practices of the miracle worker to persuade people of his ethical teachings (see also Ben-Amos and Mintz 1970). 'There can be little doubt' argues Sharot (1982), 'that the Besht's reputation for miracle making was accepted as an important proof of his charisma and of his teachings.' While he generally employed recognized physical methods such as herbal remedies or bleeding with lancet and leeches, like other local healers and magicians (*baalei shem*), he would sometimes use a prayer or the secret names of angels to exorcize a *dibbuk* (earthbound spirit) from the body of a sick person or out of a house (Trachtenberg 1977). *Baalei shem* protected the individual against sickness, and against such misfortunes as infertility, miscarriages, fire, theft and the evil eye. They reframed non-Jewish folk therapies in a Jewish idiom and employed the sacred writings of the rabbinical tradition for practical magic, together with the names of God and the angels and prophets, sometimes as anagrams, acronyms, acrostics and inversions derived from them. The *mezuzot* had originally been amulets of this sort, and they retained their thaumaturgical function despite rabbinical attempts to transform them into simple emblems. When a child was ill or a woman in obstructive labour, the Torah scroll was laid on top of them. Psalm

20 was read over the mother to alleviate the pains of childbirth, for its nine verses corresponded to the nine months of pregnancy and its seventy words to the seventy pangs of labour. The Besht himself was famous for his blessed coins and psalms of the other formulae written on parchment enclosed in a small mental case which contained the names of angels and imprecations against malevolent powers (Ben-Amos and Mintz 1970). Fifty years after his death, the *Shivhei ha-Besht*, a book compiled by a follower, relates many stories of his ability to heal:

> I heard from the Rabbi of our community that Rabbi Leibush of the holy community of Meserich visited the Besht for the Days of Awe. Before Rosh Hashanah [the New Year] he became sick. The Besht was busy curing him on the eve of Rosh Hashanah and the entire night as well. When he went to the beth hamidrash (study hall) at the time for prayer, Rabbi Leibush became faint and felt very weak. They tried to tell the Besht, but they were afraid to shout, and he did not hear them. When Rabbi Isaac of the holy community of Meserich saw that the Besht did not respond, he shouted to him in a loud voice. The Besht answered, 'Why didn't you tell me?' He hurried home and found the Angel of Death standing at the head of the bed. The Besht scolded the Angel of Death severely and he ran away. Th Besht then held Rabbi Leibush by the hand, and he recovered immediately. (Ben-Amos and Mintz 1970: 116)

The Besht's teaching was systematized by his biographer, Dov Ber of Mererich (1719–1772), known as the Magid (Preacher), who took the existing term *zaddik* (righteous man) for the local leader of a Hasidic group (Dresner 1974). The founder of Lubavitch, Rabbi Schneur Zalman of Ladi (1745–1812), who studied under Dov Ber, later commented: 'we drew up a holy spirit by the bucketful, and miracles lay around under the benches, only no-one had time to pick them up' (Wiener 1969). According to Epstein (1959), Hasidism would not have spread with such rapidity nor attained such dimensions but for the 'extraordinary galaxy of saintly mystics' it produced during its first fifty years. Hasidism holds that only the zaddik can attain the highest form of *devekut* (attachment to God at all times with one's thoughts always on him). Other Jews have to attach themselves to a zaddik through whom in turn they can become attached to God. (The term *rebbe* is now used virtually synonymously with *zaddik*.) The zaddik develops the spirituality of his adherents whilst at the same time, through his mediation with God, he can secure favours for them in both mundane and divine matters.

After Dov Ber's death, groups following various zaddikim developed in Ukraine and Poland, each known by the name of their centre of activity. Their leaders are now recalled through a particular quality or activity: some were distinguished for their fervent devotions, others for their ecstatic visions, spiritual insight or miraculous healing. Their surviving texts are characterized by an accessible popular style rooted in folklore: anecdotes, homilies, marvellous tales, puns, jokes and sematic paradoxes. Despite accusations of antinomianism and even pantheism, Hasidism spread rapidly in Poland and was introduced to Lithuania by Schneur Zalman who developed the variant called Chabad which reintroduced the more intellectual elements of Kabbalah – but now into more general accessibility, through his Tanya (Book of Teaching), the major text of Lubavitch.

Both orthodox Judaism and secular Zionism have maintained an ambivalent relationship to Hasidim, at times critical of their overt emotionalism and dependence on miraculous Rebbes (Dresner 1974), on other occasions taking them as the authentic voice of Jewish spirituality and identity. Hasidic folk tales have now become widely accessible through the popularizations of Martin Buber (1848). By the nineteenth century, Lubavitch was recognized as the 'rationalist' form of Hassidism which could appeal to the educated. It fought to secure economic and political benefits for all Jews in Eastern Europe and developed a number of charitable and educational projects. Discouraged from migrating to America because of the dangers of secularism, the majority of Hasidim were to die in the Holocaust, but the 6th Lubavitch Rebbe organized communities outside of Eastern Europe from which in 1948 most of the survivors settled in New York (Mintz 1992). Today, the major Lubavitch centres are in New York (Brooklyn), London (Stamford Hill), Israel (Jerusalem and Kefar Chabad), Canada (Montreal) and Belgium (Antwerp). It has been generously estimated that by the 1980s there were perhaps 250,000 adherents and close sympathizers worldwide (Sharot 1991).[9]

The Stamford Hill Lubavitch

Stamford Hill is an inner-city area in north-east London, with a population of around 27,000 people in an area of three square miles. There are now nearly a thousand Hasidic families living here, about two hundred of them Lubavitch. Other local Hasidic groups include Satmar, Belzer and Gur.[10] Although today 'Stamford Hill' is virtually synonymous with Jewish ultra-orthodoxy, this was not always the case. Before the Second World War many local congregations were United Synagogue or Sephardic, who later moved out to the more affluent suburbs (Kupfermann 1976). Today, less than half of the population of Stamford Hill are Jews, mainly lower middle-class tradesman, religious teachers and small businessmen.

The number of Lubavitch families increases every year, not only through the encouragement of large families but through conversion.[11] The majority of the adult Stamford Hill community are British converts from non-orthodox Judaism who are more likely to speak English than Yiddish. Some informants have even been adherents of Western-based Buddhist and Hindu sects although they were born Jews. Many had already been familiar with popularized accounts of the Kabbalah (e.g. Wiener 1969) or with the continuing counter-culture interest in matters Jungian and Hermetic (e.g. Hall 1962). Rarely a Christian may convert to orthodox Judaism to then join Lubavitch. The community conduct mass campaigns to reclaim 'stray' Jews: public meetings where rabbis preach, *mezuzot* campaigns (checking local Jews have kosher *mezuzot* on their doors) and, perhaps the most striking of all, the 'mitzvah tank', a truck going round the streets inviting male Jews to enter and lay *tefillin*.[12] Besides encouraging every Jew to be more observant, Lubavitchers attempt to attract into their group educated young single adults and campaigns are sometimes held on university campuses. 'Conversion' is less a sudden accession of faith than a gradual process in which the individual 'returns', employing more and more Jewish rituals in their daily life. Joining may cause conflict with the families of the converts, especially when a student gives up university studies or career.[13]

Daily activity within a Hasidic group is determined in principle by *Halacha* (the Way), largely derived from the Talmud, the rabbinical compilation of legal, ethical and historical writings. Minimum standards of observance for all the community include strict *kashrut* (food must be ritually pure; milk must neither be cooked nor eaten with meat), together with Sabbath and festival observance. For men there is regular attendance in the prayer house and daily study of the sacred texts, with conservative clothing, beard and covered head. For women, an enthusiastic attitude to childbearing is expected, with modest dress including covered hair (married women cut their hair short and cover their head with a *sheitl* or wig), and in most groups, regular prayer (not always in the synagogue) and some religious learning. Marriage and parenthood are sacred acts, and couples are expected to adhere to the laws governing family purity. Marriage of members is arranged by a *shidduch* maker and agreed by their fathers, and at least nominally by the Rebbe; choice of spouse depends on their families' wealth, lineage and learning (*yihus*). Children are educated in single-sex Jewish schools, with secular education valued less than Jewish learning; in their late teens some are sent to residential seminaries. Rarely university education may be considered appropriate. As for other orthodox Jews, the Hasidic injunction to study affirms it as a religious experience which brings the scholar ever nearer to God.

Lubavitch do not have careers, they earn a living. Favoured occupations include small businesses, especially those serving the wider orthodox community such as food stores or teaching and other religiously linked occupations, slaughterer (*shohet*), beadle (*shammes*) or circumcizer (*mohel*), and the rabbinate. Families tend to be large; one couple has sixteen children living in two adjoining houses. The average number of children per family is seven; parents are expected to trust in God to help them provide, educate and care for large families. During fieldwork it was found that people usually adhered strictly to the orthodox public norms. Occasionally a degree of flexibility is agreed in the interpretation of religious law; one woman from the community went to live in the north of England far from the nearest synagogue so the Rebbe allowed her to travel by vehicle on the Sabbath, or so we are told.

Although there is some association with other local Hasidic groups and occasional intermarriage, there are frequent tensions: the Satmar, who retain the kaftans and hanging sidelocks of the East European *shtetl* (Zborowski and Herzog 1962), argue the Lubavitchers adaptation to 'modernity' has been too enthusiastic, while some orthodox Jews accuse the current Rebbe of messianic ambitions (Beeston 1992). To an extent, one may take these other Hasidic groups as continuations of small *shtetl* communities linked by descent and endogamy, now concerned with preserving the group's traditions and boundaries in the modern world, while Lubavitch's use of new communication technologies, its public profile and emphasis on conversion, argue for many similarities with contemporary 'new religious movements'.

In a study of another Hasidic group, derived like the Lubavitch from the pre-war world of the *shtetl*, we noted that the mundane and the religious remained 'tied together' through the mediating symbolisms of everyday actions (Littlewood 1983). The term 'kosher' was applied simultaneously to food, clothes, non-menstruating women, books and ideas. The geography of community prayer house, home, room, clothes and body were carefully ordered, each commenting on and reflecting the others. Prayer books were divided into sections which corresponded with the rooms of a house and the parts of the body. The Torah (Law) gives contemporary Hasidim explicit norms for all daily activities. In addition, through a complex numerology employing the numerical value of words and letters, cardinal number (the number of good and bad deeds, gifts, objects, alms) and ordinal number (sequence of a text or family birth order), it inscribes the social and physical worlds in a tight network. There is no act or event, good or bad, which is arbitrary or neutral. Indeed, it can be said that contemporary Hasidim aspire to have no 'secular' life in that all everyday events and actions are aligned to a divine reality which is always to be held in mind. Members of the community isolate themselves where possible from the non-Jewish world. They argue a practical advantage in their distinctive attire which makes them less likely to go into sinful places. Mixing with the non-Jews (Goyim) is minimal except for business purposes for they are said by some to be impure and polluting: a not uncommon idea is that their souls are somehow inferior. Douglas (1970; cf. Gilman 1992), following Durkheim, has argued that the orthodox Jewish concern with the boundaries of the physical body – with its entrances and exits, with food, purification after excretion and menstruation, and masturbation (whence semen provides embodiment for evil powers) – follows a concern with the boundaries of the body politic faced with the ever-present threats of assimilation and intermarriage. Certainly, for Lubavitch, return to orthodoxy is primarily through ritual actions which inscribe a gradually increasing sanctity onto the individual body marking it off from the world of the Goyim.

Hasidic wives, *akeres habayis*, are the mainstay of the family; their domestic role is praised, particularly in guaranteeing the purity of food and household, and thus their family's health. These tasks are not recognized as 'symbolic' in the vernacular sense – as not instrumental – for failure to perform, for example, the prescribed cleaning of the house of bread before Passover allows sickness to intrude (e.g. Littlewood 1983). Whilst Lubavitch women argue that household tasks are sacred, many consider themselves more independent than other Hasidic women and to have a higher level of education, and some claim a responsibility equal to that of the men in doing the Rebbe's work. Several women are involved in 'reclaiming' other Jewish women to religious orthodoxy and compared with women of other Hasidic groups, they are less discouraged from attending the synagogue.

The Rebbe

Every room in a Lubavitch house has several pictures of the current Rebbe on the walls, as a young man and as a nonagenarian. Families take great pride in showing pictures of their visits to him, especially at the dollar ceremony (a weekly ceremony when he distributes a dollar – signifying charity – to every one of the hundreds who visit him in Brooklyn on Sunday mornings).

Menachem Mendel Schneersohn has led the group since the 1950s. Lubavitch describe him as 'the most phenomenal Jewish personality on our time' and it is through his direction that Lubavitch has developed its distinctive outward orientation. Born in Russia in 1902, he became a 'Torah prodigy', is said to be fluent in ten languages, and – unusually for Hasidim of his generation – received a secular higher education, a degree in engineering from the Sorbonne. Many miraculous stories are told about him during the fourth meal by which Hasidim seek to prolong the Sabbath: he sleeps for just one hour a day, and fasts for three days in the week; he 'give Torah' for several hours without needing a break; he meditates weekly at the grave of the 6th Rebbe with whose soul he communicates; he predicted the end of communism in Eastern Europe a year before it occurred. Although he has never visited Israel, nor indeed left Brooklyn for the past forty years, the Rebbe is widely credited with single-handedly halting at least one set of

Middle East peace talks, and with directly influencing the 1988 Israeli elections. Many of these 'miracle tales' (Mintz 1968) have personal resonances.[14] Those told about earlier zaddikim recall European fairy-tales – stories of lost children, secret parentage, tribulation and reward, buried treasure, ghosts and *dibukkim*, miraculous escapes from Cossacks and Nazis (see Mintz 1968 and the stories of Bashevis Singer). A common theme is the fundamental distinction between Jew and Goy, and the near impossibility of passing from one to another.

Succession to a Rebbe is usually dynastic. Menachem Schneersohn is the son-in-law of the previous Rebbe, and in his father's line, the descendant of the Alter Rebbe (Schneur Zalman). Under his leadership Lubavitcher institutions and activities have been established throughout the world to cater for the educational needs of the alienated Jew and 'late beginners' who would otherwise be unable to attend a *yeshiva* or girls' school.

The process of joining Lubavitch is characterized not only by the use of ritual objects, but by an increasing attachment (*hutjashrut*) to the Rebbe and to his work. Among the most important gatherings of the community are those that commemorate the deaths and key events in the lives of past zaddikim (*yohrstait*). Lubavitch are expected to be familiar with their lives, works and teachings (*hasides*), and the movement's sense of itself is a moral history understood principally through their written works and stories about them. In its shallow chronology, Hasidic Rebbes are recognized as the incarnations of previous Rebbes or of biblical prophets, and scriptural events have a contemporary action or significance; biological evolution is denied. Children are taught to revere the zaddik, and in everyday conversation Lubavitchers frequently discuss his objectives and his teachings, particularly his extraordinary personal powers and wisdom. Couples engaged in marital intercourse on the Sabbath are enjoined to fix their minds on him. Through him mundane happenstances take on new, deeper, meanings: what might otherwise be seen as 'coincidences' are to be understood as brought about by the Rebbe's intervention. He is the guide on matters of spiritual and physical health, education, marriage and business.

Miriam Hirsch had always intended to visit the Rebbe in America for the dollar ceremony but had never had the necessary money. One Sabbath, her American sister in Brooklyn went to see him. Mrs Hirsch was unaware of this but admitted that on that particular day she had thought a lot about the Rebbe. Her sister didn't mention Miriam to the Rebbe but was unexpectedly given two dollars. She sent one to London. Mrs Hirsch understood that the Rebbe was aware of the thought of every Jew; he knew how she was worrying and therefore gave her sister two dollars: 'Truly a miraculous man.'

Lubavitch are prepared for the arrival of the Messiah (*Moshiach*). They envisage a time very soon when the world will change fundamentally, for sickness, envy, greed and hatred will disappear. Several rabbis argue that many existing institutions will probably remain, a commonly mentioned instance being capitalism. The appearance of *Moshiach* is now imminent: 'If he does not come today, he will come tomorrow.' When asked why he has not yet come, the following explanation was often given to us: in each generation there are thirty-six righteous (but hidden) men, one of who is a potential Messiah, but not enough merit by Jews has been acquired for him to emerge. Many Lubavitchers suggested that perhaps now there is enough merit and admitted that they thought Rebbe Schneesohn might be the Messiah, an idea which he, like other rebbes, has done little to contradict (Beeston 1992). They point out that he is the seventh rebbe, and that Moses was the seventh generation after Abraham.

The Mystical Body

Through daily readings of the Tanya, Lubavitch makes accessible the once esoteric knowledge expounded in the texts know as Kabbalah. The term *kabbalah* (tradition, 'that which has been received') had been used since the eleventh century CE for the diffuse traditions of Jewish mystical thought said to be hidden in the religious Law and which was received from the remote past, from Ezekiel, or even, in some accounts, through Adam from the angels before the Fall. Gershom Scholem, the major historian of Jewish mysticism, has argued for a continuity with Jewish Gnosticism which had sought to reconnect the immediate and divine worlds which rabbinical Judaism so austerely divided: 'the Kabbalah was a mythical reaction in realms which monotheistic thinking had with utmost difficulty wrested from myth,' and an 'eruption of subterranean forces' which attempted 'to construct and describe a mythical world by means of thinking that excluded myth' (Scholem 1965: 98, 99): a return back across the 'abyss' which had developed between the registers of the physical and the spiritual (Scholem 1954) (see Note 2). Scholem (like Bulka 1979) suggests that the rabbinical tradition of established institutions and canonical texts had provided no help in dealing with disaster and sickness, or indeed with the spiritual vacuum left by the Sabbatian apostasy. Kabbalists however have never seen themselves in opposition to rabbinical orthodoxy but rather as its commentators and developers.

Kabbalah is said to have first been communicated as secret teaching only to a privileged few, but by the early modern period it had become a more open pursuit, a trend particularly evident in Hasidism. It speaks of the ultimate ultrahuman order as now manifest in Man, and as one which can be directly known through study or ecstatic experience, and upon which we can call and obtain practical power in this world. We may argue, as does

Scholem, affinities with South Asian religious systems, Christian and Islamic mysticism, and particularly with the sort of Western theosophico-astrological tradition currently recognized under the rubric of New Age thinking (Hall 1962; Beckford 1985; Tambiah 1990; Littlewood 1993). The material world of our experience is to be understood as an imperfect reflection of hidden, 'deeper' (or higher) underlying principles, knowledge of which serves as a practical key to confer insight and sometimes power over everyday events. Instead of the rigorously dualistic cosmogony in which the inscrutable and austere Hebrew deity suddenly creates the material world out of nothing, and across which gap occasionally pass angels or the souls of the dead, we have here a mythic narrative gradually unfolding in cosmic time through which the progress of individual souls can be mapped, with infinite gradations of being between God and Man. This metaphysical reality is often figured in anthropomorphic, if sometimes explicitly allegorical, terms: as gendered and embodied, emanating in physical space, with impulses and motivations not entirely dissimilar from those of humankind.

The most important of the more than three thousand extant texts is the Zohar, the bulk of which was probably written in Spain by Moses de Leon (died 1305); its themes were elaborated by Isaac Luria (1514–1572) in Palestine among the Iberian Jews exiled in 1492, in what is generally known to scholars as the Lurianic Kabbalah. The Zohar, a lengthy collection of tales, anecdotes, homiletics and commentaries, is in late literary Aramaic with occasional Hebrew, Arabic and Spanish expressions, the whole interwoven with paraphrases, neologisms, allegories, oxymorons, verbal paradoxes and invented quotations. There are frequent digressions retelling popular tales (*aggadahl*) and on medical and demonological questions (Preis 1928; Trachtenberg 1939). According to Epstein (1959), it is, after the Talmud, the post-scriptural book which has exercised the profoundest influence on Judaism. Its recurrent themes are the nature of the Deity and the way He made Himself manifest in the universe; the mysteries of the divine names; the soul of man, its source and destiny; the nature of evil; the importance of the written and oral Torah; and the promised Messiah and out future redemption.

According to the Zohar, the infinite (*En-Sof*), who has in Himself neither qualities nor attributes, made His existence perceptible by projecting ten successive channels of light which served as media for His manifestation of the finite. These ten channels are the Sefirot (numbers, elements, spheres), which in the Zohar are understood as the names, indeed the actual qualities and agencies, of God: the intelligible divine attributes which make up all existence. The Sefirot are figured in different patterns but may be divided into three triads or dimensions. The first triad represents the immanent intellectual power of the universe, the second triad the moral world, and the third the physical universe. The tenth Sefirah is the female aspect of divinity, the Shekhinah, now manifest in the physical world, and which Adam, the first man, mistook for the whole of divinity. The human individual is to be understood as a microcosm of the whole universe by which each person reproduces what is above in the celestial worlds. The Sefirotic structure of man simultaneously reflects and is reflected onto that of the universe, and the Sefirot may be represented as concentric circles, as the Tree of Being, or as the Cosmic Man (the lower parts being the outer circles of the first representation).[15] They may be identified with certain numbers, letters and colours, and they are gendered: in the first triad, Wisdom – masculine, the father, the giving element – is counterposed to Understanding – feminine, the mother, the receiver; the offspring of their conjunction is Knowledge.

Later Kabbalists describe four distinct realms corresponding to different orders of Sefirot: in descending order of divinity, Aziluth (emanation), Briah (creation), Yetzirah (formation), Asiyah (making, the divine archetype of the material world). The four are both simultaneous and successive (Scholem 1965), structured by the Sefirot in a similar pattern and subject to common influences. Anything which involves one level cannot fail to involve all others for 'from an activity below there is stimulated a corresponding activity on high' (Zohar 1934). There is an intrinsic relationship between what we may gloss as the 'material' and 'spiritual' worlds, each not only influencing but continuously participating in the others as prefigurings and memories (Bloom 1984). And these relationships may be understood through complex but variable numerology in which the twenty-two letters of the alphabet are exchanged (*temurah*) or substituted for their numerical value (*gematria*). The absence of numerals, vowels or punctuation in the written Torah (the first five books of the scriptures) leave it open to a bewildering number of interpretations. Some have argued that there are actually 600,000 possible interpretations of the Torah, corresponding to the 600,000 holy souls each of whom has a letter in the Torah.[16] The scriptures begin with the second letter, *beth*, to show that God's manifestation is on both levels, for the Hebrew alphabet is itself the direct manifestation of the divine, as are the shape of the letters and even the spaces between them, each possible pair of consonants forming a 'gate' for the passage of divine energy. The Torah (and the alphabet) is represented variously in Kabbalistic writings as the individual physical body, the body of the Jews as a whole, or even that of God: some maintained it existed before the creation of the physical world (Scholem 1973).

A rigid distinction between 'material' and 'spiritual' is hardly perceptible given the everyday as an immanent unfolding of the divine language. 'The Torah is to [Jewish mystics] a living organism animated by a secret life which steams and pulsates below the crust of literal meaning; every one of the innumerable strata of the hidden region corresponds to a new and profound meaning of the Torah' (Scholem 1954: 14). Kabbalistic texts embody a variety of complex, sometimes playful, shifts and crosscuttings between 'depths' of interpreting the Torah, from the referential to the figurative: literal reference (*peshatl*), conscious allegory (*remez*), Talmudic commentary (*derasha*) and mystical (*sod*) (cf. Feinberg 1990; Barrett and Lucas 1993). These four levels are known by the acronym *pardes* (orchard).

There is no unfettered speculation: even *sod* remains closely constrained by adherence to the literal interpretations of the Law and the authority of the Rebbe, and its sources lie within the religious texts and practices of all Jews. There have been no radical innovations in Jewish mysticism since the seventeenth century but, in Buber's words, Hasidism transformed the once esoteric Kabbalah into a 'folk ethos.' Unlike most other orthodox Jews, the Stamford Hill community have immediate knowledge of Kabbalah for, as part of their education, every Lubavitcher child studies the Tanya (Kehot 1981) which is based on Lurianic concepts. The Tanya (*Likutei Amarim*) was compiled by Rabbi Zalman, the founder of Lubavitch, and is regarded as 'the written law of Chabad.' Other orthodox groups adhere to the old Talmudic ruling that only married men over forty with a good knowledge of the Talmud may proceed to Kabbalah. (Much of the Zohar employs erotic imagery in figuring the exile and eventual reconciliation of divine and mundane: the human conjunction of husband and wife on the Sabbath night is a realization of the union between God and His exiled Shekhinah.)

Another name for Lubavitch is *Chabad*: an acronym from the Hebrew words *HokhmahI*, *Binah* and *Da'at* (the first triad: see above). They refer simultaneously to personal experiences and to the Sefirotic realm where there are reflected. Anything occurring in the mind mirrors that occurring in the universe as a whole. Indeed, like other systems which approach pantheism (e.g. Horton 1983; Tambiah 1990), the Sefirot are as much a psychology as a cosmology. Hokhmah (wisdom) is the intuitive flash by which an idea emerges into the mind. Once it has come into being, the thought becomes actualized through deep reflection as Binah (understanding). When the idea becomes an aspect of the person engaged in contemplation, the third stage of Da'at (knowledge) is attained. The psychological and spiritual body of man 'participates in' (Lévy-Bruhl's term), rather than 'represents', the same principles and structural counterparts as his physical body. 'If we want to know something about the ultimate reality of the world we live in, and how God the creator manifests himself through this reality, we must begin with a study of the human being' (Mindel 1974). In Jewish mysticism, our phenomenological world is far from illusory (as it is in Buddhism) but one end, as it were, of ultimate reality.

The Lubavitch speak of the Sefirot, not only as symbols or allegories (Kehot 1981: 820) or even resonances, but as immanent in bodily experience. 'We were formed after the supernal pattern, each limb corresponding to something in the scheme of wisdom' (Zohar: ii, 212; cf. Genesis 1:27). One young rabbi describes how the Torah is figured thus in the Zohar as the 'blueprint' (his words) with which God provided Himself for the physical creation: the Torah comprises 248 positive and 365 negative injunctions (*Tanchuma ha Kadum*) and these 'upper roots' have their respective manifestations in the 248 'limbs' and 365 'sinews' (or blood vessels) of the male body. Each limb of the body embodies one of the commandments, and each sinew and each day of the year embodies self-restriction. (The Tanya argues that the spiritual aspect of these 613 parts comprise the individual soul.) In this way each observance (or breach) of the commandments of the Torah directly causes, through its counterparts in the human body, a reaction in the corresponding portion of the world of Sefirot: in Zoharic terms, each is the 'clothing' of the other. In his Tanya, Schneur Zalman associated specific parts of the body with other psychological and moral attributes: 'the evil spirit is in the left ventricle of the heart, and the love of God flames in the right ventricle.' While there are intrinsic homologies between the two realms, the correspondence is realized practically not only through mystical computation but through such objects as the *tallit* (see Note 12).

Exile and Restitution

Sickness has its place in the divine schema. Luria's development of Zoharic cosmology postulates an initial voluntary contraction (*Zimzum*, self-limitation) of the Infinite to make room for the finite world of phenomena. Into the vacuum thus formed the Infinite projected His light, providing it at the same time with the 'vessels' which were to serve as the media for its manifestations in creation. Some of the vessels, unable to endure the inrush of light, gave way and broke. The breaking of the vessels caused a deterioration in the worlds above, together with chaos and confusion in the worlds below. Instead of uniform distribution throughout the universe, the light emitted by the Infinite was broken up into sparks illuminating only certain parts of the material world; other parts were left in darkness, their sparks trapped in matter. This confusion was aggravated by the failure of Adam to restore the fragments, and thus human history is born in exile. The universe remains in a state of disharmony, and the mission of every Jew, say Lubavitchers, is to restore (*tikkun*) the scattered divine sparks back to the Godhead through performing *mizvot* (divine commandments and this ritual and charitable deeds): 'the perfection of the upper worlds waits on the perfection of the lower worlds'.[17] The distinction between the more divine and the more human elements in the cosmic unfolding may be understood as one of dimension, distance, time, quality, procedure, potential, or indeed sometimes identity. Sickness and evil thus refer not to some malevolent power external to the created world of experience, evil in a strong sense (Parkin 1985), but to a lesser state of being of this world which can be redeemed in this life or in another incarnation:

> 'How, Reb Zusya, do you explain evil?' [his] students asked. 'What evil?' said rabbi with wide wondering eyes. The students pointed out that Reb Zusya was himself suffering from illness, pain and poverty. 'Oh that,' replied the rabbi, 'surely that is what my soul needs.' (Wiener 1969)

The Lurianic cosmogony – the 'great myth of exile' as Scholem (1954) calls it – informs Lubavitchers' explicit concepts of 'health' as knowledge and order obtained through following Talmudic teachings (Weisel 1978). It refers simultaneously to physiological and psychological dysfunction, to failure to perform ritual correctly, to disharmony and conflict within the family, and to the historical exile of the Jews – all as a separation from the divine. The original 600,000 souls have become fragmented and now seek to be restored (Mintz 1968). To recover one's health is, in some small measure, to restore our alienated world. Stamford Hill Lubavitch commonly argue that the 'universe itself is now in need of healing' for which they quote the Lurianic cosmogony. Since the shattering of the vessels God Himself is in exile. If there is a single image, a core symbol (Ortner 1973) which incorporates and subsumes others (Laughlin and Stevens 1980), and which captures the manifold connotations of sickness and misfortune, what Victor Turner termed a 'root paradigm,' it is that of exile and restitution.[18] 'The very nature of man. . . makes him an admirable intermediary between the material things spiritual. By means of these religious acts, not only are the material things spiritualised, but the infinite light is, at the same time, diffused in the physical world' (Mindel 1974). While not answerable to the Mosaic Law, the Goyim too are subject to the covenant God made with Noah, and thus have some small role in *tikkun*. It is the Rebbe who is to do most, for he alone can safely descend into our material world among the shattered vessels to redeem the exiled divinity, to mediate evil into good, ignorance into knowledge, sickness into health.

The Rebbe's Healing

> 'I do not ask to suffer. I ask only that there is a reason for my suffering.'
> (Hasidic rabbi cited in Weiner 1969)

The conventional understanding of a 'myth' is that it is some narrative about ultimate reality to which we have particular recourse when everyday cause-and-effect explanations are inadequate (when 'overloading the rational device triggers a symbolic processing' – Sperber 1980: 29, following Malinowski but see Toren 1983); and which to the observer exemplifies our society's fundamental values. Social anthropology continues to debate the relationship of normative myth to everyday praxis, the representational of the instrumental (Caws 1974; Sperber 1975, 1985; Sahlins 1976; Bourdieu 1977; Holy and Stuchlik 1981; Godelier 1986; Tambiah 1990). Laughlin and Stephens (1980: 335), like Sperber, argue in Malinowskian terms that myth is 'the quintessential form of a symbol system, operating to organise experience around a society's core symbols. A society's core symbols are invariably orientated upon the zone of uncertainty – that is, the set of events giving rise to significant effects for which there exists no readily perceivable cause for a large number of society's members.' Certainly, the Jewish myth of exile and restitution has served as a 'template' (Ardener 1980) to articulate the destruction of the Temple and the subsequent Diaspora, antisemitic pogroms, the Holocaust and the establishment of Israel. Yet, as a written text it has a continuing existence through time while provides an 'archive' (Foucault 1969) from which individuals take elements to figure their collective history and their personal dilemmas – and as the non-arbitrary and referential exemplified by instrumental Kabbalah (see Note 4).

In spite of his earlier Marxism, Scholem takes Jewish mysticism as a major determinant of modern rationalism. Defending it against accusations of superstition, he argues that practical Kabbalah and magic (and indeed Hasidism) are degenerate forms: shifts, as we might say, from the figurative to the concrete and the instrumental. Indeed, Hasidism emerges not only from Kabbalistic texts but through the everyday medical practice of early modern *shtetl* communities. Zoharic passages were used before Hasidism to cure sickness or to serve as protective amulets against the evil eye of envious neighbours and against *dibbukim* (Trachrenberg 1939). They can be read in multifarious ways: not only as a divine unfolding – a type of contemplative field theory – but as a pluripotent map of direction by which the dualism of everyday life, the material and the divine, can be practically transcended.[19]

Public accounts given by Lubavitch of their healing retain a normative 'top-down' textual structure akin to the structuralist accounts of Lévi-Strauss and Dow: individuals suffer apparently arbitrary affliction here below, and then, through some recourse to the transcendent world, are healed. It was initially difficult in fieldwork to look through these narratives to see how individual experiences and social relations might simultaneously embed the mythic structure.[20] The multitude of possible (and conflicting) correspondences between the physical and spiritual worlds which the Zohar theory offers are hardly accessible to every contemporary Hasid: as with other apparently closed nosologies based on correspondences (Foucault 1970; Littlewood 1993), quite variant explanations are volunteered for a particular crisis, from a fairly abstract theodicy to the concrete and immediate efficacy of transactional objects. Among Lubavitch, it is through the person of the Rebbe that Zoharic cosmology is usually operationalized in immediate situations to be used as an exemplary account. Compared with the other Hasidic groups in London (Littlewood 1983), individuals seem less likely to employ practical Kabbalah; our informants are reluctant to talk of possession by *dibbukim* (a potential consequence of failed conjurations), but this explanation is occasionally volunteered in cases of consistently deviant personal actions. One local rabbi was prepared to tell us he had witnessed it but was reluctant to give details. Another rabbi has elaborated his own treatment of jaundice using a white dove based on Zoharic complementarities.

How the do the Lubavitch of Stamford Hill act when they become ill? Their first thoughts, they say, are always about immediate pain and disability, then they consult their family or friends for a practical remedy to alleviate it, and later perhaps a Jewish physician sympathetic to the community: one of the two orthodox, but non-Hasidic, general practitioners who live locally. According to one of these doctors, their medical treatment is generally accepted but a common practice is to write a letter to the Rebbe asking why one became ill. Not every illness episode results in a *kvitl* being written. This is done, say some, when the illness is judged to be life-threatening by patient or doctor, or when the patient does not like the treatment given by the doctor: Mrs Goldstein explained that she wrote to the Rebbe only because her doctors' advice had been 'too simplistic.' The Rebbe is consulted particularly when the patient does not get better despite receiving physical treatment.

The Rebbe does not respond to every letter although it is said that he reads them all. Even when he does not reply, Lubavitchers maintain that he still sends out a *bracha* (blessing) to the person writing to him. Not infrequently, he advises against surgical interventions for 'they make their living by cutting, I make my living by not cutting' (Rebbe Schneersohn, cited by Wiener [1969]).

Samuel Drazin is a thirty-five-year old married man who was interviewed on several occasions in Lubavitch House. He had written to the Rebbe about a persistent toothache which he had experienced for some months. He had visited two dentists, but no obvious physical cause had been found. The first dentist told him that he could not see anything immediately wrong with his teeth – 'in fact, for someone of your age, your teeth are in very good condition.' He could certainly not account for the pain. The second dentist asked if Mr Drazin was under a lot of stress and he left with the impression that the dentist though it was in his mind. 'I've never had much faith in dentists,' he says, 'they cannot do a lot for you.'

The pain became so bad that he could not sleep. It affected his concentration at work. He tried several types of proprietary painkillers without much effect. His wife suggested that he visited a homeopath which he thought was a good idea although he knew very little about them. Homeopathic remedies did not alleviate the pain although he felt more relaxed.

Born in East London in 1957, Mr Drazin had grown up in Stoke Newington on the borders of Stamford Hill. His father, who had died three years earlier, had worked as a baker for most of his life, a calm gentle man, in contrast to his mother who was 'very anxious' and fussed over his childhood ailments (she had died suddenly two years earlier). An only child, he recalls his childhood as generally happy; after leaving school with few qualifications, he completed a two-year catering course. Although he had a non-orthodox Jewish upbringing (indeed he rejected religious ritual and only fitfully observed Sabbath), he had met several Lubavitchers as an adolescent, but had not paid much attention to them. After leaving college at the age of twenty, he was unemployed for two years – 'there was not much work about and I wasn't very interested in doing catering jobs.' Having a lot of free time and 'lacking in direction,' he started to visit the Lubavitch centre in Stamford Hill 'in order to learn more about my religion.' Over several months his participation in Jewish ritual increased. Starting with daily laying of *tefillin*, he soon began to attend thrice-daily religious services.

He brought several *mezuzot* and put them up on his doors to his flat. His nights were now spent at *shiurim* (study lessons) where he learnt the Tanya. After a year Samuel Drazin moved in with a Lubavitcher family who introduced him to his future wife Rachel who also came from a non-orthodox background. They now have eight children aged from six months to ten years.

Mr Darzin now works as an administrator in Lubavitch House, the administrative centre of the community. A friendly and charming man, always immaculately dressed in a white shirt and tie and wearing a Homburg hat, with a long flowing grey beard, he speaks openly about his health, emphasizing that he is certainly not one to be preoccupied with minor aches and pains, but this toothache was very bad. He had never been 'really ill' before. Mr Drazin had written to the Rebbe on several occasions in the past for in his early days as a Lubavitcher he had some doubts about becoming orthodox. The Rebbe reassured him that this was the right thing to do and encouraged him to perform further *mitzvot*. He met the Rebbe last year at the dollar ceremony and recounts how his 'heart was filled with joy.' Now, quite despondent, he sent a *kvitl* to the Rebbe asking about his toothache. The Rebbe responded by offering a blessing and emphasizing that one should check one's *tallit*. Mr Drazin examined his prayer shawl to find that one of the strands was distinctly worn. Here indeed was the explanation of his toothache, for the thirty-two strands of the *tallit* correspond to the thirty-two teeth. A worn strand may cause pain in a tooth. He triumphantly emphasized again how the physical and spiritual worlds reflected each other, for after replacing his *tallit* his toothache had disappeared in a few days. For him the episode of illness and the Rebbe's response recalled his original 'spiritual healing' on joining the group.

Our second instance, like that of the misspelt *mezuzah*, provides a formal homology between the words of a text and the physical body.

Earlier this year Mrs Halpern, aged forty-one asked her daughter in Brooklyn to contact the Rebbe about the 'unbearable and unrelenting' back pain she had experienced since the birth of her eleventh child. Although the pain had started late in her pregnancy ('probably due to the baby pressing on my spine'), it got much worse following the delivery. It was so bad that she could not sit still for longer than a few minutes. Lying down did not help either. She consulted the family doctor who 'after a very brief examination' recommended bed rest and analgesics. Mrs Halpern was not happy with this advice: for one thing, it prevented her giving her son, Isaac, the care and attention a new-born baby required. Over the next couple of weeks the pain got worse: 'my legs felt weak and my feet were tingling.' She recounted that 'although it was the Shabbat, the pain was so bad that I asked my husband to phone for an ambulance.' (It is permitted to use a phone on Sabbath in the case of an emergency.) She was seen in the local hospital casualty department by an orthopaedic surgeon who told her that she needed to be admitted for absolute bed rest and, if the pain did not settle in a few days, she would need an operation to remove a slipped disc. She reluctantly agreed to go into hospital but was perturbed by the thought of an operation: 'I had heard of someone having a similar operation who was permanently paralysed, I knew that these operations are not always successful.' As soon as the Sabbath had gone, her husband phoned their daughter Sarah and asked her to see the Rebbe's secretary and obtain a blessing for her mother.

Mrs Halpern is a short plump lady with a large blonde *sheitl* who looks somewhat older than her forty-one years. Her personality can only be described as 'motherly.' Born locally, her parents were orthodox Jews who had contact with Lubavitch. An only child (unusually for an orthodox family), she attended a Lubavitcher school in Stamford Hill where she did well and at the age of eighteen went to a seminary in France for two years. 'Although I could have gone to 'Sem' in Israel or America my parents told me to as the Rebbe's advice first. Whatever he says, you must do.' Following her return to England she was introduced to her husband Shmuel, himself a Lubavitcher who works as a printer. Mrs Halpern now works in a local group providing religious activities for children.

The Rebbe responded to her daughter's request by faxing a reply within a few hours (she was particularly keen to impress on us that 'he received several hundred letters each day, yet he responded to mine so quickly because he knew it was important: surely no ordinary man could do this!'). The Rebbe suggested in his reply that all the household *mezuzot* were checked. (He had underlined the word 'all'.) This was done by a local scribe who found a crack across the words 'when you sit in your house' (Deuteronomy 6:7). Mrs Halpern pointed out that she had the worst pain when sitting for any length of time. The scroll was replaced and after a week in hospital she was almost pain free and did not require an operation. How did the Rebbe know about the *posul* (unkosher) *mezuzah*? 'The Rebbe has a connection with HaShem [God]. He has a feeling for holiness because his soul is more spiritual than that of other men and the power of his prayer is greater. Because of this he can know these things.'

Sometimes the Rebbe's explanation is not validated so immediately: Rabbi Nifield is now sixty years old. He recently had a small stroke which left him paralysed in his left arm (although it did not impair his walking or speech). He has suffered from hypertension for some years but admitted that he had not taken it as seriously as he should have although he had been in hospital on several occasions with angina. Following the stroke, he spent a week in his local hospital where he was given physiotherapy which only slowly helped his weakness. Being a rather impatient man, as he put it, he wrote to the Rebbe.

Born in Poland, Jacob Nifield came to Britain in 1936 at the age of four, the third of ten children; his parents were a rabbi, 'a very learned man who spent all his time studying', and an 'ideal Jewish mother, a very quiet women.' Both parents died several years ago. Jacob grew up in an ultra-orthodox environment and carried out the prescribed rituals from a very young age. He spent a year in a Jewish seminary in northern England and became a rabbi at the age of twenty-six and has been teaching since in Lubavitcher schools. He is married with ten children ranging from eleven to thirty-two years old. His wife is reputedly a distant relative of the Rebbe, whom they have visited in America on a number of occasions.

He is a rather austere sixty-year-old man, dressed like many older Lubavitch in a long black coat and broad-rimmed Homburg. He has a particularly long beard, is serious in manner and always rather impatient. 'When do you think I will get better?' he asked repeatedly. Rabbi Nifield has written to the Rebbe in the past about the education of his children, especially as to whether his sons should proceed to rabbinical training. He was impressed by the Rebbe's wisdom in this matter and several of his friends had been helped after writing about health and financial problems. He proudly recalled that he had visited the Rebbe on three occasions for the dollar ceremony: 'Every day you hear more stories about his miraculous power'.

The Rebbe now responded to Rabbi Nifield's letter by offering a blessing and suggesting that he check his *mezuzot*. His wife took the *mezuzot* to a scribe who thoroughly checked the scrolls and casing, only to find they were ritually pure. He could not understand this. Could the Rebbe be wrong? 'No, the Rebbe is never wrong; if he says the *mezuzot* are not kosher, they really are not kosher.' He sent a second letter to the Rebbe telling him of the first scribe, but the Rebbe responded by suggesting the *mezuzot* were checked again. A second scribe was found but he too found them to be kosher. A third letter to the Rebbe brought the same reply. The third scribe spent a long day examining the *mezuzot*, working until the early hours of the following morning. It was only then[21] that, holding up one scroll, he found the problem: a small beam of light shone through a hole in one of the letters. The hole rendered the *mezuzah* unkosher. Rabbi Nifield had the scroll replaced and immediately regained some movement of his left side. Three months after his stroke he had only some slight weakness in his left arm.

Several people were asked about this healing. How did the Rebbe know that there was a problem with the *mezuzah*? Rabbi Nifield himself responded immediately: 'the Rebbe's soul represents the soul of the whole Jewish nation. He is aware of the life of every Jew. Every Jew's actions are known to him.' When we asked if it could possibly be a 'coincidence', he objected: 'Of course coincidences occur but I have heard too many accounts of the Rebbe's healing for my healing to be a coincidence.' He likened the *mezuzah* to 'a suit of armour in the spiritual realm. It protects a person from influences which can cause illness. An unkosher *mezuzah* simply makes a person more vulnerable.' Again, Rabbi Nifield took the opportunity to emphasize that the physical and spiritual realms were interrelated: the woman who fails to take the prescribed monthly bath (*mikveh*) after her menstruation may bear a defective child.

Mr Bright wrote to the Rebbe not about himself but about his two-month old son. Shortly after his birth Daniel had developed 'rattling breathing' about which the parents were very worried. The baby's breathing sounded much worse at night: 'like an old man with bronchitis.' A visit to their family doctor did not prove helpful: 'I cannot find much wrong with the baby, it's just his throat, I'm sure he will grow out of it.' The family were not happy with this reply, and they discussed whether or not to take Daniel to a private hospital. Mrs Bright suggested to her husband that perhaps the Rebbe's advice should first be sought.

Chaim Bright was born in Manchester and moved to Stamford Hill in 1980. He is now in his late forties. Brought up in an orthodox household, he always had close links with Lubavitch for, although his parents were not Hasidim, they attended a Lubavitch synagogue. After doing well at school he went to university to study computing and now works as a computer analyst for an insurance company. He teaches the Talmud part-time in the local boys' school where his wife Leah also teaches. In addition to Daniel, the couple have six other children aged from two to nineteen, Mr Bright proudly adding that Isaac, his eldest son, was in a seminary in Brooklyn, the home of the Rebbe.

The family had experienced much illness in the past. One child had died several years ago in a cot death: 'I suppose that's why we were so concerned about Daniel.' Two children suffered with asthma and were hospitalized on a number of occasions. In 1986 their daughter Hannah, then aged seven, had a mysterious illness and was dangerously ill in hospital. 'First the doctors said it was a virus, then they said a kidney infection. We did not know what to believe. I wrote to the Rebbe on this occasion who suggested I got a second opinion from a well-known Jewish paediatrician. He found that she had an abnormal kidney. The Rebbe always gives good advice.'

In reply to the *kvitl* about Daniel, the Rebbe wrote offering a blessing and suggesting that Mr Bright check his *mezuzot*. He did this but all were found to be kosher. He discussed the matter with a rabbi who noticed that the *mezuzah* in Daniel's room, although kosher, was much older than the others. He suggested it should be replaced. Mr Bright did this, and after several weeks Mrs Bright commented on how much better Daniel's breathing had become.

The Rebbe is consulted on a number of health-related issues apart from immediate sickness. A serious concern is infertility which is considered disastrous for Lubavitchers with their emphasis on large families.[22] Whilst the Rebbe himself is childless he is considered to have particular foresight about infertility.

Rabbi Lehrman was very concerned about his wife who had still not become pregnant after five years of marriage. Repeated hospital tests had not demonstrated any physiological abnormality either in himself or his wife so he wrote to the Rebbe. About a week later when (rather unexpectedly on a business trip) he was able to visit the Rebbe in person, the Rebbe told him 'your fears are irrelevant.' He was surprised by this and asked what the Rebbe meant, to be told 'your wife is already pregnant.' He telephoned home to learn that his wife was indeed pregnant.

The Rebbe's replies may indicate that he has talked with the petitioner's deceased parent's soul, and they frequently cite well-known texts and aphorisms, employing puns and rhymes in Hebrew or English (such as health/wealth) and logical paradoxes, as well as explicit instructions. Do the Rebbe's words themselves have power or does he just have a better knowledge of divine matters? When questioned by sympathetic observers, the Lubavitch Rebbe has agreed he has personal power to help others unite the seen and unseen realms[23] for he argues 'there is a continuous relationship between the creator and the creation.' (cited by Wiener 1969). He can cure by physical touch, or through a *mezuzah* he has blessed (Mintz 1968: 111, 125).[24] The imagery employed by Rabbi Nachman, the founder of the Bratislav Hasidim, was that of a 'banker' who could receive the bad qualities of the supplicant and exchange them for good. Woocher (1979) prefers the analogy of a 'mirror', whilst one Lubavitcher rabbi who has studied psychology likens the Rebbe to a mediating archetype who lowers himself to the petitioner's level of spirituality; Rebbe and Hasid 'invest' in each other, spiritually as well as financially (Schachter 1979).[25] Strikingly, he argues that for the Rebbe to teach someone who does not absorb the knowledge is like masturbation – indeed the Rebbe may actually experience a nocturnal emission as a consequence. He thus rematerializes what Schachter calls, in the language of psychoanalysis, the 'transference' of therapy (cf. Lutsky 1989): the Lubavitcher Rebbe psychically takes on and redeems the transgressions of the Hasid.[26]

Representation and Embodiment Across the 'Double Register': Towards a Zoharic Reading of Medical Anthropology

> The secret world of the Godhead is a world of language, a world of divine names that unfold in accordance with a law of their own. . . Letters and names are not only conventional means of communication. They are far more. Each one of them represents a concentration of energy and expresses a wealth of meaning which cannot be translated, or not fully at least, into human language. (Scholem 1965: 36)

If the 'efficacy' of the *kvitl* and its response may be regarded as an illocutionary manipulation of transactional symbols which stand for events in the material world, then it is difficult to find a formal system of healing in which the two can at times be so closely tied together. Our informants say that even our transcriptions of the healing miracles printed in this book have some power to heal. We have here an elision of the material and its divine representation so profound that it is not easy to imagine any Hasidic observance which is not a type of physical healing.

Scholem (1965: 124) argues that 'those who carry out the *mitsvah* always do two things. The *represent* in a concrete symbol its transcendent essence, through which it is rooted in, and partakes of, the ineffable. But at the same time they transmit to this transcendent essence (which the later Kabbalists called the 'upper root' of ritual action) an influx of energy' [emphasis in the original]. If psychiatrists and anthropologists have postulated correspondence between, or actual casual effects across, a 'double register', the Zohar and hence the Tanya are perhaps unique in the extent of mutual influence. Man has two souls, argues the Tanya, the animal and the divine, each dialectically constituting the other (Mindel 1974); the divine spiritualizes the material as the material spiritualizes the divine (Kehot Publications 1981: 778). Language is not an obstruction, nor even the path, to ultimate reality, but rather its actual nature (cf. Stoller 1984; Wagner 1986). The letters of the Torah are not just God's Law, but the very name of God; indeed, they *are* God, the upper roots of our physical world. The ten Sefirot together form that great, unutterable Name of God which is the act and goal of creation, and hence of human history. Representation (upper root) and embodiment in the sensible world (lower root) necessarily participate in complementary causalities.

All 'mystical' ideas developing within Western monotheism are, like miracles, concerned with reconciliations of the two registers. Rather than just representing matters as two qualitatively distinct registers, the divine and the physical, with certain rare passages between them, the concentric spheres of the Zohar allow participation in either the divine or the physical directions – a stereomorphic cosmos but one in which any event or entity is located simultaneously at the centre and the periphery.[27] A 'miracle' in the sense of a radical but temporary resonance across the two registers, a local drama of the structural anthropologist's or psychotherapist's transaction of the bodily through the symbolic, is thus hardly novel – for, in a sense, here everything and nothing is miraculous. In Zoharic theory physical healing and spiritual healing are the same event, even if the contemporary Hasid visiting his family doctor hardly has the latter foremost in mind. If the Zohar, as a theory of representation, anticipates the 'interpretive turn' in medical anthropology in its concern with directions and procedures rather than with entitles (howbeit with what Bloom [1982] terms its 'wandering meaning'), in recondiling structural order with moral agency (*cf.* Bourdieu 1977), it goes further in retaining the physical as valid as the representation. Representation itself is an aspect of the natural world.[28] Where all is symbolic, in that everything both represents and embodies everything else, there are, in a sense, no 'symbols': everything is concrete reality, everything 'works'.

In everyday practice, things are rather different. Scholem (1954), here surprisingly akin to countless guardians of religious orthodoxy, warns us against too deep a Kabbalistic immersion in the Infinite, in which everyday actions become translated as the ineffable and back again. Explaining why he had not written down his ideas, Luria is supposed to have said, 'It is impossible, because all things are interrelated. I can hardly open my mouth to speak without feeling that the sea bursts forth its dams and overflows' (Scholem 1971). The Rebbes, ever aware of the eruptions of the Kabbalah embodied in the antinomian madness of Sabbatai Svi (Littlewood 1995), set firm rules for the incorporation of Zoharic speculation into the practice of everyday life, always subordinate of the precedent rabbinical ordinances. To attempt to coerce rather than supplicate the upper register (theurgy) was of course sorcery, and if Hasidim still sought access to the strong dangers of ultimate power, it was to be only through the circumscribed intercession of the Rebbe. While scholarly Lubavitch may endlessly argue about the minutiae of the

Kabbalah, their founder disdained such miraculous interventions (Sharot 1982), yet it is through the person of their current Rebbe that ultimate redress is mediated. Hasidim refer to him as a 'channel' between the physical and the spiritual registers (Sharot 1982), an idiom which recalls the 'passages' of Moerman's (1979) somatosocial anthropology.[29] In his mediations the Rebbe reorders the everyday experiential dualism which the Kabbalah always threatens to banish: in the terminology of this chapter, a double-register now re-emerges in a distinction between material experience and its ultimate meaning, between the physical world and some determining transcendent reality.

If we are justified in talking of the Kabbalah as a 'folk model', then it is one with a close reflexive engagement with wider Western knowledge including new biomedicine. Contemporary Lubavitch do not live in an eighteenth-century enclave, and their emphasis on conversion constantly invokes the individual remaking of secular and sacred worlds. Their exemplary illness narratives do not simply articulate Zoharic cosmology and personal suffering but justify the normative rules of a small community, one always preoccupied with its own continuity and boundaries, and with its vulnerability in the wider political world. Yet for these rules individuals may argue quite various religious justifications; for no single interpretation of sacred texts can ever be taken as completely valid (Scholem 1954). Judaism is characteristically praxis, not doxa.

In conclusion, we would recommend a reading of medical anthropology through the Zohar.[30] Western monotheism's double register of immanent and transcendent has, we have argued, formal and historical continuities with that of material and representational in contemporary science. Both Kabbalah and contemporary anthropology essay an epistemological turn away from such a dichotomized universe in which the meaning of one world was simply to be read as the reality of the other. The complex correspondences and isomorphisms between lower and upper 'roots' in the Zohar certainly allow for Hasidic recourse to an ultimate reality by which immediate suffering occurs and is resolved but only imperfectly as a distinct realm we may recognize as 'otherworldly'. If this healing is itself amenable to the conventional procedures of sociological inquiry, as we have attempted here, the mythic corpus to which it refers is nevertheless one which articulates problems of reconciling embodiment and representation identical with those of anthropology. It thus constitutes an 'interpretive turn' so radical that it is able to encompass our material reality as reality, albeit a reality dialectically constituted through its own representations.

Acknowledgements

We are grateful for comments on earlier drafts of this chapter from Audrey Cantlie, Byron Good, Bruce Kapferer, Laurence Kirmayer, Britt Krause, Murray Last, Godfrey Lienhardt, Maurice Lipsedge, Margaret Lock, David Parkin, Edward Schieffelin, Bernard Wasserstein, James Watson, Allan oung, David Zeitlyn and anonymous *Culture, Medicine and Psychiatry* referees, and to participants in seminars at the School of Oriental and African Studies, the Oxford Institute of Social and Cultural Anthropology, and the Department of Humanities and Social Studies in Medicine at McGill.

Notes

1. Earlier fieldwork in Stamford Hill (1990–1992) by one of the authors (S.D.) has been briefly described in Dein (1992). The Rebbe died in 1994 and the ethnographic present here refers to 1991–1993. The personal names of informants are pseudonyms, and we have generally used here the Hebrew rather than Yiddish transliteration; interviews were in English. Many informants were rabbis who comprise about a fifth of the male adults.
2. 'Dualism' is used variously to refer to distinctions between immanent and transcendent; between corporal and spiritual (and thus temporal and religious authority); or between what we may term evil and good (Parkin 1985). In Pauline Christianity, as in Kabbalah, these three 'slid together' (Brown 1989: 48). In this chapter we are using the term primarily in the first usage, one which is closely allied to the second whilst not altogether independent of the third. In the second and third senses, Judaism is arguably less dualist than Christianity: 'I form the light and create darkness: I make peace and create evil: I the Lord do all these things' (Isaiah 45:7). For a more extended consideration of how the various scriptural and post-scriptural texts did, or did not, distinguish between *nephesh* ('soul', 'spirit') and *basar* ('body'), and for possible Hellenistic influences, see Preuss (1978), Bottomley (1980), Rubin (1988), Gilman (1992), Eilberg-Schwartz (1992).
3. Lock and Scheper-Hughes (1990) comment that 'a singular premise guiding Western science and clinical medicine is its commitment to a fundamental opposition between spirit and matter, mind and body, and underlying this real and unreal.' This remained true of anthropological structuralisms even if these abandoned direct one-to-one correspondences between the registers (A::B) in favour of relational patterns (A1:A2::B1:B2).
4. To argue for the primacy of a semantic approach is problematic given that meaning itself refers to a multitude of types of understanding (see the chapters in Parkin 1982), and interpretation is a residual anthropological category (Sperber 1985). If biomedicine is relegated as merely one local interpretation of the physical world, then 'experience near' anthropology remains an academic interpretation of a (local) interpretation (ibid.), and one that still offers an intellectualist metanarrative in proposing that humans are essentially driven by their quest for meaning. (The interpretive genre paradoxically enhances dualism through displacing the truth claims of medicine onto that discipline itself.) We do not argue here for a particular sense of 'meaning' or 'symbol', let alone a psychological or linguistic explanation of human signification and representation, except to say that we favour the observations of many of the authors in Foster and Brandes (1980) that one can locate the same 'symbolizations' on a spectrum between the expressly referential and

the figurative, the shallow and the deep (Barrett and Lucas 1993), and that movement between the two modes seems mediated by intention, context or affect. As we argue below, movement in the referential direction may be such that lexical representations become objectified as entities in themselves, less meanings to be unravelled than themselves directly gaining ontological status in the cognized world (McGuire 1983; Wagner 1986; Lakoff 1987; Tambiah 1990: cf. Foucault 1966): whether in everyday life (Berger and Luckman 1966) or in anthropological theory (Boyer 1986).

5. Not altogether surprisingly, given anthropology's earlier organicist analogies of social structure. This is not to say that individual agency could not be recognized in such tightly ordered schemata (Bourdieu 1977; Godelier 1986), but that some implicit sense of the overdetermined complex was always assumed to be born in mind by – or rather to constitute – individuals; and any innovation by them took place through various combinations of identification and negation (Littlewood 1984, 1993). We would argue that the demise of such tight structuralist isomorphisms is not only an attribute of changing intellectual fashion or the demise of colonial objectification but that everyday life in the 'timeless small-scale societies' with which anthropologists have been concerned has generally become more pluralistic and subjectively instrumental (cf. Bourdieu 1977; Featherstone 1990): certain religious groups expected.
6. Taking 'myth' in its restricted sense as a narrative about personages in a sacred world and time akin to some ultimate reality (cf. Kirmayer 1993), it may be argued that Western biomedicine offers no such narratives but simply paradigms of sickness reality which only implicitly recall the ultimate justification of our world (Lock and Gordon 1998).
7. For accounts, see Buber (1948), Dresner (1974), Katz (1961), Mintz (1968) and Sharot (1982). The attribute Hasid (pious one) had previously referred to the Jewish rebels against Antiochus Epiphanes (second century BCE) and to the German followers of Rabbi Yehuda the Hasid (thirteenth century CE).
8. Scholem (1974) argues that the Sabbatian attack on the literal law through an antinomian enactment of Kabbalah both reflected and amplified the development of secular Judaism, opening up the ghetto to more universalized and psychologized ideas as the medieval Jewish accommodation with feudal power collapsed through the growth of local nationalisms (Katz 1961). Like Sharot (1982), he (1954) sees Hasidism as a 'neutralization of messianic elements into mainstream Judaism,' whilst Bakan (1958) goes so far as to talk of a 'dialectical synthesis'. For a review of the debate, see Sharot (1982).
9. On Lubavitch in New York, see Mintz (1968); in Montreal, Shaffir (1974); in London, Kupferman (1976), Wallach (1977); on ultra-orthodoxy in Jerusalem, Bilu et al. (1990).
10. The Satmar who generally settled in Williamsburg do not recognize the state of Israel, arguing that the Hebrew nation cannot be restored before the advent of the Messiah. The Gur live mainly in Israel, as do the Belzers. The Breazlav are unusual in having no living rebbe.
11. The idiom of conversion is somewhat inappropriate: rather Lubavitch 'reclaim' Jews to orthodoxy (cf. Wallace's [1958] term 'revitalization').
12. For orthodox Jews, relations between the mundane and the ultrahuman are mediated through a number of objects. At one level the whole household may be said to be 'sacred' in opposition to the Gentile world (Littlewood 1983) but additionally there are three more specific 'ritual' (transactional) objects to which this chapter refers. *Tefillin* are phylacteries, worn during prayer on the head and on the arm near the heart, which contain scriptural texts written on parchment exhorting the Jew to love God and to subject to Him everyday life, thoughts, feelings and actions (Exodus 3: 1–10, 11–16; Deuteronomy 6: 4–9, 11: 13–21). Similar texts, affixed in a case to the door frame of the

main entrance of every living room of the house as well as the *mezuzah*, summon the Jew to consecrate his home, making it an abode worthy to be blessed by the presence of God. The *tallit*, a prayer shawl donned by adult males during morning and additional prayers, has eight fringes at each of its four corners.

13. Joining involves a gradual detachment from significant others outside the group with increasing interaction with established members, approximating to the general model of conversion proposed by Lofland and Stark (1965). This is not the place to argue why, in a generation after Auschwitz, certain Westerners should seek to 're-enchant' their secular world.
14. Mrs Lévy visited the Rebbe for the dollar ceremony some ten years ago and asked for a blessing for a *shidduch*. She was carrying several books which she dropped accidentally in front of him. On her second visit last year he looked carefully at her and said, 'Be careful with your books!' Another informant approached the Rebbe about his son who was physically handicapped and for whom he was unable to arrange a *shidduch*. The Rebbe gave him two dollars, one for himself and one to take to Israel; not understanding the reason behind this, he went nevertheless to Israel taking the second dollar with him. In Jerusalem he happened to speak to a Hasid on a bus sitting opposite him and recounted the problem of his son. The other was astounded, for he himself had a disabled daughter and had written to Rebbe Schneersohn to find her a partner: the Rebbe had given him the identical advice. Subsequent friendship led to the marriage of their two children.
15. A common representation, allied to that of the circles, is that of a nut: sensible experience is the shell which has to be broken to reach the 'real' essence. This is common figuring in any system in which, as in biomedicine (Littlewood 1991), a distinction is made between 'reality' and 'appearance'; in biomedicine, the physical is the kernel, in Hasidic medicine it is the husk. Other systems of Kabbalah offer either a more personified deity or a more ethereal one who, as in Gnosticism, is counterposed to the demiurge mistakenly represented in Genesis as the Creator.
16. This requires further complexities as there are only 3,400,000 physical letters in the Torah.
17. Scholem (1954) suggests that the scattering of the sparks may be read directly as the historical exile of the Jews, restitution as redemption. Sharot (1982) points out that whilst Luria himself did not expressly relate his schema to the Iberian expulsion of 1492, we, as observers, can note a Weberian (or euhemerist) affinity between historical event and subsequent myth. Certainly, there is occasional explicit reference to this by others, together with a shared idiom. In prayer, Hasidic men tie a cord around their waist to separate the spiritual upper part of their body from the mundane lower half, for aliyah [to go up] is physical height as well as ascent to the divine, and more recently the term for secular migration to Israel (Jacobs 1973). In the arguably manic-depressive illness of Sabbatai Svi, aliyah described his period of elated mood, and thus his messiahship (Littlewood 1995).
18. Sullivan (1987) proposes that the 'most important figure or symbol in any given religious tradition is the source of healing.' Our identification of an overarching representation is of course likely to reflect immediate concerns: in which case his observation is tautologous. Yet the heavy semantic load embedded in 'core symbols' (enabling symbols – Lawson and McCauley 1993) is perhaps fully accessed only in particular situations.
19. Whilst we have emphasized here a linear image of exile, this can be figured also as a three-dimensional containment and catharsis, well represented in public and household ritual (Littlewood 1983).

20. Fieldwork with conversionist groups is distinctive in that they continue to offer presentationalist justifications of normative actions (Littlewood 1993). Unlike other illness narratives (Good 1994), these have a fixed and formal (Lawson and McCauley 1993; cf. Early 1982) tripartite pattern – appeal to the Rebbe about a problem, the Rebbe's response, resolution of the problem – which recalls the exemplary legends Hasidim recount of past zaddikim. They may be taken as standardized and edifying testimonials, emblematic self-presentations for other Hasidim and for the anthropologist as a potential convert: to use Crapanzano's (1992) term, they have become 'meta-pragmatic'. Thus the story described above of the misspelt *mezuzah* has already been recorded among Brooklyn Lubavitch in very similar terms but there about a *tefillin* (Mintz 1968: 334).
21. The early dawn is the best time to study Kabbalah and kindred matters: the Hebrew words for 'mystery' and 'light' are equivalent in gematria (a way of interpreting texts by assigning numerical values to letters, words, or phrases).
22. Margolin and Wiztum (1989), in their discussion of Sephardic interpretations of infertility and impotence, suggest that a common explanation is having been 'tied' by jealous sorcery. In the accounts cited here the petitioners argue that they expect, through the Rebbe, to effect some definite change in the natural world: in Ahem's (1979) terminology, following Austin, their petitions were, like spells (Tambiah 1990), performative, 'strong illocutionary acts.' Although offered retrospectively as efficacious, it is likely that at the time many were 'weak,' simply performed as immediately appropriate or 'felicitous' (Lloyd 1990) or little more than wishes, Wittgenstein's 'actions of instinct' (Tambiah 1990: 56); and they of course have a perlocutionary context which we do not detail in this chapter.
23. Although our narrative emphasizes the Rebbe's knowledge, collections of exemplary stories published by Lubavitch emphasize something more like instrumental power over the physical world. The term 'miracle' is commonly used. An eighteen-year-old boy, Rafi, is seriously ill with leukaemia (Lubavitch Publications 1992). The hospital doctor advises an immediate operation, but Rafi's tearful brother tells his teacher who contacts the Rebbe only to advise the operation must be delayed until he has prayed on the Sabbath. The doctor, an atheist who is furious at this interference, decides to proceed. He arrives late at the hospital after being held up with a burst tyre, the nurses report the instruments have gone missing, and he has to postpone the operation. The boy's condition suddenly improves, and the operation is no longer necessary. Many Lubavitchers offered us the work 'charisma' for their Rebbe's power, the term suggested by Weber (1947) to designate situations where an individual who embodies a group's concerns through 'extrasocial qualities' leads them independently of tradition, physical coercion or role-bound status. Sociologically, charisma is less an explanation of social action than a description, one defining element in a typology; what is significant is not the 'personality' of the leader, but their social function as symbol, catalyst and message bearer (Littlewood 1993). He or she may be relatively unimpressive as a practical leader, serving like Sabbatai Svi as the locus on which current preoccupations are placed. In the popular sense, however, 'charisma' refers to something like 'strength of personality' or even 'ultrahuman power'. The Rebbe approximates better to Weber's 'traditional authority' or even the 'divine king' of Oxford Africanists. In Hasidic stories, he recalls another anthropological figure – the trickster of folk tales, outwitting the powerful official or greedy peasant, on occasion ironically defeated through his own stratagems.
24. Which recalls the presentation of food and money offered by the *shtetl* Hasid to his Rebbe which the latter then redistributed (Zborowski and Herzog 1962).

25. Like Christ. One rabbi reading an earlier draft of this chapter argued that the emission was impossible. See also Hoffman (1981). A more appropriate image may be that of a 'condenser' or 'container' (Parkin 1992; Lutzky 1989), an idiom which becomes a little clearer when we consider the converse of a miracle – the 'scandal' of medieval Christian terminology. In February 1992 the Rebbe, then aged ninety, had a stroke. The medical details were unclear, although local newspapers such as the *Jewish Chronicle* reported that it was minor, and he was making a good recovery. Lubavitch House requested that all Jews recite psalms once a day. Although apparently not seriously ill, the Rebbe was unable to give out dollars, nor to respond to petitions. Members of the community were asked why he himself had become sick, and what they thought this sickness meant. Among the explanations given was this one from a young rabbi: 'The soul of the Rebbe represents the group soul of the Jewish people. His suffering represents the suffering of every Jew. It is like a body and head, the Rebbe being the head of the Jewish body. The two cannot exist independently. If the body is sick, it can give rise to a headache. If the brain does not work, how can the body function? If every Jew does not perform good deeds the Jewish body will become sick and in turn the Rebbe. If more Jews perform these deeds the Rebbe will recover.' In order to heal their leader a new Torah was written in New York, and every Jew asked to donate a pound towards a letter in it. Another rabbi explained: 'All Jewish souls are tied to the Rebbe's soul. In the Torah there are 600,000 words (328,000 complete words and 272,000 incomplete words). In the world there are 600,000 general souls which divide up into many more souls. These general souls are linked to the Rebbe's soul. By writing a perfect Torah the Rebbe's soul becomes perfect again and this will affect his body.' He described how the Rebbe must first undergo a descent into a shattered vessel before he can ascend to a higher level, taking with him some of the hidden sparks. This descent is associated with a decay in the physical body. The rabbi intimated that perhaps this was a prelude to the messianic arrival. He admitted that it was quite possible that the current Rebbe was indeed the Messiah. 'Every descent of the Zaddik means an elevation of divine light' (cited by Scholem 1954). (Before the Rebbe's death in June 1994 Lubavitch intensified a public 'Moshiach campaign' implying he was the Messiah, and expectations of some sort of 'resurrection' surfaced throughout late 1994.)
26. The Cosmic Man is made up of all men (Ben Shimon Halevi 1974), 'members and parts of various ranks all acting upon each other so as to form one organism' (Zohar). If we need a figuring, the notion of a fractal (in which each part replicates the whole – Mandelbrot 1977) is more apposite than of a single spiritual-physical dyad: perhaps Pribrams's hologram or Wagner's (1986) holograph, the linguistic trope of synecdoche or the participatory symbols of Lévy-Bruhl's primitive mentality. Compare Notes 15, 19.
27. In Bolinger's (1980) words, 'the culture inserts a sign and gets back a symbol,' as the increasingly referential word itself becomes materialized as an independent entity, Tambiah's (1990) 'objectified charisma'. (See Note 4.) Whilst a similar potential exists in Christianity – 'the word made flesh' – we might argue it is more esoteric theology than instrumental practice, although there are analogues in the sacraments and in popular healing (Cramer 1993; McGuire 1983), and of course in Islamic medicine (Parkin 1992).
28. Bloom (1984) proposes that the deity of the Kabbalah may be (mis)read as language; for Scholem (1954) He exists as a theory of representations. Foucault (1970) takes the late medieval 'signatures' (in which natural object and name were intrinsically linked, as in Hermetic and Kabbalistic typologies) as not properly a theory of representation at all but rather one of resemblance through sympathy, mimesis, repetition and transforma-

tion: representation proper requiring the Renaissance distinction between an object and its name which itself is not of the natural order but arbitrary (and hence the natural world cannot be replicated or coerced through such devices as numerology or alphabetic order). He notes the primacy given in the European systems of signatures to Hebrew, the universal language spoken by Adam which retained something of the material creation. The recovery of this or some other language which directly embodied (or later, represented) reality was a recurring Renaissance preoccupation (Eco 1993). The more figurative numerology of religious texts by Kabbalists proceeded from already existing referential practices: Hebrew lacks numerals, so numbers have always been represented by a letter of the alphabet (on which see Crump 1990), and there had long been a popular tradition that misspelling the paraphrases of the divine name in the Torah was likely to visit serious sickness and misfortune on the community (Trachtenberg 1939). Even a misspelt Torah was too powerful to be safely destroyed and was buried in a vault.

29. Or the 'channels' of structuralism (Laughlin and Stephens 1980). Any dualist epistemology, whether religious or scientific, has difficulties in justifying the nature of the links between the two registers. Again, we have to be wary of assuming a uniform local understanding: for the less scholarly or recently 'reclaimed' Hasid, the Rebbe is often not so much a channel as a thaumaturge. (Contrariwise, most people regularly check their *mezuzot* anyway.) If mediation between the two registers occurs typically through a particular individual, it is difficult not to locate in them some personal 'magical' power (Tambiah 1990; cf. McGuire 1983): what Scholem and Bastide, following Andrew Lang, term a 'degeneration' of religion as a cosmological figuring. Frazerians would argue the converse – for the figurative as a degeneration of the instrumental: as does Robertson-Smith (1972) in his account of the origins of Jewish religion.
30. In Bloom's (1982) terms, a misprision or creative misreading, analogues of Freud's physiological readings of Brentano, or Lévi-Strauss' sociological reading of Jakobson. Arguably this is less of a 'misreading' for both Kabbalah and contemporary anthropology offer not dissimilar epistemologies of signification, and Ellen (1977) proposes that 'analytical classifications' such as the Zohar are particularly amenable to the procedures favoured by structural anthropologists.

References

Ahem, E.M.1979. 'The Problems of Efficacy. Strong and Weak Illocutionary Acts', *Man* (n.s) 14: 1–17.

Alexander, F. 1939. 'Psychoanalytic Study of a Case of Essential Hypertension', *Psychosomatic Medicine* 1: 139–52.

Ansel, A. 1982. *Judaism and Psychology*, 3rd edition. New York: Felshelm.

Ardener, E. 1980. 'Some Outstanding Problems in the Analysis of Events', in M.L. Foster and S.H. Brandes (eds), *Symbols as Sense: New Approaches to the Analysis of Meaning*. New York: Academic Press.

Barrett, R.J.J. and R.H. Lucas. 1993. 'The Skulls are Cold, The House is Hot: Interpreting Depths of Meaning in Iban Therapy', *Man* (n.s) 28: 573–96.

Beckford, J. 1985. 'The World Images of New Religious and Healing Movements', in R.K. Jones (ed.), *Sickness and Sectarianism: Exploratory Studies in Medical and Religious Sectarianism*. Aldershot: Gower.

Beeston, R. 1992. '"Messiah" Arouses Rival Rabbi's Wrath', *The Times* (London), 29 February.

Ben-Amos, D. and J.R. Mintz (trans. and eds). 1970. *In Praise of the Ba'al Shem Tov (Shichei ha-Besht).* Bloomington: Indiana University Press.

Ben Shimon Halevi, Z. 1974. *Adam and the Kabbalistic Tree.* London: Rider.

Berger, P.L. and T. Luckman. 1966. *The Social Constriction of Reality.* New York: Doubleday.

Bilu, Y., E. Witztum and O. Van Der Hart. 1990. 'Paradise Regained: "Miraculous Healing" in an Israeli Psychiatric Clinic', *Culture, Medicine and Psychiatry* 14: 105–27.

Blacking, J. (ed.). 1977. *The Anthropology of the Body.* London: Academic Press.

Bloom, H. 1984. *Kabbalah and Criticism.* New York: Continuum.

Bolinger, D. 1980. 'Intonation and "Nature"', in M.L. Foster and S.H. Brandes (eds), *Symbols as Sense: New Approaches to the Analysis of Meaning.* New York: Academic Press.

Bottomley, F. 1980. 'Ideas of the Body in the Old Testament', in F. Bottomley, *Attitudes to the Body in Western Christendom.* London: Lepus.

Bourdieu, P. 1977. *Outline of a Theory of Practice.* Cambridge: Cambridge University Press.

Boyer, P. 1986. 'The "Empty" Concepts of Traditional Thinking: A Semantic and Pragmatic Description', *Man* (n.s.) 21: 50–64.

Brown, P. 1989. *The Body and Society: Men, Women and Sexual Renunciation in Early Christianity.* London: Faber and Faber.

Buber, M. 1948. *Tales if the Hasidim (2 vols).* New York: Schocken.

Bulka, R.P. (ed.). 1979. *Mystics and Medics: A Comparison of Mystical and Psychotherapeutic Encounters.* New York: Human Sciences Press.

Caws, P. 1974. 'Operational, Representation and Explanatory Models', *American* Anthropologist 76: 1–10.

Clifford, J. 1988. *The Predicament of Culture: Twentieth Century Ethnography, Literature and Arts.* Cambridge, MA: Harvard University Press.

Cramer, P. 1993. *Baptism and Change in the Early Middle Ages c.200-c.1150.* Cambridge: Cambridge University Press.

Crapanzano, V. 1992. *Hermes' Dilemma and Hamlet's Desire: On the Epistemology of Interpretation.* Cambridge, MA: Harvard University Press.

Crump, T. 1990. *The Anthropology of Numbers.* Cambridge: Cambridge University Press.

Csordas, T.J. 1988. 'Elements of Charismatic Persuasion and Healing', *Medical Anthropology Quarterly* 2: 445–69.

______. 1994a. *The Sacred Self: A Cultural Phenomenology of Charismatic Healing.* Berkeley: California University Press.

______. 1994b. 'Introduction', in T.J. Csordas (ed.), *Embodiment and Experience: The Existential Ground of Culture and Self.* Cambridge: Cambridge University Press.

______. 1994c. 'Words from the Holy People: A Case Study in Cultural Phenomenology', in T.J. Csordas (ed.), *Embodiment and Experience.* Cambridge: Cambridge University Press.

Dein, S. 1992. 'Millennialism, Messianism and Medicine', *International Journal of Social Psychiatry* 18: 262–67.

Douglas, M. 1970 [1966]. *Purity and Danger: An Analysis of Concepts of Pollution and Taboo.* Harmondsworth: Penguin.

______. 1973 [1970]. *Natural Symbols: Explorations in Cosmology.* Harmondsworth: Penguin.

Dow, J. 1986. 'Universal Aspects of Symbolic Healing: A Theoretical Synthesis', *American Anthropologist* 88: 56–69.

Dresner, S.H. 1974 [1960]. *The Zaddick.* New York: Schocken.

Durkheim, E. and M. Mauss. 1963. *Primitive Classification.* London: Cohen and West.

Early, E.A. 1982. 'The Logic of Well-Being: Therapeutic Narratives in Cairo, Egypt', *Social Science and Medicine* 16: 1491–97.

Eco, U. 1993. *La Ricerca Della Lingua Perfetta nella Cultura Europea*. Rome: Laterza.

Ehrenwald, J. 1979. 'Precognition and the Prophetic Tradition: from ESP to the Effective Myth', in R.P. Bulka (ed.), *Mystics and Medics: A Comparison of Mystical and Psychotherapeutic Encounters*. New York: Human Sciences Press.

Eilberg-Schwartz, H. (ed.). 1992. *People of the Body: Jews and Judaism from an Embodied Perspective*. New York: State University of New York Press.

Ellen, R. 1977. 'Anatomical Classification and the Semiotics of the Body', in J. Blacking (ed.), *The Anthropology of the Body*. London: Academic Press.

Featherstone, M. (ed.). 1990. *Global Culture: Nationalism, Globalisation and Modernity*. London: Sage.

Feinberg, R. 1990. 'Spiritual and Natural Etiologies on a Polynesian Outlier in Papua New Guinea', *Social Sciences and Medicine* 30: 311–23.

Foster, M.L. and S.H. Brandes (eds). 1980. *Symbols as Sense: New Approaches to the Analysis of Meaning*. New York: Academic Press.

Foucault, M. 1970 [1966]. *The Order of Things: An Archaeology of the Human Sciences*. London: Tavistock.

Gellner, E. 1992. *Postmodernism, Reason and Religion*. London: Routledge.

Gilman, S. 1992. *The Jew's Body*. New York: Routledge.

Godelier, M. 1986 [1984]. *The Mental and the Material: Thought, Economy and Society*. London: Verso.

Good, B. 1994. *Medicine, Rationality and Experience: An Anthropological Perspective*. Cambridge: Cambridge University Press.

Good, B. and M. Good. 1986. 'The Cultural Context of Diagnosis and Therapy: A View from Medical Anthropology', in M. Miranda and H. Kitano (eds), *Mental Health Research Practice in Minority Communities: Development of Culturally Sensitive Training Programmes*. Washington, DC: Department of Health and Human Services, pp. 1–27.

Grunbaum, A. 1984. *The Foundations of Psychoanalysis: A Philosophical Critique*. Berkeley: University of California Press.

Hage, P. and F. Harary. 1983. *Structural Models in Anthropology*. Cambridge: Cambridge University Press.

Hall, M.P. 1962. *An Encyclopaedic Outline of Masonic, Hermetic, Qabbalistic and Rosicrucian Symbolic Philosophy*. Los Angeles: Philosophical Research Society.

Heelas, P. and A.M. Haglund-Heelas. 1988. 'The Inadequacy of "Deprivation" as a Theory of Conversion', in W. James and D.H. Johnson (eds), *Vernacular Christianity*. Oxford: JASO.

Hobart, M. 1982. 'Meaning and Moaning? An Ethnographic Note on a Little Understood Tribe', in D. Parkin (ed.), *Semantic Anthropology*. London: Academic Press

Hoffman, E. 1981. *The Way of Splendor: Jewish Mysticism and Modern Psychology*. New York: Shambala Press.

Holy, L. and M. Stuchlik (eds). 1981. *The Structure of Folk Models*. London: Academic Press.

Jackson, M. 1983. 'Knowledge of the Body', *Man* (n.s.) 18: 327–45.

Jacobs, L. 1973. *Hasidic Prayer*. New York: Schocken.

Kapferer, B. 1993 [1983]. *A Celebration of Demons: Exorcism and the Aesthetics of Healing in Sri Lanka*. Oxford: Berg.

Katz, J. 1961. *Tradition and Crisis: Jewish Society at the End of the Middle Ages*. New York: Free Press.

Kehot Publication Society. 1981. *Tanya (Likutei Amarim-Tanya, bilingual edition)*. Stamford Hill, London.

Kirmayer, L. 1993. 'Healing and the Invention of Metaphor: The Effectiveness of Symbols Revisited', *Culture, Medicine, and Psychiatry* 17: 161–95.

Kleinman, A. and L.H. Sung. 1979. 'Why Do Indigenous Practitioners Successfully Heal?', *Social Science and Medicine* 13: 7–26.
Kupferman, A.J. 1976. *The Lubavitch Hasidim of Stamford Hill.* M.Phil. thesis, University of London.
Laderman, C. 1987. 'The Ambiguity of Symbols in the Structure of Healing., *Social Science and Medicine* 24: 293–301.
Lakoff, G. 1987. *Women, Fire and Dangerous Things: What Categories Reveal About the Mind.* Chicago: Chicago University Press.
Last, M. 1981. 'The Importance of Knowing About Not Knowing', *Social Science and Medicine* 15: 387–92.
Laughlin, C.D. and C.D. Stephens. 1980. 'Symbolisation, Canalisation and P-Structure', in M.L. Foster and S.H. Brandes (eds), *Symbols as Sense: New Approaches to the Analysis of Meaning.* New York: Academic Press.
Lawson, E.T. and R.N. McCauley. 1993. *Rethinking Religion: Connecting Cognition and Culture.* Cambridge: Cambridge University Press.
Lévi-Strauss, C. 1949. 'L'Efficacité Symbolique', trans. as *The Effectiveness of Symbols,* in C. Lévi-Strauss (1968), *Structural Anthropology – 1.* Harmondsworth: Penguin.
______. 1970 [1964]. *The Raw and the Cooked: Introduction to a Science of Mythology – 1.* London: Cape.
Littlewood, R. 1983. 'The Antinomian Hasid', *British Journal of Medical Psychology* 56: 67–78.
______. 1984. 'The Individual Articulation of Shared Symbols', *Journal of Operational Psychiatry* 15: 17–24.
______. 1991. 'Artichokes and Entities: Or, How New is "The New Cross-Cultural Psychiatry"?', *Transcultural Psychiatric Research Review* 28: 343–56.
______. 1993. *Pathology and Identity: The Work of Mother Earth in Trinidad.* Cambridge: Cambridge University Press.
______. 1995. 'Psychopathology and Religious Innovation: An Historical Instance', in D. Bhugra (ed.), *Psychiatry and Religion.* London: Routledge.
Lloyd, G.E.R. 1990. *Demystifying Mentalities.* Cambridge: Cambridge University Press.
Lock, M. and D.R. Gordon. 1988. 'Relationships between Society, Culture and Biomedicine', in M. Lock and D.R. Gordon (eds), *Biomedicine Examined.* Dordrecht: Kluwer.
Lock, M. and N. Scheper-Hughes. 1990. 'A Critical Interpretative Approach in Medical Anthropology: Rituals and Routines of Discipline and Dissent', in T. Johnson and C. Sargent (eds), *Medical Anthropology: A Handbook of Theory and Practice.* Westport, CT: Greenwood Press.
Lofland, J. and R. Stark. 1965. 'Becoming a World Saver: A Theory of Conversion to a Deviant Perspective', *American Sociological Review* 30: 82–75.
Lubavitch Publications. 1992. *A Collection of Stories on the Lubavitcher Rebbe.* New York: Lubavitch Printing House.
Lutzky, H. 1989. 'Reparation and Tikkun: A Comparison of the Kleinian and Kabbalistic Concepts', *International Review of Psycho-Analysis* 16: 449–58.
Magolin, J. and E. Witztum. 1989. 'Supernatural Impotence: Historical Review with Anthropological and Clinical Implications', *British Journal of Medical Psychology* 62: 333–42.
Mandelbrot, B.B. 1977. *Fractals: Form, Chance and Dimensions.* New York.
Mauss, M. 1979 [1950]. *Sociology and Psychology.* London: Routledge and Kegan Paul.
McDougall, L. 1977. 'Symbols and Somatic Structures', in J. Blacking (ed.), *The Anthropology of the Body.* London: Academic Press.

McGuire, M.B. 1983. 'Words of Power: Personal Empowerment and Healing', *Culture, Medicine and Psychiatry* 7: 221–40.

McMullin, E. 1978. 'Structural Explanation', *American Philosophical Quarterly* 15: 139–47.

Mindel, N. 1974. *Philosophy of Chabad.* New York: Kehot Publication Society.

Mintz, J.R. 1968. *Legends of the Hasidim.* Chicago: Chicago University Press.

______. 1992. *Hasidic People: A Place in the New World.* Cambridge, MA: Harvard University Press.

Moerman, N. 1979. 'Anthropology of Symbolic Healing', *Current Anthropology* 20: 59–80.

Munn, N. 1973. 'Symbolism in a Ritual Context: Aspects of Symbolic Action', in J. Honigmann (ed.), *Handbook of Social and Cultural Anthropology.* Chicago: Rand.

Ortner, S. 1973. 'On Key Symbols', *American Anthropologist* 75: 1338–46.

Parkin, D. (ed.). 1982. *Semantic Anthropology.* London: Academic Press.

______. 1985. *The Anthropology of Evil.* Oxford: Blackwell.

______. 1992. *Dispersing Problems: Muslim Medical Practitioners on the Kenya Coast* (unpublished manuscript).

Piaget, J. 1968. *Le Structuralisme.* Paris: Presses Universitaires de France.

Preis, K. 1928. 'Die Medizin im Zohar', *Monatsschrift Für Geschichte und Wissenschaft Des Judentums* 72: 241.

Preuss, J. 1978 [1957]. *Biblical and Talmudic Medicine.* New York: Hebrew Publishing.

Rivers, W.H.R. 1924. *Medicine, Magic and Religion.* London: Kegan Paul, Trench and Trubner.

Robertson-Smith, J.S.R. 1927. *Lectures on The Religion of the Semites: The Fundamental Institutions,* 3rd edition. London: A. and C. Black.

Rorty, R. 1980. *Philosophy and The Mirror of Nature.* Oxford: Blackwell.

Rubin, N. 1988. 'Body and Soul in Talmudic and Mishnaic Sources', *Koroth* 9: 151–64.

Sahlins, M. 1976. *Culture and Practical Reason.* Chicago: University of Chicago Press.

Samuel, G. 1990. *Mind, Body and Culture: Anthropology and the Biological Interface.* Cambridge: Cambridge University Press.

Schachter, Z.M. 1979. 'The Dynamics of the Yehidut Transaction', in R.P. Bulka (ed.), *Mystics and Medics: A Comparison of Mystical and Psychotherapeutic Encounters.* New York: Human Sciences Press.

Scheper-Hughes, N. and M. Lock. 1987. 'The Mindful Body: A Prolegomenon to Future Work in Medical Anthropology', *Medical Anthropology Quarterly* 1: 6–39.

Schieffelin, E.L. 1985. 'Performance and the Cultural Construction of Reality', *American Ethnologist* 12: 707–24.

Schochet, J. 1979. *Mystical Concepts in Hasidism.* New York: Kehot.

Scholem, G.C. 1954. *Major Trends in Jewish Mysticism,* 3rd edition. New York: Schocken.

______. 1965. *On The Kabbalah and Its Symbolism.* New York: Schocken.

______. 1971. *The Messianic Idea in Judaism and Other Essays in Jewish Spirituality.* New York: Schocken.

______. 1973. *Sabbatai Zevi.* London: Routledge.

Seager, W. 1991. *Metaphysics of Consciousness.* London: Routledge.

Shaffir, W. 1974. *Life in a Religious Community: The Lubavitcher Chassidim in Montreal.* Toronto: Toronto University Press.

Sharot, S. 1982. *Messianism, Mysticism and Magic: A Sociological Account of Jewish Religious Movements.* Chapel Hill: University of North Carolina Press.

______. 1991. 'Hasidism in Modern Society', in G.B. Hundert (ed.), *Essential Papers in Hasidism.* New York: New York University Press.

Sperber, D. 1975. *Rethinking Symbolism*. Cambridge: Cambridge University Press.
______. 1980. 'Is Symbolic Thought Pre-Rational?', in M.L. Foster and S.H. Brandes (eds), *Symbols as Sense: New Approaches to the Analysis of Meaning*. New York: Academic Press.
______. 1985. *On Anthropological Knowledge*. Cambridge: Cambridge University Press.
Spero, M.H. 1979. 'On the Nature of the Therapeutic Encounter Between Hasid and Master', in R.P. Bulka (ed.), *Mystics and Medics: A Comparison of Mystical and Psychotherapeutic Encounters*. New York: Human Sciences Press.
Stoller, P. 1984. 'Sounds in Songay Cultural Experience', *American Ethnologist* 11: 559–70.
Tambiah, S.J. 1968. 'The Magical Power of Words', *Man* (n.s.) 3: 175–208.
______. 1990. *Magic, Science, Religion and the Scope of Rationality*. Cambridge: Cambridge University Press.
Toren, C. 1983. 'Thinking Symbols: A Critique of Sperber 1979', *Man* (n.s.) 18: 260–68.
Torrey, E.F. 1971. *The Mind Games: Witchdoctors and Psychiatrists*. New York: Emerson Hall.
Trachtenberg, J. 1977 [1939]. *Jewish Magic and Superstition*. New York: Atheneum.
Wagner, R. 1986. *Symbols That Stand for Themselves*. Chicago: Chicago University Press.
Wallace, A.F.C. 1958. *Revitalisation Movements*. New York: Random House.
Wallach, M. 1977. 'The Chassidim of Stamford Hill', *Jewish Chronicle Magazine*, 27 May: 11–19.
Weber, M. 1947 [1923]. *The Theory of Social and Economic Organisations*. New York: Free Press.
Weisel, E. 1978. *Four Hasidic Masters and Their Struggle Against Melancholy*. London: Notre Dame.
Wiener, H. 1969. *9 1/2 Mystics: The Kabbala Today*. New York: Collier.
Winter, J.A. 1973. 'The Metaphoric Parallelist Approach to the Sociology of Theistic Beliefs: Themes, Variations, and Implications', *Sociological Analysis* 34: 212–29.
Witztum, E. and D. Greenberg. 1990. 'Mental Illness and Religious Change', *British Journal of Medical Psychology* 63: 33–41.
Woocher, J.S. 1979. 'The Kabbalah, Hasidism and The Life of Unification', in R.P. Bulka (ed.), *Mystics and Medics: A Comparison of Mystical and Psychotherapeutic Encounters*. New York: Human Sciences Press.
Young, A. 1976. 'Some Implications of Medical Beliefs and Practices for Social Anthropology', *American Anthropologist* 78: 5–24.
Zborowski, M. and E. Herzog. 1962. *Life Is With People: The Culture of the Shtetl*. New York: Schocken.
The Zohar. 1934. (Selections translated by H. Sperling, M. Simon and P. Levertoff). London: Soncino.

Chapter 2

Cultural Performance – Lubavitch Messianism

Introduction

Millennial convictions – the promise of a paradise on earth with an end to all evil and suffering – have been widely documented in diverse religious contexts throughout human history. The predominant focus of the academic literature on millennialism has been on predictive millennialism (where religious believers make clear predictions of the timing of the apocalypse) and the various strategies deployed by such believers to deal with the 'failure of prophecy'. This literature is highly influenced by two seminal texts – Cohn's (1993) and Festinger, Riecken and Schachter's (1956).

There are abundant historical accounts suggesting that such failure is associated with severe disappointment (see for instance O'Leary 1994 on the Millerites, Festinger et al. 1956 on the Seekers). The various forms of rationalization that have been adopted to assuage such feelings of disappointment have been described by Stone (2000), who argues that when a prediction fails, believers retreat to a more ideologically defensible position, which often involves non-empirical reinterpretations of the original prophecy. The scholarly literature generally postulates 'failed' millennialism as a crisis of belief whose solution is cognitive. The discrepancy between what ought to be and what actually is constitutes one source of tension or cognitive dissonance for believers. Those who experience such tensions may choose to relinquish their religious activities altogether. Alternatively, they may change or moderate their religious convictions in accordance with the situation at hand. They perform what Bennett Berger (1981) calls 'ideological work' – the process of aligning belief and practice that is necessary to keep people's convictions in a viable relationship with their interests, behaviour and circumstances. A large number of studies cited in the sociological and anthropological literature suggest that, despite empirical disconfirmation, millennial beliefs persist, or may even intensify, among religious groups (e.g. Dawson 1999; Stone 2000).

The standard paradigm for understanding responses to failed prophecy is Festinger's (1956) well-known theory of cognitive dissonance, which argues that such dissonance is assuaged by reinterpretation of beliefs and increased proselytization. Although many studies in diverse religious contexts uphold the basic assumptions of cognitive dissonance theory (Bainbridge 1997), it has attracted much criticism on both empirical and theoretical grounds. In many instances, the suggested behavioural manifestations of dissonance reduction, such as increased proselytization, simply do not occur.

Some scholars have criticized the theory for its failure to take account of the emic perspectives of believers and the capacity of religious meaning systems to accommodate illogical and conflicting religious beliefs (Tumminia 1998; Zygmunt 1972). Others have argued that cognitive dissonance cannot capture the variety and richness of the historical manifestations of failed prophecy (Kravel-Tovi and Bilu 2008; Kravel-Tovi 2009). Finally, it has been argued that cognitive dissonance may be less of a problem for the believer than for the researcher (Bem 1970). Unlike believers in science, many religious believers do not require consistent and frequent confirmatory evidence. Beliefs may withstand the pressure of disconfirming events not because of the effectiveness of reducing strategies but because disconfirming evidence may simply go unacknowledged. But cognitive dissonance theory purports to explain how some beliefs are reinforced, not why they persist.

Cultural Performance

The literature on 'failed' prophecy has to date focused upon cognitive factors to the neglect of other social practices which construct alternative realities.

As Dein and Dawson (2008: 175) argue. 'The authoritative provision of a plausible rationalisation, communicated promptly and persuasively, can offset the cognitive dissonance initially experienced by individuals. If further actions are taken at this juncture to reaffirm the group's cohesion, such as special rituals, ceremonies, and educational events, the dissonance can be significantly dissipated.' In many contemporary religious groups, leaders and their followers have to persuade potential believers as to the truth of their claims and address the discrepancy between their cognitions and empirical reality. They deploy diverse cultural practices to this end. These practices include various communication media: television, radio, the internet and newspaper print alongside 'ritual' performances.[1]

The past decade has seen an emerging literature examining the relationship between communication media and religion. One area of increasing interest relates to the relationship between media and ritual (Hoover and Clark 2002; Grimes 2002). After a discussion of the diverse ways in which ritual and media are related, Grimes (2002) argues that performance-related theories offer the most provocative approaches to the interface of ritual and media. He deploys Richard Schechner's definition of performance: the 'showing of a doing'. In this respect, both ritual and media are species of performance having much to do with each other. Like that of ritual, the power of media lies in its ability to mediate the rhetorical and psychological power of performers and in turn to persuade by argument and suggestion. Both can be transformative in the Turnerian sense – making a transition from the everyday world to an alternative context. But Grimes (2002) cautions that although media and ritual share similarities, they are not the same thing.

In recent years, the study of rituals has moved away from seeing their enactment in terms of structures of representation to seeing them rather as processes of practice and performance (Schechner and Appel 1990; Schieffelin 1985). Rather than conceptualizing ritual as a set of symbols or a structure of meanings that formulate or 'make sense of' particular, often problematic, cultural or psychological situations, the performative perspective sees rituals as being effective on account of their non-discursive, dramaturgical and rhetorical characteristics. The performative perspective is concerned with experience-near aspects of social phenomena; with actions rather than text, with illocutionary rather than with propositional force and with the social construction rather than the representation of reality. What renders the performance compelling is not primarily the meanings embodied in the symbolic materials but the ways in which the symbolic materials emerge in interactions between actors and the audience. It is concerned with creating a sense of presence and verisimilitude, which is able to alter moods, attitudes, social states and states of mind. Rituals not only reflect everyday and cosmological realities, they construct these in the first place.

Bell (1997) lists the general characteristics of ritual-like activities that mediate a sense of the sacred as multi-sensory experience, framing, formalism, traditionalism and invariance, all of which facilitate the production of a sense of an authoritative order that lies beyond the mundane world.

Rituals are multi-sensory performances involving visual imagery and dramatic sounds in which not only is seeing believing, but doing is believing (Moore and Meyerhoff 1977). The power of performance lies in the heightened multi-sensory experience it affords: participants are pulled into a complex sensory experience that can also communicate a variety of messages and generate specific religious experiences by eliciting emotions. Some authors, such as Alcorta and Sosis (2005), argue that ritual not only serves as a forum for signalling godly commitments; it also inculcates religion by generating affirming religious experiences. These ideas echo Emile Durkheim's theory of 'collective effervescence' (Durkheim 1964).

Various aspects of ritualistic practice, such as music, dancing and monotonous repetition, might suppress common sense perspectives on the world by facilitating the experience of 'trance' (Rouget 1985). For instance, in his classic text *The Interpretation of Cultures*, Clifford Geertz (1973: 90) observes that ritual transports participants into another mode of existence, which relies on the suppression of the common sense perspective of the everyday world. These thoughts are echoed by Etzel Cardeña (1989: 14), who writes that ritual operates via repetition toward the elimination of critical thought. Thus, counter-intuitive beliefs may be more likely to be accepted during ritual.

The second characteristic of ritual is framing – a term used to describe the ways in which some activities or messages set up an interpretive framework for understanding other subsequent or simultaneous acts or messages. By virtue of this framing, performance is understood to be other than mundane reality and in turn shapes people's experiences and cognitive ordering of the world. Intrinsic to performance is the communication that this activity is 'different', 'significant' and 'deliberate'. Ritual literally constructs a sense of the sacred by explicitly differentiating this realm from the profane one. Rituals are also characterized by their temporal features: they are special in terms of the schedules associated with them. Scheduled periodicity renders the rituals deliberate and meaningful in contrast to other activities.

The third characteristic – formalism – refers to the fact that rituals often employ more formal, or restricted, codes of speech and action than people use in everyday life. This may enhance the 'power' of ritual.

Fourth, ritual emphasizes traditionalism – the attempt to make a set of activities identical to or consistent with cultural precedents. Such traditionalism is a powerful tool of legitimation and includes the near-perfect repetition of activities from an earlier period, the adaptation of such activities in a new setting or the creation of practices that simply evoke links with the past.

The final characteristic discussed by Bell is invariance – a disciplined set of actions marked by a precise repetition and physical control. While traditionalism emphasizes the authority of the past, and subordinates the present, invariance is concerned with ignoring the passage of time altogether and emphasizes the timeless authority of the group, its doctrines and its practices.

Thus, ritual achieves transformations by virtue of its dynamic, diachronic and physical characteristics in contrast to the acting out of tradition or cognitive maps. Specific sites are rendered sacred by virtue of the rituals performed there. It is ritual-like activity which gives form to the specialness of a site, distinguishing it from other places in ways that evoke highly symbolic meanings. What makes activities ritual-like is twofold: the way in which they differentiate some places from others by means of distinctive acts and responses, and the way in which they evoke experiences of a greater, higher or more universalized reality.

Lubavitcher Messianism

Over the past twenty years, we have been conducting ethnographic fieldwork among Lubavitcher Hasidim in Crown Heights, Brooklyn, USA. Lubavitch is a worldwide movement of Hasidic Jews, whose main centre is in Brooklyn, New York. The organization is also called Chabad, an acronym deriving from the first three Kabbalistic sefirot, *Chochma, Binah and Daath.* It is estimated there are about 200,000 members of Lubavitch worldwide, the main communities being in Israel, Great Britain, the United States and Belgium. This group is differentiated from other Hasidic groups by its efforts to return secular Jews to religious observance, an activity which Lubavitchers hold will hasten the messianic redemption. Recently, Lubavitch has become known for its messianic fervour and the conviction that the 'current' Rebbe is Moshiach – the Jewish Messiah (see Dein 2001; Dein and Dawson 2008; Ehrlich 2004).[2]

Rachel Elior (1998: 385) argues that the development of Chabad messianism was a response to the Holocaust and constituted an attempt by the sixth Rebbe, Rabbi Yosef Yitzhak Schneerson, to account for the catastrophe by viewing it as the final stage of pre-messianic tribulations, which would lead to divine redemption in the near future. Death and hopelessness were to be transformed into a spiritual birth and future hope, the meaningless torment and impotence being in effect messianic birth pangs. However, by 1945 it had become clear that the anticipated physical redemption would not take place and that the pre-messianic tribulations had brought only further torment and grief. Nevertheless, these emotions were channelled into an outreach programme influencing the whole Jewish community; messianic hope was transformed into practical activity. Scott-Green and Silverstein (2003) argue that earlier generations of Lubavitch emphasized individual redemption rather than speaking of the possibility of collective messianic redemption. Today, the movement is characterized by explicit messianic discourse and fervour. Menachem Schneerson, the seventh Rebbe, led the movement from 1950. Upon his assumption of leadership, he assured his followers that this was the 'last generation' before the redemption and that the coming of Moshiach was imminent. The Rebbe commenced his leadership on the theme of 'the seventh': that Lubavitch was ready to finally accomplish what had been prepared by the preceding six generations. For him, the seventh generation was without doubt the generation of redemption; the time had arrived. He constantly referred to his deceased father-in-law, the previous Rebbe, assigning to him the role of Moshiach, which was understood by all his followers to be a model for himself. In 1991 Schneerson stated:

> What more can I do to motivate the entire Jewish people to clamour and cry out and thus actually bring about the coming of Mashiach [sic]? All that has been done now has been to no avail. . . . all that I can possibly do is to give the matter over to you. Now, do everything you can to bring Mashiach here and now, immediately . . . I have done whatever I can: From now on, you must do whatever you can.

Following this statement, Lubavitch replaced the general expectation of imminent redemption with an expectation of a personal Messiah embodied in the figure of the Rebbe, who would reveal himself in the present. Messianic tension was increasingly focused on the Rebbe, his forceful proclamations being taken to signify that he was Moshiach. His messianic discourse in 1991 was punctuated by references to recent world events – the fall of the Soviet Union and Israel's escaping extensive harm from Iraqi missiles. These events were deployed as signposts toward the imminent redemption.

The campaign to present Schneerson as Moshiach was reinforced through the widespread use of mass media, the publication of books and pamphlets, and the use of bumper stickers on cars proclaiming that 'Moshiach is Here Now: Let's be Ready!' For instance, Shandler (2009) describes how one print advertisement produced in the early 1990s proclaimed: 'it's OK to get excited about Moshiach'. The advertisement explained that 'many prominent authorities' had identified Schneerson as the 'Presumed Messiah'. Less observant Jews were exhorted not only to increase their religious observance but also to engage with the advert itself by filling in their name and address, and a list of commitments to the Rebbe, such as increasing Torah study. Responding to the advert was taken as an act that would implicitly hasten the redemption.

In the early 1990s, Chabad Hasidim became more vocal about Schneerson being Moshiach, even submitting a petition to him asking that he reveal himself as the long-awaited Messiah. In 1991, Hasidim began singing a new song, *Yechi*, proclaiming him to be the Messiah. On several occasions, after first ignoring the song, the Rebbe appeared to gesture his approval. In 1992, the Rebbe had his first stroke. Despite his profound incapacity, messianic fervour in the Lubavitch community intensified, culminating in plans to crown him as Mosiach. Lubavitchers referred to Isaiah 53, 'a man of sorrows, and familiar with suffering', and argued that his illness was a prerequisite to the messianic arrival. In the autumn of 1992, on Rosh Hashanah, Schneerson was brought to a window constructed on the upper level of the synagogue at

770 Eastern Parkway overlooking the main sanctuary. Hasidim sang the full version of *Yechi*, and he made encouraging motions with his left hand (his right side had been paralysed by the stroke). As he was no longer able to speak, his gestures were open to interpretation and there was subsequently heightened scrutiny of his public gestures and appearance. It was no longer what the Rebbe said, but rather what his followers saw which was important for them. The Rebbe became more like his familiar presence in photographs, visible but silent (Shandler 2009).

The messianic fervour reached a climax in 1993, when a rally of over 8,000 people was organized in Crown Heights, where the Rebbe was to be crowned as 'King Messiah' under the leadership of a senior Lubavitcher Rabbi, Shmuel Butman. Prior to the rally, Butman had informed the press that it would culminate in the coronation of the Rebbe as King Messiah. The Rebbe himself stated on many occasions that the Messiah was already here and that the process of redemption was beginning to unfold. Given the Rebbe's charisma, it is unsurprising that his followers believed him.[3] Although he appeared to publicly approve of the messianic attributions to him, we can never know with certainty whether or not he himself believed he was Moshiach.

Death of the Rebbe

In 1994, the Rebbe suffered a second stroke, which rendered him comatose. His faithful followers saw this as a prelude to his messianic revelation and the arrival of the redemption. At one point, as he lay dying in intensive care, around 2,000 followers assembled outside the Beth Israel Medical Centre, singing and dancing – anticipating the imminent arrival of the redemption. Supporters and believers signed petitions to God, demanding that he allow their Rebbe to reveal himself as the long-awaited Messiah and rise from his sickbed to lead all humanity to their redemption. He died on 12 June 1994 and was buried next to his predecessor. His funeral procession was televised across the world by satellite. To outsiders, his funeral was something of a paradox – while his coffin was being lowered into the ground, international audiences were able to see Hasidim in Crown Heights dancing and singing in anticipation of his resurrection. His followers' expectations of his immediate return were heightened.

After the Rebbe's death, Chabad rapidly divided into two groups, broadly labelled *meshichist* (messianist) and anti-*meshichist* (anti-messianist) (Dein 2001; Ehrlich 2004; Dein and Dawson 2008). This split, however, is more socio-political than it is ideological; the boundaries are far from clear, and the two groups should perhaps be seen more as the extremes of a spectrum. The main division is around whether or not the Rebbe's messianic status should be publicly proclaimed. The *meshichistim* maintain that the Rebbe's public discourses in the early 1990s constituted an almost formal declaration and acceptance of his messiahship, that he authorized the campaign to publicize this claim, and that this authorization is still valid today. There is generally little social interaction between the groups, with intra-group marriages, but there are some exceptions. Messianists typically wear yellow lapel pins adorned with crowns and fly matching yellow flags on the façades of their homes. The views of this group are represented in a magazine published by them called *Beis Moshiach*.

The *meshichistim* nevertheless differ widely in their attitudes to the Rebbe's death. Some maintain that he died but will be resurrected as the Messiah. Others hold that he is still physically alive and is still the Messiah just as he was before 1994, and assert that he is not present in the coffin that was buried in the cemetery in Queens. A prominent Lubavitcher rabbi stated: 'now the Rebbe is also alive and affects us here physically. [That] after *Gimmel Tamuz* [the Hebrew date of the Rebbe's death] 1994 no change has occurred in the relationship between the Rebbe and *chassidim* – no change as the Rebbe relates to *chassidim* and no change as *chassidim* relate to the Rebbe'.[4] Some Lubavitchers within the *meshichistic* camp are even more radical and insist that in order for the Rebbe to be revealed, everybody must acknowledge his messiahship. Those who oppose public declarations of this belief are seen as deliberately delaying his revelation and must therefore be dealt with forcibly and even violently. A small minority hold that he has divine powers or is the 'creator' himself. As one *Boreinunik* (the name applied to those who hold this belief) explained: 'There is no place where the Rebbe ends and [God] begins.'[5]

The other camp, loosely called 'anti-*meshichist*', vehemently opposes all public claims that the Rebbe is the Messiah. All major Chabad organizations, including Agudas Chasidei Chabad and Merkos L'Inyonei Chinuch, adopt this position, but there are varied opinions concerning the Rebbe's messianic status. Some anti-messianists hold that the Rebbe could have been Moshiach if God had willed it, but they disagree vehemently that Moshiach could come from the dead. For them, Schneerson was the best candidate for the Messiah in his generation but now that he is dead, they say, his claim is no longer viable. They appear to accept the Rebbe's death as final. As one anti-*meshichistic* Lubavitcher stated shortly after the funeral, 'Sure I felt disappointment, but you have to move on.' They hold that the Rebbe, although physically dead, still has a spiritual influence on the world.

Media Propagation of the Rebbe

The use of various media to bring forth their deceased zaddikim is far from new in Hasidic groups. Music is considered as a powerful force in Hasidic life, with the ability to elevate souls. Traditionally, Hasidim attest to the power of *niggunim* – a body of paraliturgical, folk and popular melodies, repetitive in nature and sung to vocables or simple text – to render present their original composers, and many state that during performances they can feel or even see the presence of their Rebbe (Koskoff 2000: xi). Television and internet broadcasts render such 'seeing' more modern.

There is little doubt that the Lubavitcher messianic campaign has benefitted from the use of modern media technology from the arrival of the sixth Lubavitcher Rebbe in the United States in 1940 through to the death of the 'current' Rebbe and continuing into the present. Lubavitch has forged a new spiritual relationship with the Rebbe through innovative and provocative media practices: print advertising, photography, radio, the internet, television and radio (Shandler 2009). Unlike other Hasidic groups in the USA, Lubavitch has a commitment to visibility in the public sphere and this commitment is central to its mission of fostering increased religious observance and propagating its messianic ideas.

Shandler (2009) discusses the use of visual technology to propagate the presence of the Rebbe since his death. On 31 January 1996, the messianic faction of Lubavitch broadcast a television programme commemorating Menachem Schneerson's assumption of leadership in 1951. The aim of this programme was to declare the Rebbe as King Moshiach, and to pray for his immediate revelation. During the broadcast, Rabbi Shmuel Buttman, chairman of the International Campaign to welcome Moshiach, described how he was 'inviting the Rebbe to this great *farbrengen* [Hasidic gathering]'. Viewers were shown the Rebbe's table and his chair. There followed brief footage of the Rebbe entering the same ritual space amid a crowd of Hasidim with a soundtrack of the Rebbe speaking of Moshiach's imminent arrival. The broadcast then moved on to a series of live connections with Chabad congregations in Russia, South Africa, Israel, France, Australia and the United States, where local rabbis exhorted their congregations to call for the Rebbe to reveal himself as the Messiah.

These live segments alternated with archive audio and video of the Rebbe at his first *farbrengen*, where he discussed Lubavitcher messianism in front of his enthusiastic followers. The broadcast ended with a display of multiple images of Chabad communities worldwide chanting '*Yechi Adoneinu Moreinu V'Rabbenu Melech Hamoshiach L'olom Vo'ed*' [Long live our lord, our teacher, our master, King Messiah for ever and ever]. The television performance conflates past and present and attempts to portray a sense of the Rebbe's continuing presence to his followers through the properties of televisibility, simultaneity and verisimilitude. These images allowed for a subjunctive engagement with the Rebbe, albeit with his virtual presence.

I shall now examine how such technology, alongside ritualistic performance, is used in Crown Heights, the messianic centre of Lubavitch.

Ethnographic Fieldwork in Crown Heights

Crown Heights is a neighbourhood in the central portion of the New York City borough of Brooklyn. The neighbourhood is an ethnic and social melange of three groups: orthodox Jews, African Americans and Haitians. The focus of my fieldwork has been on 770 Eastern Parkway, the administrative centre of the Lubavitch movement.[6] The building contains a large synagogue, a *Kollel* (institute for advanced study of the Talmud), and the community's library. The secretariat of the Lubavitch Movement and other related offices are also based there. Lubavitchers refer to the building as '770'. The synagogue is used for three purposes: it is a place of daily prayer services, a study hall for advanced students, and an assembly hall for Chabad gatherings (*farbrengens*). Besides being a synagogue, the site is considered especially holy, as it served as the home and offices of the last two Lubavitcher Rebbes. The synagogue's official name is Congregation Lubavitch of Agudas Chasidei Chabad, although it is referred to by several other names throughout the worldwide Chabad community: *Beis Moshiach* (Messiah's House), the numerical value of 770, and *Beis Rabeinu Sheb'bovel* (the Babylonian House of our Teacher). Like other Hasidic headquarters, 770 is a major destination of pilgrimage by Lubavitchers and non-Lubavitcher Jews from around the world and attracts thousands of visitors each year.

Outside 770 are bookstalls selling Jewish literature, including books about the Lubavitcher Rebbe. Lubavitcher men stand in groups outside the entrance chatting, some on mobile phones, some waiting for the regular buses which transport the Rebbe's followers from 770 to the Rebbe's tomb in Queens. In the streets immediately adjacent to the synagogue, a large number of shop windows display pictures of the late Lubavitcher Rebbe with the word Moshiach inscribed underneath. This image also appears on car bumper stickers. Parked on every corner are *Mitzvah* tanks (mobile educational units) carrying billboards stating 'Moshiach is here now. Let's be ready.' Shops sell souvenirs such as watches with the Rebbe's face on them. It is virtually impossible to turn a corner without seeing a picture of the Rebbe. The streets are bustling with Lubavitcher men running to and from services, many wearing badges on their lapels with the word Moshiach inscribed on them.

Many of the local school classrooms have a picture of Schneerson on the eastern wall (towards which Jews pray). Students and children are instructed to 'direct their hearts and thoughts' to Rabbi Schneerson, who is 'omnipotent' and 'omniscient', and will fulfil all of their wishes when they pray to him. Typically, pictures of Rabbi Schneerson are displayed in every room of Lubavitcher homes, where bookcases are filled with copies of his teachings and directives. In many households, there are photographs of visits to 770 for the ceremony of dollars (a weekly ceremony attended by thousands of people who would seek blessings from the Rebbe and who would receive a dollar from him, symbolizing charity).

Meshichistic Lubavitchers typically refer to Schneerson as 'The Rebbe King Messiah who lives forever' and use the phrase '*Chai veKayam*' (He is alive). They refer to his 'apparent passing', a phrase that reveals the questionable ontological status of his death, vehemently reject epithets usually ascribed to the dead, such as 'may his memory be for a blessing', and frequently use expressions wishing him a long life. Different terms are used to refer to his continued existence. Some refer to resurrection – the Rebbe has risen from the dead and therefore is even more powerfully at work than before – whereas others refer to his 'occultation' or 'concealment'. Despite the fact that he cannot be seen, he is still held by his followers to be aware of their desires and to know their thoughts. Most importantly, he is held to possess agency and to influence the physical world. During my fieldwork many Lubavitchers reported how the Rebbe had miraculously intervened in their lives. Some recounted instances in which he had brought about cure in times of serious illness. According to one story, a young woman had decided to undergo a termination of pregnancy, having found out that her unborn baby suffered from severe congenital heart defects. The night before the termination she dreamed that the Rebbe had visited her and said, 'I came here for you; don't do this!' She did not undergo the termination and shortly afterwards gave birth to a healthy baby.[7]

Rituals to Embody the Rebbe

In recent years the messianists have assumed ownership of the 770 synagogue, hanging messianic banners inside and in several instances physically attacking anti-messianists who tried to remove them; they have also vandalized the dedication plaque on the building's facade, scratching out the Hebrew acronym for 'Of Blessed Memory' after the Rebbe's name. The synagogue itself, in the basement of 770, can only be described as decrepit, with its peeling paint, dirty linoleum floors, wooden benches and unidentifiable odour. It is here that hundreds of Lubavitcher Hasidim commune with the Rebbe on a daily basis.

Since the Rebbe's death, things have hardly changed in the synagogue. Everything appears stage-managed to replicate the living presence of the Rebbe. Pictures of the Rebbe are to be seen everywhere, his staring eyes signifying the fact that the Rebbe can see into his followers' innermost selves, a fact commonly mentioned by those who visited him while alive. A DVD plays in the entrance hall, showing the Rebbe distributing dollars at the dollar ceremony. These visual signifiers give the sense that everything continues just as it has always done when the Rebbe was alive.

Inside the prayer hall, hundreds of men stand or sit on benches praying or intensely discussing various Jewish tracts. The activity in 770 is never ending and the study hall is a continuous hive of activity. Many of the Rebbe's followers study, pray and even sleep in the synagogue. The sound of men reciting tracts from the Rebbe's books and other discussions on Jewish literature is ongoing throughout the day and night, interrupted only by eruptions of loud, repetitive clapping and singing of 'Long live our master, our teacher and our rabbi, King Messiah for ever and ever', signifying the start of the thrice daily public prayer sessions. Many in the congregation appear to enter a state of ecstasy as the singing intensifies.

At the front of the synagogue stands the Rebbe's empty velvet-covered chair with its cushions unruffled for more than fifteen years. The chair is kept as it was during his lifetime. Before the daily afternoon prayers, a number of the men meticulously perform the ritual of opening out a Persian rug, moving the Rebbe's chair out from under a desk, and preparing his prayer shawls and books as if he were about to walk in and take his seat. At the start of the service, the Rebbe's followers stand on either side of a red carpet to create a pathway leading from the stairs to the podium. His Hasidim look towards a balcony in the distance as if expecting the Rebbe to emerge and take up his place on a platform just as when he was alive. This is accompanied by loud singing of Hebrew prayer. In major rituals, the Rebbe is honoured by utterances of the first verse of the prayer, and the gaze of the congregation is focused upon the vacant chair. The congregation then recites the subsequent verses. At the end of the service, the carpet is rolled up and the Rebbe's chair is put back under the desk, these activities being accompanied by song and dance as the Rebbe 'exits'. The dancing suddenly stops and the room is silent. Four young boys, each carrying a large yellow flag bearing the Rebbe's crest, part the dancers and move alongside the platform that supports the Rebbe's chair and desk. Raising the flags high in the air, they chant in unison: 'We want Moshiach now! We want Moshiach now! We want Moshiach now!"

Menachem, a thirty-year-old Lubavitcher, reported his experience of being present during this ceremony:

> The Rebbe is here with us now. I can feel a definite presence. No, I cannot see him but I feel overwhelmed. You can definitely feel his power. I know that it is he who is leading the service. A few people can see the Rebbe. People tell me, 'Just open your eyes and you can see him.' A few spiritually developed people have seen him – in body and in flesh looking as he did before his passing. It's not happened to me yet. Perhaps one day it will, I don't know, I hope so.

On further questioning, he explained that many who attend the services can feel this 'spiritual presence'. A person can learn to open his eyes by studying the Tanya (an early work of Hasidic philosophy by Rabbi Shneur Zalman of Liadi, the founder of Chabad Hasidism, first published in 1797) and the Rebbe's teachings. 'Eyes' refers to both the spiritual and the physical sensory organs. He recounted that one man had a video recording of the late Rebbe walking towards the podium. I was unable to interview this man.

On the Sabbath and High Holidays there is a *farbrengen*, at which, prior to his death, the Rebbe presided and gave his discourses on Hasidic matters, frequently alluding to the 'imminent' redemption. The Rebbe's table is kept covered with a white tablecloth and is set with *halla* (bread), a bottle of wine and a wineglass. A watch is placed on the table to 'count down to the redemption', as one man explained. The Rebbe's chair is brought to the table and his Hasidim sit in front of it. At the conclusion of the meeting, a Hasid cuts the *halla* and pours wine into the wineglass. These are then distributed among the Hasidim.

On the Day of Atonement (Yom Kippur), a mobile staircase is placed upon the podium so that the Rebbe 'can watch from above' and direct the traditional singing as he had done in previous years. During the Harvest festival (Succoth), a tabernacle is built for the Rebbe with the 'four species' laid out for him inside. Some eagerly extend their hands to receive the Rebbe's *lekah* (cake), a custom which was carried out when he was alive.

Going into the Rebbe

In Hasidic groups where a Rebbe dies without heirs and without publicly naming a successor, the cult of the zaddik often focuses upon pilgrimages to the grave of the late zaddik.[8] For example after the death of Aron Rokeah, the Belz zaddik who died in 1957, his followers made regular pilgrimages to his tomb in Jerusalem to pray together, renew acquaintances and deposit *kvitlim* (petitions) while pronouncing their personal supplications. These were followed by joyous banquets at which the men praised and honoured their Rebbe. It is common for followers of Rabbi Nahman of Bratslav to visit his grave once a year on Rosh Hashanah.

Just as the Rebbe once visited the *Ohel* (the tomb of the Rebbes) to commune with his deceased father-in-law when he was alive, his followers now travel to the *Ohel* to commune with him and ask for his intercession in life issues: marriage, business, health and education. Typically, women who experience infertility will ask to become pregnant. Others plead that a sick child will recover or that a marriage will work. Paradoxically, although they maintain that the Rebbe is alive, many *meshichistim* regularly visit the Rebbe's grave. While some vehemently deny that he lies there, and do not visit his grave, others go to the graveside to communicate with him and ask for his intercession. One Lubavitcher explained this paradox:

> Terms like 'living' and 'dead' do not easily apply to a zaddik. They are not ordinary people. It is possible for the Rebbe to be alive and dead. It is not logical but there is no contradiction. Yes, we hold that the Rebbe is alive, but his physical body is in the *Ohel* and his spirit is there. The Rebbe can be in many places at once, both spiritually and physically. His soul is in *Gan Eden* (Heaven) but manifests itself in the physical world. We cannot understand this. What is important is that we are connected to him.

The tomb has expanded, and close to it is a Lubavitch house consisting of an anteroom, a kitchen where those leaving the cemetery can wash their hands, and a library/study hall containing a large body of the Rebbe's numerous talks and published letters. Inside the study hall are rows of tables resembling the interior of 770. Blank papers and pens are placed on the tables for visitors to write requests to the Rebbe. In the corner is a continuous supply of biscuits and coffee.

Two fax machines churn out a constant stream of requests for blessings. Every hour or so, one of the Rebbe's assistants collects them from the machines to take them to the Rebbe's grave, where he reads them and places them on top of the pile of notes. The pile is a foot high, evenly covering the eight-foot-square area of the grave. Lubavitchers maintain that their deceased Rebbe's spirit hovers over the grave and that his spiritual interaction with his followers has been increasing since his death.

Each day, large numbers of visitors exit from the Lubavitch house and slowly and silently walk the short distance to the Rebbe's grave. There are numerous observances related to visiting the Rebbe's resting place, such as refraining from food (though not drink) before the visit and removing leather shoes before entering the mausoleum (as did Moses before approaching the burning bush). But most important is the mental preparation of charity, learning and spiritual stock-taking. Prior to entry, visitors wash their hands and light candles. After taking off their shoes, they enter the mausoleum and take their place among the assembly of people fervently praying and requesting the Rebbe's intercession. Though *ohel* means 'tent', the mausoleum is like a *chuppah* (wedding canopy) in reverse: closed on all sides but open to the heavens. Inside, there is an inner wall about waist high that dozens of people lean on as they recite prayers over the graves.

One young man from London recounted that shortly after a visit to the Rebbe, whom he had asked to help him with financial problems, he received money from a distant relative in Brazil, whom he had never met. Another man recounted how his terminally ill grandmother made a full recovery after he visited the *Ohel*. Lubavitchers and non-Lubavitchers travel there, often from abroad, and deposit requests written on pieces of paper on the grave. For insiders, a visit to the *Ohel* was not 'going to a grave'. Visitors referred instead to their 'going into the Rebbe'. They reported the distinct impression that the Rebbe had responded to them, as he did when he was alive. 'It's kind of a recharging of your spiritual battery,' said one woman, who had flown in from Melbourne. 'I always feel a little more connected.'

The 'Miracles' Continue

The occurrence of 'miracles' testifies to the existence of a supernatural agency. In line with their belief in his persisting influence, Lubavitchers maintain that the Rebbe is still able to advise his faithful followers, who still write, fax or email him for advice relating to health, wealth, marriage or education. If anything, he is now even more accessible than before his 'apparent passing'. Believers are urged to open his 29-volume collection of letters (*Igrot Ha Kodesh*) at random in their quest for guidance. These often, they testify, address their specific problems with amazing accuracy and provide an automatic reply from the invisible Rebbe. Those who are unable to understand the Rebbe's response are urged to consult a Chabad expert, who will interpret the passage.

Internet technology enables the *meshichistim* to transmit the messianic ideology rapidly around the globe, creating a sense of community and potentially bringing new members to the movement. The Rebbe's living status is reinforced on numerous websites that *meshichistim* have created. Some examples are www. LivingWith MoshiachOnline, www.LongLiveTheRebbe KingMessiahForever.com, YechiHaMelech.org, Moshiach.tvBlog, www.king messiah.com, www.770live.com and www.moshiach.net. These sites present detailed 'proofs' of the fact that the Rebbe is not physically dead.

Many of the websites contain information about how the Rebbe can be 'accessed' through his teachings and describe the numerous 'miracles' that the Rebbe has engineered. It is even possible to submit a question, which a computer programme automatically inserts into the appropriate page of the Rebbe's writings before providing a written response in terms of a passage from the *Igrot Ha Kodesh*. Those who participate in this online activity report how they feel close to the Rebbe; cyberspace becomes a sacred space. Some of the websites contain video clips of the Rebbe distributing dollars and sound recordings of his followers singing the *Yehi*. All of this adds to the sense of the Rebbe's continuing presence. A recent addition to the repertoire of the Rebbe's 'miracles' relates to the use of water from his *mikvah* (ritual bath) for healing purposes. According to a story quoted by Gotfryd and Branover (2000: 115), an elderly man who nearly lost his right arm following an angioplasty was miraculously healed by drinking this water.

Discussion

I have argued that the literature on 'failed prophecy' has focused upon cognitive factors to the neglect of other social practices that can construct alternative realities. For Lubavitch, like many groups whose messianic expectations fail to materialize, resort is made to eschatological hermeneutics to explain and reinforce the messianic ideology.[9] However, there are other strategies for assuaging disappointment and creating a sense of the Rebbe's continuing presence based upon ritualistic performances and the deployment of modern media including television, radio and the internet. For this group, the acting out of the predicted event represents a ritualized reaffirmation of belief – a collective experience of symbolic fulfilment that provides disappointed followers with social and psychological support to render such an experience less cognitively distressing (see Stone 2000: 19; Palmer and Finn 1992).

So, to what extent do the various rituals deployed by the *meshichistim* to bring the Rebbe to life show the general characteristics of ritual-like activities that mediate a sense of the sacred: multi-sensory experience, framing, formalism, traditionalism and invariance – all of which facilitate the production of a sense of an authoritative order that lies beyond the mundane world (Bell 1997)? Do those involved see themselves not as creating specific realities but rather as responding to those realities?

In the Rebbe's synagogue, the Rebbe is repeatedly brought into existence by the performance of stylized, repetitive and stereotyped performances, which literally embody the Rebbe. The movements of the Hasidim, their formation of a symbolic pathway for the Rebbe and their deferential posture create a symbolic space in which the Rebbe 'appears'. Their gestures, words and physical delineations of space and time actually accomplish what a ritual ought to do, namely shape attitudes. As Bell (1997) has argued, as the body moves about, marking off space and time, it defines even the most complex ritual environment by simple acts such as kneeling, circumambulation, and procession. Rappoport (1999) has echoed these ideas by similarly arguing that the oral and bodily gestures performed in a ritual generate 'statements' about reality that communicate both information and attitudes, especially acquiescence to the reality so defined. In the case of 770, the repetitive singing and dancing induces a state of ecstasy akin to a trance, where it is possible to accept alternative realities and 'feel' the presence of the Rebbe. The structure of the song, with gaps between verses. provides spaces in which the Rebbe appears. All of this occurs 'just as it was' before the Rebbe's death, lending a sense that nothing has changed in 770. In Bell's sense, this ritual is characterized by traditionalism – both evoking and legitimating the past.

It is the ritual activities performed at the Rebbe's grave that render it sacred: the hand-washing, the removal of shoes and the lighting of candles. This is reinforced by the sense of formality. The fact that the sixth Lubavitcher Rebbe is buried there next to Schneerson signifies a link with tradition (the Rebbe's regular visits to his father-in-law's grave). This ritual evokes both the past and the present. At the *Ohel* the *mechichistim* are 'cut off' from everyday reality. Their being inside the tomb creates a feeling of separateness from the outside world. The solemn atmosphere reinforces a sense of separation from the triviality of the outside world. The walls of the *Ohel* create a symbolic space; the fact that the *Ohel* has no roof makes it possible for the Rebbe literally to 'come in from above'. The singing at the graveside creates a heightened sensory state in which the Rebbe 'appears'.

But it is the continuing 'miracles' that most strongly reinforce the sense of the Rebbe's presence. His followers never fail to receive answers to their requests. He does not just exist in some transcendental realm, outside their everyday experience, but is actively involved in a pragmatic way in the mundane world and he continues to work to bring about the redemption.

Notes

1. Ritualization in the widest sense may be one way of dealing with failure of prophecy. Palmer and Finn (1992), examining the Ottawa-based Institute of Applied Metaphysics, postulate that if millenarian activity is approached not as a set of beliefs but rather as a collective ritual of initiation into a new type of religious organization, then an important factor in the survival of millenarian movements is the quality of the ritual experience: 'waiting for world's end is a symbolic act and it requires the presence of ritual actors and the organization of sacred time and space' (1992: 409).
2. Hasidism originated from seventeenth-century Polish Jewry. It differs from other forms of Judaism in its emphasis on the zaddik – the spiritual leader of the group, who is held to be an intermediary between God and mankind and is often seen as a 'miracle' worker, to whom regular appeal is made at times of crisis. The most recent Rebbe, Menachem Mendel Schneerson, has been described by Lubavitchers as 'the most phenomenal Jewish personality of our time' (Lubavitch Publication 1989). He was born in Nikolaev in Russia in 1902 and was well known as a Torah prodigy (a young person with

an exceptionally good knowledge of the Torah). He became the leader and seventh Rebbe of Lubavitch in 1951. Until his death in 1994, he resided in Brooklyn at 770 Eastern Parkway and for forty years did not leave New York.

3. Charismatic authority involves the attribution of superhuman powers or the ability to perform 'miracles'. As Weber has pointed out, it is inherently fragile and often becomes routinized (accommodated to the routines of everyday life), eventually being mixed with traditional and bureaucratic authority (Craib 1997: 134).
4. From an article entitled 'The Rebbe is Alive and Well and Living in 770'. http://failed messiah.typepad.com (accessed 12 February 2007). No author is credited.
5. Not surprisingly, these new beliefs have attracted a lot of derision from the wider Jewish community and, on account of their proclamations of the imminent resurrection of Schneerson, some have labelled meshichistim 'Christians' (Berger 2001). The prevalence of these views within the movement is disputed, although it appears that the major institutions in the three Lubavitcher population centres, in Crown Heights (USA), Kfar Chabad (Israel) and Safed (Israel), are either dominated by believers in the Rebbe's messiahship or influenced to a considerable extent by this belief (Berger 2001). With the exception of Sabbatianism, followers of the Rebbe have spawned the largest and most long-lived messianic movement in Jewish history since antiquity.
6. Since 1992, I have been conducting ethnographic fieldwork in Crown Heights, which I have visited on four occasions (1992, 1994, 2008, 2010) as a participant observer of messianic activities, attending religious services and visiting the Rebbe's grave. In all, I interviewed 30 messianic Lubavitchers (aged 16 to 76), asking them about the Rebbe's messianic status and their understandings of his 'apparent' death. I kept detailed field notes concerning my interviews and observations. Additionally, I consulted a number of websites devoted to the Rebbe as Moshiach. On account of gender divisions within the community, I generally interviewed men but through links with a local Lubavitcher family I was able to interview three women.
7. A few members of the congregation reported having dreams in which the Rebbe appeared to them, and several recounted stories of those who had seen the Rebbe. In one instance, a young Lubavitcher student in Israel claimed to have seen the Rebbe following an argument at school. The Rebbe apparently castigated her for being disrespectful to her teachers. One website publishes stories of those who claim to have seen the Rebbe after his death (http://seeingtherebbe.wordpress.com/).
8. Pilgrimage to the tombs of Jewish saints is not uncommon in Sephardic Judaism, although it is rarer among Ashkenazis (see Ben Ami 1998 for a discussion). Hasidic Jews visit the tombs of the Baal Shem Tov and the second-century Kabbalist Simeon Ben Yochai.
9. The *meshichistim* devote much of their time to distributing texts affirming the fact that the Rebbe is alive and is Moshiach. These ideas are reinforced at public meetings where these texts are discussed. It was not difficult for the *meshichistim* to immediately affirm that the Rebbe had not really died by appealing to a range of eschatological hermeneutics deriving from biblical verses and rabbinic literature such as Sanhedrin 98b, the basic Talmudic commentary, which explains: 'If Moshiach is from those who are alive now, surely he is Rabbeinu Hakadosh [Rabbi Yehuda HaNassi], who suffers sicknesses and is an absolute saint . . . If he is from those who have already died, he is Daniel, the delightful one, who was condemned to suffer in the lions' den and was an absolute saint.' Lubavitcher theology is monistic and acosmic: everything that exists is a direct revelation of the infinite divine essence. Lubavitch has always held to the paradoxical nature of the divine presence – a paradoxical spirituality – perceiving the divinity as a mystical unity of opposites, simultaneously revealed and concealed, present and absent, being and non-being, a dual

process of creation and annihilation, transcending all constraints of time, place and conventionally perceived reality (Elior 1998: 404). Not surprisingly, for his followers the Rebbe could be physically present but concealed.

References

Alcorta, C. and R. Sosis. 2005. 'Religion, Emotion and Sacred Symbols: The Evolution of an Adaptive Complex', *Human Nature* 16(4): 323–59.

Bainbridge, W. 1997. *The Sociology of Religious Movements*. New York: Routledge.

Bell, C. 1997. *Ritual Perspectives and Dimensions*. New York: Oxford University Press.

Bem, D. 1970. *Beliefs, Attitudes and Human Affairs*. Belmont, CA: Brooks and Cole.

Ben Ami, I. 1998. *Saint Veneration among the Jews in Morocco*. Detroit: Wayne State University Press.

Berger, B. 1981. *The Survival of a Counterculture: Ideological Work and Everyday Life among Rural Communards*. Berkeley: University of California Press.

Berger, D. 2001. *The Rebbe, The Messiah and the Scandal of Orthodox Indifference*. London: Littman Library of Jewish Civilisation.

Cardeña, E. 1989. 'The Varieties of Possession Experience', *Association for the Anthropological Study of Consciousness Quarterly* 5(2–3): 1–17.

Cohn, N. 1993. *The Pursuit of the Millennium: Revolutionary Millenarians and Mystical Antichrists of the Middle Ages*. London: Pimlico.

Craib, I. 1997. *Classical Social Theory*. Oxford: Oxford University Press.

Dawson, L. 1999. 'When Prophecy Fails and Faith Persists: A Theoretical Overview', *Nova Religio* 3: 60–82.

Dein, S. 2001. 'What Really Happens When Prophecy Fails: The Case of Lubavitch', *Sociology of Religion* 62(3): 383–401.

Dein, S. and L. Dawson. 2008. 'The Scandal of the Lubavitch Rebbe: Messianism as a Response to Failed Prophecy', *Journal of Contemporary Religion* 23(2): 163–80.

Durkheim, E. 1964. *The Elementary Forms of Religious Life*. London: George Allen and Unwin.

Ehrlich, M.A. 2004. *The Messiah of Brooklyn: Understanding Lubavitch Hasidism Past and Present*. Jersey City, NJ: Ktav Publishing House.

Elior, R. 1998. 'The Lubavitch Messianic Resurgence', in P. Schafer and M. Cohen (eds), *Toward the Millennium: Messianic Expectations from the Bible to Waco*. Leiden: Brill, pp. 383–408.

Festinger, L., H. Riecken and S. Schacter. 1956. *When Prophecy Fails*. Minneapolis: University of Minnesota Press.

Geertz, C. 1973. *The Interpretation of Culture*. New York: Basic Books.

Gotfryd, A. and H. Branover. 2000. *Living in the Age of Moshiach*. Toronto: Mendelsohn Press.

Grimes, R. 2002. 'Ritual and the Media', in S. Hoover and L. Schofield Clark (eds), *Practicing Religion in the Age of the Media: Explorations in Media, Religion and Culture*. New York: Columbia University Press, pp. 219–34.

Hoover, S. and L. Schofield Clark. 2002. *Practicing Religion in the Age of the Media: Explorations in Media, Religion and Culture*. New York: Columbia University Press.

Koskoff, E. 2000. *Music in Lubavitcher Life*. Urbana, IL and Chicago: University of Illinois Press.

Kravel-Tovi, M. 2009. 'To See the Invisible Messiah: Messianic Socialization in the Wake of a Failed Prophecy', *Chabad Religion* 39(3): 248–60.

Kravel-Tovi, M. and Y. Bilu. 2008. 'The Work of the Present: Constructing Messianic Temporality in the Wake of Prophecy Among Chabad Hasidim', *American Ethnologist* 35(1): 64–80.

Moore, S. and B. Myerhoff. 1977. *Secular Ritual: A Working Definition of Ritual.* Amsterdam: Van Gorcum.

O'Leary, S. 1994. *Arguing the Apocalypse: A Theory of Millennial Rhetoric.* New York: Oxford University Press.

Palmer, S.J. and N. Finn. 1992. 'Coping with Apocalypse in Canada: Experiences of Endtime in La Mission De l'Esprit Saint and the Institute of Applied Metaphysics', *Sociological Analysis* 53(4): 397–415.

Rappoport, R.A. 1999. *Ritual and Religion in the Making of Humanity.* Cambridge: Cambridge University Press.

Rouget, G. 1985. *Music and Trance: A Theory of the Relations Between Music and Possession.* Chicago and London: University of Chicago Press.

Schechner, R. and W. Appel. 1990. *By Means of Performance.* Cambridge: Cambridge University Press.

Schieffelin, E. 1985. 'Performance and the Cultural Construction of Reality', *American Ethnologist* 12(4): 707–24.

Scott, Green, W. and J. Silverstein. 2003. 'The Doctrine of the Messiah', in J. Neusner and A. Avery Peck (eds), *The Blackwell Companion to Judaism.* Oxford: Wiley-Blackwell.

Shandler, J. 2009. *Jews, God, and Videotape: Religion and Media in America.* New York: New York University Press.

Stone, J. 2000. *Expecting Armageddon: Essential Readings in Failed Prophecy.* London: Routledge.

Tumminia, D. 1998. 'How Prophecy Never Fails: Interpreted Reasoning in a Flying Saucer Group', *Sociology of Religion* 59(2): 157–70.

Zygmunt, J. 1972. 'When Prophecies Fail: A Theoretical Perspective on Comparative Evidence', *American Behavioural Scientist* 16(2): 245–68.

Chapter 3

Did Christianity Lead to Schizophrenia?

Paul, you are beside yourself, too much study is sending you mad.
—Acts 26.24

This chapter proposes that schizophrenia has not been universal, either culturally or historically, but that nevertheless its current near ubiquity would argue for some approximately universal predisposition. This we would seek in Christian monotheism's reflexive consciousness and in its later secular successors. We have previously argued that the possibilities of religion and of psychosis have evolved together, through a common evolutionary trajectory (Dein and Littlewood 2011),[1] but what in modern times and Westernized societies has got us from the human possibility of schizophrenia ('proto-schizophrenia') to frank schizophrenia?

Before considering evidence for the non-universality of schizophrenia, we have to bear in mind that any attempt to search for the illness beyond its current perspective leads to the obvious objection that overt schizophrenic symptoms, though present elsewhere, may be apparent only within an already modern and Westernized perspective. Thus when C.G. Seligman, a physician and anthropologist, argued that severe mental illness was unknown in early contact New Guinea except in situations of considerable Westernization (Seligman 1929), he was criticized by anthropologists for ignoring psychosis which might be 'concealed' in local patterns of ritual performance (apart from the likelihood that any cases of severe mental illness which came to colonial medical attention were only likely to be already in a situation of considerable contact and dominance by the Europeans – and thus 'contact' was over salient). Similar objections make the popular argument that shamanism or possession ritual conceals or 'compensates for' schizophrenia (cf. Fabrega 1982).

Fabrega has argued in a caveat that the 'first rank symptoms' of schizophrenia, taken in modern comparative psychiatry as an accurate manifestation of unequivocal schizophrenia, really necessitate 'basic Western assumptions about human action and social reality,' particularly cultural conventions of the autonomous self (Fabrega 1982: 56). He cites such conventions that persons are independent beings whose minds and bodies are separated from each other and function autonomously; that under ordinary conditions external influences do not affect an individual; that thoughts are recurring inner happenings that the self 'has'; that thoughts and feelings are rather different things but that both are silent and private; that one's body is independent of what one feels or thinks; and that body and feelings have a purely naturalistic basis and cannot be modified by external suprahuman agents (Fabrega 1982). Barrett (2004), finding that the Iban of Borneo have difficulty understanding his questions about two first-rank symptoms, thought insertion and thought broadcasting, argues in a related way. His three Iban individuals (contrasted with thirty-nine European Australians in a matched psychotic sample) who experience these symptoms are all converts to Christianity. He suggests an association with education and reading, and a familiarity with the idea of an omniscient God who can tell what is in one's mind. (But equal numbers of Iban and Australians experienced auditory hallucinations.) Traditional Iban notions of thinking, he proposes, are much more embodied, tied closely to emotion, will, and desire: their word for 'thought' also denotes 'speech.'

Given the absence of any objective measures of the psychobiology of 'proto-schizophrenia', are we then compelled to go round in circles when considering the universality of schizophrenia in other societies and historical epochs? In this chapter, we propose a fairly broad perspective of what the 'eventual' symptoms of schizophrenia might be, taking into account the apparent overlap with other patterns such as mania or delirium: and thus in intention at any rate avoiding the category mistake of assuming that all the manifestations of schizophrenia are and have been universal. Nevertheless, past commentators have inevitably made judgements in relation to their own categories of illness, and putting their own conclusions together can never be fully persuasive: we have to move in and out of presumed uniformity and less certain family resemblances.

Cultural Variation

The idea that Westernization resulted in a higher incidence of schizophrenia was common in the nineteenth and twentieth centuries and was discussed by Kraepelin in 1919 (1971). In 1810 Richard Powell had noted insanity was 'considerably on the increase' whilst Andrew Halliday (1828) wrote 'we seldom meet with insanity among the savage races of men; not one of our African travellers remark their having seen a single madman' (as cited in Hunter and Macalpine 1963: 821–22). We can take these comments with a degree of caution. This was not only a case of colonial prejudice and Victorian anxieties: the travellers were hardly looking for mental illness, nor were the early modern doctors attempting to methodically search out and register all insane people in any community. Imperial psychiatrists in Africa like Tooth and Carothers (as, more recently, Lopez in Brazil, Beaglehole in Hawaii, and Dhunjibhoy in India) later commented on the infrequency of schizophrenia among communities relatively untouched by colonialism or Westernization (as reviewed by Torrey in 1979) but on the high frequency of toxic, confusional, or organic symptoms found in apparent schizophrenia (the primary illnesses here may of course have been an infection), but we have to be aware of their fairly prejudicial colonial mindset. Yet the Nigerian psychiatrist Adeoye Lambo (1965) agrees that schizophrenia among non-literate Yoruba is less likely to be associated with systematized chronic delusions and is more confusional, anxious, transitory, and affective, whilst urban Yoruba have the same pattern of schizophrenia as educated modern Europeans.

It is perhaps better to rely on anthropologists (taking into account the local concepts of personhood and illness) who draw rather similar conclusions. Ackernecht (1943) cites some early field studies. In Ghana, Field (1960) however argues that the association between education and schizophrenia is simply that the former makes the illness more visible, but Fortes in 1969, in a different and more administratively remote area, argues rather differently. He carried out his initial fieldwork among the Tallensi of northern Ghana in the 1930s, and then revisited them with his wife, a doctor and medical psychologist, in the 1960s. The Tallensi recognized a chronic pattern called *galuk* characterized by unintelligibility, confused, and erratic behaviour, an incapacity to carry out normal social and productive tasks, yet clearly distinguished from eccentricity or 'other forms of abnormality.' Among the local population of around 5,000, Fortes identified in the 1930s only one instance of *galuk* amidst plenty of eccentrics, mentally handicapped, and senile individuals. He thinks there were no others and that early death or social concealment by the generally tolerant Tallensi were unlikely. By contrast, among the same villages in the 1960s, with local missionization and some primary education, Fortes and Mayer found thirteen cases, and more in neighbouring areas: 'I had to refuse to see any more. . .' (1969: 53). Most of the thirteen had previously worked in urban Southern Ghana for a period, either as domestic servants or unskilled labourers.

Firth (1973: 224), without citing specific instances, maintains that non-industrial societies are more tolerant of the symbolizations of mental illness and are more likely to enter into a successful dialogue with them. Reviewing data from Ireland and Istria, Murphy (1982: 70) argues that high rates of schizophrenia occur in situations of 'conflicting or unduly complex demands'; considering the low rates among Tongans and Taiwanese, he speculates that their culture is less individualistic. Devereux proposes schizophrenia as a *psychose ethnique*, a product of violent processes of acculturation and oppression (Devereux 1970: 248), and identifies causal psychological detachment and fragmented or specialized lives amongst other factors. Communities in the early stages of Westernization are less common now, but the World Health Organization's various studies on schizophrenia have found in developing countries a lesser incidence, better prognosis, shorter episodes, and a more affective presentation (Hopper 2008). Leff (1981: 156) argues that the relationship of schizophrenia to the acute transient psychoses of the sort commonly described in the Third World (the *bouffées délirantes* of Franco-Cuban psychiatry: Littlewood and Lipsedge 1981) 'remains unsolved.' Working from contemporary Western symptoms, he argues that there has been a shift from bodily to psychological modes of expression; thus, the bodily equivalents of delusions of control are the symptoms of catatonia (waxy flexibility, mitgehen, echopraxia, and echolalia) more common in developing and rural societies. Jablensky (1987) argues that schizophrenia is more severe and chronic in modernized societies and with industrialization (similarly Cooper and Sartorius [1977] who favour aspects of social response); Hopper (2008) provides a critical review of such 'culture' explanations.

Historical Variation

Early Babylonian, Egyptian, Hebrew, and Indian texts refer to what we may take as insanity: 'impulsive, uncontrolled and unreasonable behaviour' (Rosen 1968: 32; also B. Clarke 1975) but not in any systematic way; there is simply a general recognition of irrational behaviour along with a demonological explanation. Ideally, the term used for this by physicians or other experts in earlier eras should be supplemented by popular lay perceptions (Macdonald 1987) and by detailed biographical descriptions (Macdonald 1987), but the early experts did not amplify their diagnoses with the sort of description we need. Without such evidence we cannot easily accept such statements as this by Zilborg (1941: 45) about the classical Greeks: 'There were certain mental disturbances, obvious even to the lay person of our day, which continued to remain unrecognised.' Were Socrates's 'voices' really schizophrenia (1941: 41)? How can we know? It appears likely that the Greeks did not clearly distinguish 'madness' (μαΐνια, μαΐνιομενου) as psychosis from 'delirium' (παράνοια, παραφρονεοτυς). The Hippocratic corpus (1923/1981: 140, 174) often places the two together and uses both to refer to something in the course of a fever. There is no word for, or description of, chronic psychosis here unless this was subsumed into acute madness or delirium, and both Simon (1978) and Evans, McGrath and Milns (2003) state there is no mention of anything like schizophrenia in Greece, and that μαΐνια (mania) simply connotes 'frenzy.' Madness in myth, epic, and tragedy relies on extremes of passion (Padel 1981), with associated temporary illusions (mistaken perceptions; Rosen 1968, Chapter 3). However, there is some idea of chronic madness in tragedy (Padel 1981), and Jeste, Del Carmen, Lohr and Wyatt (1985) argue that these are historical descriptions of something like schizophrenia but that the symptoms have changed over time, whilst Devereux (1970: 274) confidently identifies an increase during the decline of Rome. Certainly, something happens here. It is in the later Roman period that Philo recounts an actual case of a quiet and chronic madman (Rosen 1968) as does Aretaeus (Zilborg 1941: 77), and Galen and Soranus, in the early Christian era, both note that mania then occurred without fever (Diethelm 1971); by the first century CE Celsus refers to a 'third type' of insanity, characterized by false images or disordered judgement (as cited in Jeste et al. 1985) but it was often associated with inappropriate laughter and 'foolish amuse[ment]' and thus might correspond to modern mania (Evans et al. 2003).

Like Diethelm, Hunter and Macalpine (1963), in their selection of early modern and modern texts in British psychiatry, easily tag past descriptions with a label of 'schizophrenia' but it seems wiser to refer to accounts where we have some more detailed contemporary description of the patients. And here we have a long gap between Hippocrates and Galen and the seventeenth-century English divine and astrologer, Richard Napier, who kept modestly detailed records and clinical descriptions of his patients. Napier (or, rather, his biographer who examined the casebooks statistically) finds a higher than expected proportion of young adults among those severely mentally disturbed, an association with villages with a transient population and those with a higher than average proportion of Puritans and Catholics (both presumably more religiously observant than moderate Anglicans; Macdonald 1981: 40, 61, 68–69). His 'most flamboyant and recognizable kinds of insanity' (madness, lunacy, and distraction) are comparatively rare and account for 5% of consultations: they are characterized by incoherent speech and unpredictable suicides, by aimless wandering, sudden changes of mood, assaults, self-mutilation, and the destruction of others' and their own property. These are all distinguished from melancholia and from what we would now term situational and neurotic complaints. Macdonald notes that it was only later that Locke's emphasis on cognition and perception was to place delusions in madness rather than, as previously, in melancholy (thus suggesting that Napier might have underemphasized the amount of insanity by placing it under melancholia).[2]

Going back to less detailed accounts, the Anglo-Saxon literature now mentions instances of chronic insanity such as a four-year history (B. Clarke 1975: 42) but those recorded are miraculous cures and hence presumably cases with a good prognosis. Cognitive changes are sometimes noted: 'his powers of speech, discussion and understanding failed him utterly' (B. Clarke 1975: 42). De Gordon in the fourteenth century mentions talking to oneself, failure to finish sentences or explain them, meaningless remarks and aimless wandering, affective lability and attempts to grasp the impossible and irrational with poor judgement (as cited in B. Clarke 1975: 97). Clarke describes at length the case of the English King Henry VI: prudish, passive, religiously obsessed, and habitually dressed in black, at the age of thirty-one he had an illness recalling catatonia which lasted for six months, plus two relapses, some one and a half years in all.[3]

B. Clarke (1975) favours such biographical data when we can get it, to avoid the emphasis on the obviously acute and frenzied cases which in the medieval period and later were dealt with by immediate physical restriction rather than observation. By the sixteenth century chronic madmen or their imitators (Tom O'Bedlams) were commonly seen around Britain (B. Clarke 1975: Chapter 9). Thomas Willis in his *Soul of Brutes* (1674) said there was no need to give any illustrations but notes their 'incongruous notions' (as cited in B. Clarke 1975: 294; and Hunter and Macalpine 1963: 191): the pattern of severe mental illness was apparently well known. Lunacy (Latin *insania*, *furor*; Greek *mania*) now was generally distinguished from *phrenyse* which occurred only with a fever (B. Clarke 1975: 259) but there was little psychological description: simply 'like a wylde beast' (as cited in Hunter and Macalpine 1963: 14). By the nineteenth century, it was common to remark psychological symptoms like 'loss of affect' and detachment from surroundings (Hunter and Macalpine 1963: 879–80), and social and cultural explanations had appeared. Already in the seventeenth century, religious enthusiasm had been said to lead to insanity, and in the early nineteenth century it was recognized that there had been an increase in incidence in Western Europe, especially in the towns rather than the countryside, and especially in England (1963: 823–41),[4] although doubts were raised about selective bias in the statistics. In 1837, in a survey that took into account bias and data selection, rates of insanity were cited as approximately 1 in 1,000 in Europe (Scotland 1 in 574) as opposed to 1 in 262 in the United States. That until the 1700s delusions seem to have been included as melancholic rather than manic symptoms (Macdonald 1981: Chapter 4), and that it was the florid and antisocial patterns which naturally came more readily to public notice may however of course both argue that recognition of schizophrenia or proto-schizophrenia was likely to have been reduced in the earlier period, to increase in the modern era when both facilities and diagnostic patterns resemble more closely our current procedures.

Reflexive Self-Consciousness and Modernity

Nevertheless, we are left with some evidence that the transition to Western European modernity, both historically and culturally,[5] has been associated with a pattern of psychosis which, compared with its predecessors, is less 'affective,' less florid and confused, which is associated with lasting cognitive changes such as delusions, and is more chronic with a worse prognosis: in short, something resembling our current idea of schizophrenia. Among the cultural changes that have accompanied this, observers have attributed a variety of not unrelated patterns – 'social change' in general, traumatic social change, urbanization, industrialization, modern education, literacy, Christianization, individualism – and conscious self-awareness. Most medical interest has focused on the social response to psychosis: here we want to emphasize by contrast the psychological schemata in a society which might propel proto-schizophrenia into schizophrenia. Now schizophrenia is usually thought of primarily as a biological pattern, so how might 'soft' social and cultural changes affect the core symptoms (as opposed to altering prognosis through social responses like stigmatization)? Jenkins (2004) suggests that it is the individual's subjective attribution of the proto-symptoms (an attribution located in culture) which affects the eventual manifestation of the symptoms themselves – which are thus as cultural as they are biological. Given rather individualized and psychological thinking, the proto-voices[6] have now to be externally located in another person (Morrison 1999), to which we might add the obvious objection that psychopathologies (just like 'normal functioning') are a product of both biology and culture.

In this chapter we focus on Christianity, not because Christianity is the single salient influence on the modern world, but because it is a significant one that has influenced (indeed it has made possible) the appearance of the industrialized and individualized world, so much so that a history of the West without Christianity would be meaningless. All (universal at least) religions provide not only an account of extramundane beings and our ultimate justification, with prescriptive norm, for social life, but also some account of the nature of humans and how they function. Though theology is obviously a social representation rather than an internal or external account of lived experience, it will be evident from the anguished quotations below (particularly those from St Augustine's *Confessions*) that the convert is constantly trying to align themself with the public dogma, reading and experiencing life through the new conceptions. We have emphasized conversion because here the discrepancy between lived experience and theology is especially salient, at least initially: for if successful the convert's ascribed role becomes his personal achievement.

The idea of the modern self famously provided by Geertz (1983: 59) – a 'bounded, unique, more or less integrated motivational and cognitive universe, a dynamic centre of awareness, emotion, judgement and action organized into a distinctive whole and set contrastively both against other such wholes and against a social and natural background' – would be unintelligible in the absence of Christianity in which its sources may be located. A theology tells us what a person is, how people differ, how they act and are motivated; it is a theory of uniformity and difference. It offers a schema for the natural and ultrahuman worlds, for agency, and for influence, how appetites, emotions and cognitions arise, what they signify; and it offers a schema of our ultimate destination as beings. Every theology involves a practical, everyday psychology of human life. We are not arguing that Christianity contains in embryo everything that we might characterize as 'modern' (indeed, in the case under consideration, the onset of Christianity seems to have led to a temporary shift towards demonic explanations of what might otherwise be seen as illness[7]), nor that the original appearance of Christianity in a pagan world had exactly the same effects for a psychology as twentieth-century missionization; but that the secular modern world has involved certain psychological conventions of thinking which were strongly fortified by Christianity, as Marcel Mauss argued in 1938 [1979].

Sass (2004), following the work of the phenomenologist Wolfgang Blankenburg, proposes that psychological hyper-reflexivity is significant in schizophrenia: reflective self-consciousness and other patterns in which the individual comes to focus on itself and on features of its own functioning, associated with a loss of the usual taken-for-granted experience of the local world (what, following Blankenburg, he terms a 'loss of self-evidence' [2004: 305–307], akin to the well-known 'delusional mood' of schizophrenia in which the environment is no longer normal for something odd is going on). The initially tacit, including the processes of personal psychological functioning, now becomes the focus of awareness: 'a focused, introspective awareness that derealises sensations by detaching them from the unnoticed background whilst simultaneously subjecting these sensations to processes of externalisation and reification' (Sass 2004: 312–13). Aspects of the self are experienced as akin to external objects as the tacit becomes forced, artificial and awkward, and to be examined.[8] Reflecting on this only further distances the person from any sense of naturalness or capacity for spontaneous action, thus exacerbating self-alienation (Sass 2001). Living with this destabilizing cognitive slippage and the loss of the tacit is made worse, says Sass,[9] by those (modern) societies which encourage the same tendencies, in which everybody increasingly lives in a less stable external world and is plunged into idiosyncratic internalized experience, into a set of fragmented pluralistic alternatives in which the act of choice itself becomes problematic, and in which the individual self is increasingly restricted in that its processes, indeed it itself, become an object for scrutiny. Sass describes this as 'a shift from extraverted traditional societies in which emotional life, organized through myth and ritual, is at the centre, to the more introverted modern societies in which intellectual processes are far more dominant' (2001: 318), to, as we might say, the triumph of psychology as the dominant mode of personal being. It is our argument that this 'excessive' reflexive self-consciousness in part originated with Christianity and Christian conversion, and, reinforced by the Reformation and the development of popular everyday secular psychology, has grown in the modern era and is a concomitant of 'Westernization' (modernization, internalization) in non-Western societies.[10] We will now offer six instances as to how Christian theology might have provided a route to this psychology.[11]

Scrutiny of the Self in the Act of Conversion

A Delocated and Omniscient God Addressed in an Internal Conversation

To forsake other gods is not so difficult when you can move away from them and their geographical sphere of influence – if they are gods of place and nation. The popular gods of later paganism, amoral and deceivable (Origen 1869: 414), were still to be found in their place of origin, and continued their work in a local tradition, although they could relocate. While Christian universalism was to be characterized by belief, Greek and Roman religion had been orthopraxic, later with an idea that empirical knowledge of the gods was possible through divination, oracles or emergent fate: these had been generally orientated to the wellbeing of the collectivity and the gods did not communicate directly with one (Ando 2008); there was 'no proximate communication' with them (*nullo inter se propinquo communicato*) as Apuleius (1908: 11) had put it. But gods and humans were in a reciprocal relationship where the former could be benevolent when men practised the correct ritual or sacrifice: as the younger Pliny lamented, the Christians only had to burn a bit of incense and all would be well. Roman, like modern African, sacrifice was concerned with warding off disaster or achieving practical benefits (Peel 2000). Smith (1990) has made a distinction between these 'locative cults' (which were often syncretic, subsuming one local god into another more powerful one) contrasted with the new 'utopian cults' such as the Hellenistic mystery religions[12] and Christianity which demanded a fundamental change in the individual and hence something like introspection. And 'God is one,' insists the author of the early 'Shepherd of Hermas' (Anonymous A, 2003): drawing on Judaism, the Christian God now denied the very existence of other gods (Origen 1869: 429). Omnipresent, he controlled every bit of the world, not just the area around his place of origin. (Similarly, the Hebrews who migrated from Palestine to Alexandria in the late Hellenistic period had had to do without a God in his Temple in Jerusalem, as they had to, more radically, after the destruction of the Temple and the expulsion of the Jews by Hadrian.) Communication with God was now not only by a ritual of place but by an obligatory internal personal conversation – prayer. For the nineteenth-century missionaries, 'one of the proofs of the sincerity of our converts is the habit of prayer which they have acquired' (Peel 2000: 256). This God was universal, omniscient, and omnipresent: 'What torments my heart suffered in mental pregnancy, what groans, my God! . . .And though I did not know it, your ears were there,' says St Augustine, 'You knew what I endured; no human being knew' (Augustine 2008: 119–20). There was no escaping this God for He already knew what you were thinking, but one could try to plead with Him or placate Him in a silent conversation and he might respond personally: 'The Lord did not leave us alone in our affliction', says a bereaved missionary in Yorubaland (Peel 2000: 167). 'The sacrifices of God are a broken spirit. . . and to obey is better than to sacrifice. God wants our hearts', an African convert is told (Peel 2000: 185). Missionaries, evangelizing the Yoruba in the nineteenth century, consciously modelled their work on the Acts of the Apostles (Peel 2000: 155): 'Her ori [personal deity] is made of cowries and only God who made them should be worshipped' (Peel 2000: 157), just as St Clement had stated that 'We were maimed in our understanding, worshiping stones and pieces of wood. . . all of them made by humans' (Clement 2003: 165–66); and similarly Eusebius (Kofsky 2000, *passim*). Christianity pushed the pagans into a universal linear time of redemptive history and away from their cyclical local history (Leach 1961). Rather than, say, committing a particular crime in society, the Christian was born in universal sin (which could be redeemed). For the Yoruba, their concern with a deferral of death was transformed into the promise of eternal life (Peel 2000) – or damnation.

A Private Self Similarly Independent of Immediate Physical Context Yet Located in the Individual

This new deity could be encountered anywhere – 'Wherever two are gathered in my name' (Matthew 18.20) – for Christianity was universal and individual ('neither Jew nor Greek. . . bond nor free. . . male or female, for you are all one man in Christ Jesus', says St Paul). And ultimate control rested with Him, Creator and Master of the whole universe, throughout the whole universe. No longer was there any point in threatening your recalcitrant (Egyptian) idol for not coming up with the goods (Cumont 1958 [1911]: 93): as similarly in colonial Africa, at least according to the missionaries (Peel 2000). If God was independent of social context and place, then so was the individual self at least in its conversations with God (as Dilthey argues). Religious status was no longer signalled by external signs (circumcision), or social position (the higher stages of the Roman priesthood had been occupied by aspiring politicians in the course of their career: 'The internal status of the officiating person was a matter of. . . indifference to the celestial spirits', Cumont 1958 [1911]: 91). 'Now it is not our flesh that we must circumcise, we must crucify ourselves, exterminate and mortify our unreasonable desires' (John Chrysostom 1979); 'circumcise your heart', says St Barnabas (2003: 45) for religion became internal and private. Like the African or Roman self (Mauss 1979 [1938]), the Jewish self had been embedded in a functioning society, individually decentred and socially contextualized (Di Vito 1999); it survived death only through its bodily descendants: 'But Abram cried, what can you give me, seeing I shall die childless' (Genesis 15.2). To die without issue meant extinction in both religious systems (Madigan and Levenson 2008). But now an enduring part of the self, or an associate of it – the soul – had a connection to what might be called body and consciousness yet had some sort of ill-defined association with them. In its earthly body it was in potential communication with God. Like God it was immaterial and immortal. (The associated resurrection of the physical body, though an essential part of Christian dogma, has played an increasingly less important part in the Church [cf. Stroumsa 1990].) For nineteenth-century pagan Yoruba who already accepted some idea of a hereafter, each village has its separate afterlife which had to be fused by the missionaries into a more universal schema (Peel 2000: 175). If the conversation with God was one to one, then each self-aware individual had then to make up their own mind on adherence – and thus the detached observer became the surveyor of the whole world (Dumont 1985). Sacral and secular became distinct (separate 'functions' as Dumont calls them), further presaging a split between psychological faculties. The idea of the self/soul as an autonomous unit facing God became the basis, via the stages Mauss (1979 [1938]) briefly outlines, for a political philosophy of individualism (MacFarlane 1978). The missionaries in Africa constantly attempted to reach the inside of their converts but bemoaned the fact that the Yoruba did not seem to have any inward core to the self (Peel 2000: Chapter 9). Lienhardt (1985), whilst broadly sympathetic to the idea of a precolonial African 'collectivist' self, maintains that some aspects of individuality were of course already recognized ('said the king. . . it is only I who can see the dance of the tortoise: his dance is entirely inside him' – a folktale quoted in Lienhardt 1985: 143); he agrees that Christian education has developed this private self as more distinct and more drastic.

Scrutiny of the Self

If each separate person was now a potential temple for God (1 Corinthians 3.16), yet 'be you transformed in the renewing of your mind' (Romans 12.2). The everyday mundane self and experience were suspect and had to be interrogated. Introspection had been previously recommended by Plotinus ('go into yourself' [1984: 1.8.9.7–8]), and Augustine (2008: 123) recalls that 'By the Platonic books I was admonished to return into myself' – not without some struggle, for 'I did not wish to observe myself. . . And I looked and was appalled. . . Where shall I go to escape from myself?' (2008: 44, 60). 'Abase thee, abase thee, O my soul!', says Marcus Aurelius (1906: 14) similarly. Immoral acts now become a part of you rather than something circumscribed and past to be punished by illness or crop failure: 'If we say we have no sin, we are deceiving ourselves' (1 John 1.8). Christian duty now prescribed for all a rigorous, ever deeper self-examination; one had to reject the compromised past, but in doing that one inevitably doubted one's earlier perceptions and memory as having been suspect (though once tacit) and fundamentally misconceived or false. 'Renunciation and despair of it are our first steps in the direction of the truth,' says William James of evangelical Victorians (1964 [1904]: 140). 'I had become to myself a vast problem and I questioned my soul' (Augustine 2008: 57–58). 'Le moi est haissable', observed Pascal (1910). 'What is the attitude of our soul towards your neighbour?. . . Examine carefully whether your heart be sincere,' recommends St Francis de Sales (1934: 294–95, 296), '[a]fter each point of the examination you will find yourself to have failed.' And Thomas à Kempis (1952: 196) advises, 'Therefore carefully examine your conscience to the best of your ability, cleansing and purifying it by true contrition and humble confession.' A nineteenth-century mission diary in Africa (Peel 2000) similarly comments as follows: 'Depressed in spirit, felt my own depravity'. There was a shift from practice to belief (emphasized yet again in the Reformation with its particular emphasis on self-control [Max Weber]), and thus a focus on how you could believe, how you knew that you believed, and what it was to be sure (Needham 1972). (But there never could be any certainty, as Calvin notoriously noted.) Early Christianity appears to have been essentially a peasant protest movement (Horsley 2005), and such introspection only seems to have come in after its more immediate political defeat (the leader's execution) with gentile Christianity's shift to a less politically engaged internalization (compare the early modern Anabaptists and Quakers). Augustine quotes Galatians (5.17) – 'you are unable to do what you wish' – to emphasize a compartmentalized and conflicted mind in which the elements are set against each other, unknowing, a conflict particularly salient at the period of conversion, and which William James (1964 [1904]) makes sense of using the idea of an unconscious. The point of self-examination was to achieve a new self-mastery to conquer what were taken as the more bodily emotions. St Colombanus writes in a seventh-century sermon: 'Will you not beware of yourself, wretch, and have no confidence in yourself – you who are ensnared by yourself, but not set free by yourself' (as cited in Holder 2000: 113). Early monastic accounts emphasize a constant monitoring of mood and the practical management of mood, in fighting the demons of anger (Goehring 2000; Stewart 2000): 'do not let the sun go down on your anger' (Ephesians 4.26). One attempted such self-mastery away from others, in secret; similarly, good deeds should be private and hidden (Mathew 6. 1–18). Secular introspective scrutiny in printed autobiographies (as well as in private letters) can be dated from the mid-sixteenth century in England, emerging out of religious confessional literature (Skura 2008; Barker 1984; cf. Burckhardt 1945): 'In those days I would wreak mine anger altogether with pen and ink on paper'; 'I. . . thought that to dissemble with a dissembler was no dissimulation' (*c.*1569); 'as I have changed the inward affectes of my minde, so I have lured my wanton workes to effectuall labours' (1590; all three quoted in Skura 2008).

Everyday Sense Data Is Downplayed

If Hebrew salvation had been essentially this worldly, in Daniel 12 (and 1 Enoch 22) we do have some firmer intimations of a life to come (possibly under Zoroastrian influence; Madigan and Levenson 2008). In Christianity there was now a clear Platonic separation between the world of everyday experience – mundane, temporary, and compromised – and the real other world which was beyond sensory perception. 'Nothing that is visible is good' says St Ignatius (2003: 273). Origen (1872: 462) comments that 'All the Christians therefore have the eye of the mind sharpened, and the eye of sense closed.' Estranged from God, we now had to find him by estranging ourselves from our everyday life, however appealing: 'Natural good is not simply insufficient in amount and transient, there lurks a falsity in its very being', describes William James for Christian people (1964 [1904]: 140).

'Do not love the world nor the things which are in the world' (1 John 2.15). 'Such [social] amusements,' comments Edward Gibbon acerbically (1993: 527), 'were rejected with abhorrence, or admitted with the utmost caution, by the severity of the fathers'. Thomas à Kempis (1952: 33, 88) recommends that 'Man's true spiritual progress depends on denial of the [bodily] self. . . Live a dying life. . . dead to self.' St Ignatius comments that 'I no longer desire to live like a human' (Ignatius 2003: 281). Our current world was impermanent, but we had been redeemed from the sin of Adam through the Incarnation: 'Old things have passed away, all has become new', says a nineteenth-century American convert (cited in James 1964 [1904]: 200). It is particularly the immediate material aspects of our current world – food, sex, comfort, anger – that must be downplayed through fasting and self-denial, and engagement with them deprecated (Origen 1872: 460). This involved the individuals themselves who to an extent become questionable and unreal. In the seventeenth century John Bunyan recommended, 'I must first pass a sentence of death upon everything that can properly be called a thing of this life, even to reckon myself, my wife, my children, my health, my enjoyment, and all, as dead to me' (as quoted in James 1964 [1904]: 156). As the boundaries of possible experience passed beyond the human lifespan, they became separated from real life, extending on as a more abstract principle. '[Christians] live in their respective countries, but only as resident aliens', says the author of the 'Epistle to Diognetus' (Anonymous B 2003). What people actually could do in this extended life to come was left a little vague in experiential terms, but there were continued debates in the early church as to the activities and nature of the soul: was it purely intellectual as Origen (1869: 137–42) avowed? Or did Resurrection involve the body as well as the soul (with the nature of the resurrected body being left open for medieval debate)? Like other religious systems, but perhaps more so, Christianity used logical paradoxes to emphasize the value of the theorized spiritual over the experienced (the Folly of the Cross, Death of Death and Hell's Destruction, three persons in one, 'My power is made perfect in weakness,' '*Credo quia impossibile est*'). As the missionary taught when faced with materially inclined (and presumably mystified) Africans, 'to die is to gain' (Peel 2000: 166).

Conflicted Agency and Divine Grace

'And he is truly learned who renounces his own will for the will of God' (Thomas à Kempis 1952: 32). One had to surrender to God – 'break us, melt us, mould us and fill us with a love of God', as Methodists still appeal to the Holy Spirit (Heelas 1981: 41); and personal agency was anyway less to be taken for granted – 'I saw that when I acted against my wishes, I was passive rather than active' (Augustine 2008: 114). Jewish salvation and divine punishment seem to have been this worldly and collective (Exodus 20.5) although there are hints of something more individual in Ezekiel 18.1–4 (Madigan and Levenson 2008). Rather than their being natural and unremarked, the individual now had themself to focus on what it was to decide and act, and why. How did some people make the decision to reject God? Was it some malign external force yet within oneself (later to become codified as the Devil)? If God acted through you, was the active agent God or you, or somehow both? How could it have gone otherwise? How can I be sure I am saved? Can I be sure I am sure? Though the fuller development of these questions only occurred in late medieval theology, we can imagine how they pricked the minds of the more philosophical or nervous early converts like Augustine. And yet at the same time one was somehow finally responsible for one's actions: Augustine opposed astrology because it located sin as external to him (Augustine 2008: bk 4, Chapter 3). And yet the full weight of moral decision was ultimately externalized onto God as 'grace,' his gratuitous and undeserved gift (Pitt-Rivers 1992): 'one of the symbolic ways of displacing personal responsibility', comments Firth unkindly (1970: 25). God comes to Augustine without his apparent intentions and does something to him: 'I was astonished to find that already I loved you' (Augustine 2008: 127); yet 'fearing a precipitate plunge, I kept my heart from giving any assent' (2008: 94). But that final plunge is somehow involuntary and up to God's grace, for 'the mind commands the body and is instantly obeyed. The mind commands itself and meets resistance' (2008: 47). In the second century, Origen (1869: 416) comments that some 'may have been converted to Christianity, as if against their will.' The confusing idea of 'grace' somehow implies that God acts, and yet doesn't act obviously, allowing and encouraging something human to happen (and was it inevitable anyway?). If so, why was it previously blocked by our sin? Presumably this would lead to confusion over personal and divine agency in the individual: Augustine for instance is constantly uncertain as to whether God or he is the active agent of a decision or action. We might assume that for the average convert, this would have been guided and made easier by the clergy, but the internalized God/self/soul/mind relations continued to be ambiguous: 'So I was in conflict with myself and was dissociated from myself. The dissociation came against my will; this was not a manifestation of an alien mind but the punishment suffered in my own mind . . . And so it was "not I" that brought this about' (2008: 148–49). Augustine's conversion does not seem to have resolved these experiential issues, but rather they passed into relative insignificance when he surrendered, took shelter in God, and then passed the credit for all his new, now approved, actions and thoughts onto God's grace.

Decomposition and Conflict of the Self in Conversion

Conversion (followed by exorcism and baptism) was a total transformation which entailed the introduction of a split in the self which was ideally resolved through God's grace. You could be a Roman pagan, and a Neo-Platonist as well as a bit of a Manichee, as was Augustine, in a sort of 'add on' process (or consider Lucius Apuleius who collected various different pagan initiations), in which you might emphasize bits of one more than the other but you did not have to totally discard the other. Christianity, however, demanded a total renunciation of the old: 'Unless a man is born again, he cannot see the kingdom of heaven' (John 3.3). (We are here assuming a voluntary conversion, not the forced mass conversions of Saxon England or Germany, or later of Uganda, but the rationale of any conversion presumed some volition which all successful converts placed retrospectively on their past act.) In conversion, two of you are recognized and experienced: the older unregenerate you, which persists in memory (or backsliding) after the conversion, 'our old self' (Romans 6.6); and the new you, self-anticipated or imagined before conversion, whether to be then welcomed or not. In the seventeenth century, Sir Thomas Browne, speculating on salvation, similarly comments, 'There is another man within me' (Browne n.d.: 110). Pascal says, 'So man is always divided and opposed to himself' (Pascal 1910: 190). 'God grant me chastity and continence but not yet', the vacillating Augustine complains (2008: 148). His dilemma ended in his final conversion when he found an injunction from God (Romans 13: 13–14) to give up the erotic life – but through God's agency and grace, not Augustine's. At the actual moment of conversion, you are in two minds – 'the divided self', as William James (1964 [1904]: Chapter 8) called it[13] – at which point the operations of the other self may for a moment become more salient and problematic, and have to be momentarily considered, for you *are* then that other self. 'The winds blow first one way, then the other, pushing my heart to and fro' (Augustine 2008: 106). There is a dialogue between the two selves: 'Why then are you perversely following the teaching of your flesh?', he asks himself and admonishes, 'Do not be vain my soul' (2008: 62, 63). 'Because we are of two minds. . . we do not realise that we are doing evil', says St Clement (2003: 197). For Augustine the two selves were the older unregenerate self, dominated by the sensual appetites, opposed to the new spiritual self ('This weight was my sexual habit'; 2008: 137), and he finally rejected his philosophical background because it could not deal with this sort of conflict (2008: 131). The actual moment of passing over to the new self was more or less involuntary (see section on Conflicted Agency and Divine Grace, above) and might be sudden (Origen 1872: 148). At the end, although the conflict had been real, acceptance of

Christianity will mean there should be no residual doubts: 'the alternative for them will be to be converted to the true view and not to deny that in the process of deliberation a single soul is wavering between different views' (Augustine 2008: 149). Through becoming a Christian, recognition of God's Incarnation in Jesus cut short his unavailing quest for perfect Platonic forms (Stroumsa 1990).[14]

Conclusion: A Psychology of Self Awareness

Bringing these six influences of Christianity together, we have an implicit and experienced psychology of detachment from immediate embodied experience in the world, with an emphasis on scrutinizing and questioning the convoluted workings of a hidden and immaterial self, seen as distinct from other similar selves and from the natural world, now in private communication with an omniscient presence who already knows one's thoughts and emotions, and with ambiguous agency for personal actions and experience in the world which are no longer to be taken as tacit and unproblematic: all of which come to the fore in the process of conversion in which one has to disassemble one self and create another by carefully bringing one's decisions to conscious awareness yet attributing the final shift externally to the omniscient grace. This involved identification and scrutiny both of the processes of memory and cognition, and of the relations between self and outside world, and between new entities (God, soul) which had a close relation with the self, in a way that was hardly necessary for the pagan. Indeed, with the growth of the idea of heresy, to correctly align such personal cognitions with the dominant procedures became an issue of vital importance. Drawing on Hebrew religion, and on the Hellenistic mystery religions and on Stoicism and Neo-Platonism,[15] this new view could depict a more explicit hierarchy of deity, the moral soul, through the cognitive mind to animal impulses, which might all act in concert or, more usually, be in conflict.[16] We find this psychological schema in Augustine: 'I turned then to examine the nature of mind,' he says in a review of his conversion, 'vicious acts only occur if obsession has captured the mind's affective part which is at the root of the impulse to carnal pleasures' (Augustine 2008: 67–68). We are assuming that all of this gradually percolated down, through theological texts and clerical training, to the sermons and homilies preached to the ordinary populace, and thus to the way they would understand and experience themselves. With literacy, words and ideas became separate from the individual who voiced them and maintained an independent existence.

Unlike Greek philosophy, Christianity galvanizes everybody. St Gregory of Nyssa comments that:

> Every corner of the city is thronged with men arguing on incomprehensible subjects. Ask a man how many obols a thing costs, and he dogmatises on generated and ungenerated essence. Inquire what is the price of bread and you are answered the Father is greater than the Son, the Son is subordinate to the Father. Ask about your bath and you are told the Son was created out of nothing. (Kellett 1962 [1933]: 216)

Tertullian and Origen note that theology was as accessible to a workman as to a philosopher (e.g. Origen 1872: 156, 467).

The central issue in all of this seems to be the emphasis on a continued scrutiny of personal actions and inclinations amidst a multitude of alternatives, on the downplaying of the everyday physical world, and on the problematization of agency: in all, a new self-awareness and self-reference, a shifting of the centre of gravity of consciousness into the individual human being. Many habitual aspects of ourselves, and these we can presume are already enhanced in proto-schizophrenia – our bodily functioning, 'chance' thoughts, sensations, impulses, and memories – can be attributed to some source external to the experiencing self (to physiology, memory, dreams, genes, passions, habits). We cannot however now attribute agency to them. As agency is withdrawn from the natural world, from others, from animals, plants, stars, and spirits, our individual agency appears enhanced and yet there remains the uneasy balance between the 'is it me?' and the 'is it something external?'[17]

Many external causes, spirits, and stars not only no longer have agency but are no longer validated by our society, so any personal explanations of an external locus of control become increasingly idiosyncratic and divorced from our common social life (Tausk 1948 [1919]).[18] If the passage from proto-schizophrenia to schizophrenia is thus perhaps intelligible in social terms, does this offer any clues to the nature of proto-schizophrenia itself? If the attribution of agency is a general human characteristic and is integral to both religion and psychosis (Dein and Littlewood 2011), then this might suggest that both the proto-symptoms and their transformation into schizophrenia are concerned with this attribution, the transformation being related to the indigenous psychology we have considered here. This type of estrangement from experience (later reinforced by a number of secular and religious developments)[19] fits well with Sass' criteria for the reflexive self-consciousness that has perhaps propelled us into schizophrenia.

Acknowledgements

The genesis of this chapter lies in intermittent discussions over many years with Georges Devereux, Raymond Firth and Godfrey Lienhardt. We are grateful for more recent comments from Mitchell Weiss, David Napier and colleagues at the 2009 Conference on Cultural Psychiatry in Norcia, Italy, and at seminars at University College London, Durham and Oxford. Translations from the New Testament are our own; from the Old Testament those of the Authorised Version.

Notes

1. In common modules for agent hyperidentification and theory of mind.
2. For instances of non-affective delusions as Tudor melancholia, see Littlewood (2009).
3. Possibly inherited from his insane French grandfather, Charles VI, on whom see B. Clarke (1975).
4. Insanity was twice as common in England as in Piedmont or Savoy (B. Clarke 1975).
5. An obvious objection to our procedure, beyond what threatens to be an unfashionable unitary model, is that we cannot readily conflate recent cultural changes and the historical as a unitary phenomenon in what may recall a nineteenth-century evolutionist schema: recent small-scale communities are not our ancestors and have changed in time just as have European societies. Nevertheless, we would maintain that they have shared some common psychological features in the same way that, say, parliamentary democracy and feminist individualism have been a product both of Western historical development as well as of contemporary low-income countries. This chapter is not an essay in evolutionary inevitability but in social contingency.
6. It is obviously clumsy to keep talking of proto-symptoms and proto-voices, instead of symptoms and voices, but we need to bear in mind that a phenomenological description of the early stage is necessarily opaque and the 'proto-' prefix reminds us that this will emerge only finally as the experienced symptom whether this takes a classically schizophrenic pattern or not.
7. Like elf-shot in Anglo-Saxon England (B. Clarke 1975).
8. Blankenburg had not suggested that this 'loss of self-evidence' was temporally prior or causal in schizophrenia: his approach was purely phenomenological.
9. Who had previously published a comprehensive work on parallels between modern reflexive self-consciousness and insanity (Sass 1992).
10. 'Westernization' and 'modernization' are hardly unproblematic terms: we are using them here as a shorthand for relatively increased material resources, industrialization, urbanization, literacy, the absence of prescriptive marriage patterns, individualization and (more recently) lower fertility and mortality rates, a later age of marriage, the development of nationalism, and a more immediate relationship with the world economic and cultural system (Littlewood 2002: 86).
11. There are large problems of method with the sort of schema we have offered here: a conflation of the historical and the cultural, and of course a drastic summarization of an enormous field; a simplification of a complex theology across a vast chronological gap between early Christianity and more recent missionization, assuming the same

things mattered in the same way to diverse peoples; an emphasis on English material (no Petrarch or Luther, or indeed possible Indian or Chinese parallels); and a detaching of local theorizations from their immediate social context. Nor are we looking at the spread of 'Christian psychology' beyond Christianized countries through industrialization and individualization. We have ignored the specific contributions of colonialism and capitalism, the later trajectory of the self from Descartes to Kant and beyond, and the problem of reconciling a world of top-down essences with that of bottom-up experience. There is hardly an example or interpretation here which could not be qualified.

12. The seeds of gentile Christianity were located in these religions, as they were in later Greek philosophy and in the Israelite religion. Some of our 'Christian' changes are presaged or facilitated by the Stoics and Neo-Platonists: reading Plotinus, Marcus Aurelius, Augustine – or even Julian (who accepted the idea of a supreme God and an individual soul; Burr 2000) – shows us how much late paganism anticipated or paralleled Christianity: the single omniscient deity, the progress of the soul, the universality of individual moral obligations. 'God is, and cares for us and ours,' and one 'must dig within thee', recommends Marcus Aurelius (1906: 16, 94). And similarly, the indignant Yoruba of the Ibadan Empire maintained to the quizzical missionaries that they already recognized a supreme power above the gods (Peel 2000: 116–22). The choice of roles offered in Greek tragedy (Antigone) pointed the way to something approximating to a self-contained self: Momigliano (1971) argues that the Hellenistic period had biographies and thus a notion of the individual. The religion of the Hebrews showed some of the psychologization of Christianity in the emphasis on personal sin in the Book of Enoch and the Testaments of the Twelve Patriarchs, as well as the Jewish scriptures' emphasis on an omniscient deity and the possibility of a life beyond the material (Madigan and Levenson 2008). It would be unwise to speculate on the religious psychology of the Judaeo-Greek cults of Alexandria but we might presume something interesting here.
13. Later a common idiom for the schizophrenic self – e.g. R.D. Laing.
14. Conversion from paganism to Christianity of course has not always taken such a drastic and psychological form and might be motivated by economic self-interest and local loyalties, whilst still accompanied by troubling dreams or illness (for a modern missionary instance, see Firth 1973: 325–26).
15. As Bertrand Russell put it, the philosophy of later antiquity had been a gradual process of increasing subjectivity. Augustine represents of course an instance where both family background and Hellenistic philosophy pushed him into a Christian direction. His rather abstract Platonic divinity gradually developed personalistic characters under the influence of his Christian friends and mother: God now had a particular interest in him.
16. As in Aquinas. A more formal instance of something like this is found in the triventricular psychology of the medieval and Renaissance periods – sensation, reason, and memory – though this is more Galenic than Christian. See however the divine projection on to this in Robert Fludd's interesting diagram of 1619 (Clarke and Dewhurst 1972: 38).
17. In a neuro-philosophical paper, Kircher and Leube (2003) propose that our first level of consciousness (pre-reflexive consciousness) comprises such primary experiences which are tacit and 'transparent' in that while the brain constructs our reality, the mechanism of this construction is not represented in it, thus resulting in naïve realism – the assumption that the content of consciousness has a direct contact to the immediate environment. If we then reflect on primary experiences, the content enters introspective consciousness (level two). Primary self-experiences include self-agency (as well as self-coherence, self-affectivity, and autobiographical memory) – the sense that one is the author of one's

actions. Life requires a balance between anticipated action planning and control, and proprioceptive feedback: failure leads to incorrect attribution of events to the self, as in schizophrenia where self-monitoring fails. We would speculate that excessive introspective self-consciousness leading to an objectification of experience in level two, with neglect of proprioception leading to a failure in maintaining this balance.

18. Lienhardt (1961: 149) describes how pagan Dinkas' everyday emotions and memories were not experienced as subjective but as put into the person through other people and events in the environment; a memory is something external still acting on one (for Kircher and Leube's naïve realism, see Note 17 above). The dismantling of such a psychology makes 'thought insertion' and 'made affects' more problematic and abnormal, no longer shared by one's fellows.

19. A process of psychologization and abstraction continued by of course Islam in an approximately parallel development (not to mention the Reformation which did much to enhance an inner directed awareness) but also through the more secular aspects of literacy, clock time, printing, the diary and the autobiography, double-entry bookkeeping, monetarization and credit, the market, interest, industrialization, and communication technology, all of which have led to a gradual 'disembedding' (Giddens 1990) from our pagan Being in the World. All societies have some monitoring of thought and action: what is new is a 'reflection upon the nature of reflection itself' (Giddens 1990: 39).

References

Ackernecht, E.H. 1943. 'Psychopathology, Primitive Medicine and Primitive Culture', *Bulletin of the History of Medicine* 14: 30–68.

Ando, C. 2008. *The Matter of the Gods: Religion and the Roman Empire*. Berkeley: University of California Press.

Anonymous, A. 2003. 'The Shepherd of Hermas', in B.D. Ehrman (ed.), *The Apostolic Fathers* (Vol. 2). Cambridge, MA: Loeb Classical Library.

Anonymous, B. 2003. 'Epistle to Diognetus', in B.D. Ehrman (ed.), *The Apostolic Fathers* (Vol. 2). Cambridge, MA: Loeb Classical Library.

Apuleius. 1908. *Liber de Deo Socratis* [The god of Socrates], in *Apuleius, III, De Philosophia Libri*. Leipzig, Germany: Teubner.

Barker, F. 1984. *The Tremulous Private Body: Essays on Subjection*. London: Methuen.

Barnabas, St. 2003. 'Epistle of Barnabas', in B.D. Ehrman (ed.), *the Apostolic Fathers* (Vol. 2). Cambridge, MA: Loeb Classical Library.

Barrett, R.J. 2004. 'Kurt Schneider in Borneo: Do First Rank Symptoms Apply to the Iban?', in J.H. Jenkins and R.J. Barrett (eds), *Schizophrenia, Culture and Subjectivity*. Cambridge: Cambridge University Press.

Browne, T.N.D. *Religio Medici*. London: Blackie.

Burckhardt, J. 1990 [1860]. *The Civilisation of the Renaissance in Italy*. Harmondsworth, UK: Penguin.

Burr, E.G. 2000. 'Julian "the Apostate," Against the Galileans', in R. Valantasis (ed.), *Religions of Late Antiquity in Practice*. Princeton, NJ: Princeton University Press.

Clarke, B. 1975. *Mental Disorder in Earlier Britain*. Cardiff: University of Wales Press.

Clarke, E., and K. Dewhurst. 1972. *An Illustrated History of Brain Function*. Oxford: Sandford.

Clement, St. 2003. 'Second Letter of Clement', in B.D. Ehrman (ed.), *The Apostolic Fathers* (Vol. 1). Cambridge, MA: Loeb Classical Library.

Cooper, J.E. and N. Sartorius. 1977. 'Cultural and Temporal Variations in Schizophrenia: A Speculation on the Importance of Industrialisation', *British Journal of Psychiatry* 130: 50–55.
Cumont, F. 1958 [1911]. *Oriental Religions in Roman Paganism*. New York: Dover.
Dein, S. and R. Littlewood. 2011. 'Psychosis and Religion: A Common Evolutionary Trajectory?' *Transcultural Psychiatry* 43(1): 318–35.
Devereux, G. 1970. *Essais d'Ethnopsychiatrie Generale*. Paris: Gallimard.
Di Vito, R. 1999. 'Old Testament Anthropology and the Construction of Personal Identity', *Catholic Biblical Quarterly* 61: 217–38.
Diethelm, O. 1971. *Medical Dissertations of Psychiatric Illness Printed before 1750*. Basel: Karger.
Dumont, L. 1985. 'A Modified View of Our Origins: The Christian Beginnings of Modern Individualism', in M. Carithers, S. Collins and S. Lukes (eds), *The Category of the Person*. Cambridge: Cambridge University Press.
Evans, K., J. McGrath and R. Milns. 2003. 'Searching for Schizophrenia in Ancient Greek and Roman Literature: A Systematic Review', *Acta Psychiatrica Scandinavica* 107: 323–30.
Fabrega, H. 1982. 'Culture and Psychiatric Illness', in A.J. Marsella and G.M. White (eds), *Cultural Conceptions of Mental Health and Therapy*. Dordrecht, the Netherlands: Reidel.
Field, M. 1960. *Search for Security: An Ethno-Psychiatric Study of Rural Ghana*. London: Faber and Faber.
Firth, R. 1970. *Rank and Religion in Tikopia*. London: Allen and Unwin.
______. 1973. *Symbols, Public and Private*. London: Allen and Unwin.
Fortes, M. and D.Y. Mayer. 1969. 'Psychosis and Social Change among the Tallensi of Northern Ghana', in S.H. Foulkes and G.S. Prince (eds), *Psychiatry in a Changing Society*. London: Tavistock.
Francis de Sales, St. 1934. *Introduction to the Devout Life*. London: Burns, Oates and Washbourne.
Geertz, C. 1983. *Local Knowledge*. New York: Basic Books.
Gibbon, E. 1993 [1776]. *The Decline and Fall of the Roman Empire* (Vols. 1–2). London: Everyman.
Giddens, A. 1990. *The Consequences of Modernity*. Cambridge: Polity Press.
Goehring, J.E. 2000. 'The First Sahidic Life of Pachmius', in R. Valantasis (ed.), *Religions of Late Antiquity in Practice*. Princeton, NJ: Princeton University Press.
Heelas, P. 1981. 'The Model Applied: Anthropology and Indigenous Psychologies', in P. Heelas and A. Lock (eds), *Indigenous Psychologies*. London: Academic Press.
Higgins, E.S. and S. Kose. 2007. 'Absence of Schizophrenia in a 15th Century Islamic Medical Textbook', *American Journal of Psychiatry* 164: 1120.
Hippocrates. 1981 [1923]. *The Sacred Disease*. Cambridge, MA: Loeb Classical Library.
Holder, A.G. 2000. 'Sermons of Columbanus', in R. Valantasis (ed.), *Religions of Late Antiquity in Practice*. Princeton, NJ: Princeton University Press.
Hopper, K. 2004. 'Interrogating the Meaning of "Culture" in the WHO International Studies of Schizophrenia', in J.H. Jenkins and R.J. Barrett (eds), *Schizophrenia, Culture and Subjectivity*. Cambridge: Cambridge University Press.
______. 2008. 'Outcomes Elsewhere: Course of Psychosis in "Other Cultures"', in C. Morgan, K. McKenzie and P. Fearon (eds), *Society and Psychosis*. Cambridge: Cambridge University Press.
Horsley, R.A. 2005. 'Jesus Movements and the Renewal of Israel', in R.A. Horsley (ed), *Christian Origins*. Minneapolis, MN: Fortress Press.

Hunter, R. and I. Macalpine. 1963. *Three Hundred Years of Psychiatry*. London: Oxford University Press.
Ignatius, St. 2003. 'Letters of Ignatius', in B.D. Ehrman (ed.), *The Apostolic Fathers* (Vol. 1). Cambridge, MA: Loeb Classical Library.
Jablensky, A. 1987. 'Multicultural Studies and the Nature of Schizophrenia: A Review', *Journal of the Royal Society of Medicine* 80: 162–67.
James, W. 1964 [1904]. *The Varieties of Religious Experience*. New York: Mentor.
Jenkins, J.H. 2004. 'Schizophrenia as a Paradigm Case for Understanding Fundamental Human Processes', in J.H. Jenkins and R.J. Barrett (eds), *Schizophrenia, Culture and Subjectivity*. Cambridge: Cambridge University Press.
Jeste, D.V., R. Del Carmen, J.R. Lohr and R.J. Wyatt. 1985. 'Did Schizophrenia Exist before the 18th Century?', *Comprehensive Psychiatry* 26: 493–503.
John Chrysostom, St. 1979. *Discourses Against Judaizing Christians [Adversus Judaeos]*. Washington DC: Catholic University of America Press.
Kellett, E.R. 1962 [1933]. *A Short History of Religions*. Harmondsworth, UK: Penguin.
Kircher, T.T.J. and D.T. Leube. 2003. 'Self-Consciousness, Self-Agency, and Schizophrenia', *Consciousness and Cognition* 12: 656–69.
Kofsky, A. 2000. *Eusebius of Caesarea Against Paganism*. Leiden, the Netherlands: Brill.
Kraepelin, E. 1971 [1919]. *Dementia Praecox and Paraphrenia*. New York: Krieger.
Lambo, T.A. 1965. 'Schizophrenia and Borderline States', in A.V.S. De Reuck and R. Porter (eds), *Transcultural Psychiatry*. London: Churchill.
Leach, E.R. 1961. *Rethinking Anthropology*. London: Athlone.
Leff, J. 1981. *Psychiatry around the Globe*. New York: Dekker.
Lienhardt, G. 1961. *Divinity and Experience*. OxfordK: Clarendon Press.
______. 1985. 'Self: Public, Private: Some African Representations', in M. Carithers, S. Collins and S. Lukes (eds), *The Category of the Person*. Cambridge: Cambridge University Press.
Littlewood, R. 2002. *Pathologies of the West*. London: Continuum.
______. 2009. 'Strange, Incredible and Impossible Things: The Early Anthropology of Reginald Scot', *Transcultural Psychiatry*. 46: 348–64.
Littlewood, R. and M. Lipsedge. 1981. 'Acute Psychotic Reactions in Caribbean-Born Patients', *Psychological Medicine* 11: 303–18.
Macdonald, M. 1981. *Mystical Bedlam: Madness, Anxiety and Healing in Seventeenth Century England*. Cambridge: Cambridge University Press.
______. 1987. 'Madness, Suicide and the Computer', in R. Porter and A. Wear (eds), *Problems and Methods in the History of Medicine*. London: Croom Helm.
Macfarlane, A. 1978. *The Origins of English Individualism*. Oxford: Blackwell.
Madigan, K.J. and J.D. Levenson. 2008. *Resurrection: The Power of God for Christians and Jews*. New Haven, CT: Yale University Press.
Marcus Aurelius. 1906. *The Thoughts of Marcus Aurelius*. London: Oxford University Press.
Mauss, M. 1979 [1938]. 'A Category of the Human Mind: The Notion of Person, the Notion of Self', in *Sociology and Psychology*. London: Routledge and Kegan Paul.
Momigliano, A. 1971. *The Development of Greek Biography*. Cambridge, MA: Harvard University Press.
Morrison, A.P. 1999. 'A Cognitive Analysis of the Maintenance of Auditory Hallucinations: Are Voices to Schizophrenia What Bodily Sensations Are to Panic?', *Behavioural and Cognitive Psychotherapy* 26: 289–302.
Murphy, H.B.M. 1982. *Comparative Psychiatry: The International and Intercultural Distribution of Mental Illness*. Berlin: Springer.
Needham, R. 1972. *Belief, Language and Experience*. Oxford: Blackwell.

Newman, J.H.C. 1964 [1864]. *Apologia Pro Vita Sua*. London: Oxford University Press.
Origen. 1869. *The Writings of Origen*. Edinburgh: Clark.
______. 1872. *Origen Contra Celsum*. Edinburgh: Clark.
Padel, R. 1981. 'Madness in Fifth-Century (B.C.) Athenian Tragedy', in P. Heelas and A. Lock (eds), *Indigenous Psychologies*. London: Academic Press.
Pascal, B. 1910. *Thoughts of Pascal*. London: Methuen.
Peel, J.D.Y. 2000. *Religious Encounter and the Making of the Yoruba*. Bloomington: Indiana University Press.
Pitt-Rivers, J. 1992. 'Postscript: The Place of Grace in Anthropology', in J.G. Peristiany and J. Pitt-Rivers (eds), *Honour and Grace in Anthropology*. Cambridge: Cambridge University Press.
Plotinus. 1984. *Enneads*. Cambridge, MA: Loeb Classical Library.
Rosen, G. 1968. *Madness in Society*. London: Routledge and Kegan Paul.
Sass, L. 1992. *Madness and Modernity: Insanity in the Light of Modern Art, Literature and Thought*. New York: Basic Books.
______. 2001. 'Self and World in Schizophrenia: Three Classic Approaches', *Philosophy, Psychiatry and Psychology* 8: 251–70.
______. 2004. 'Negative Symptoms, Common Sense and Cultural Disembedding in the Modern Age', in J.H. Jenkins and R.J. Barrett (eds), *Schizophrenia, Culture and Subjectivity*. Cambridge: Cambridge University Press.
Seligman, C.G. 1929. 'Temperament, Conflict and Psychosis in a Stone-Age Population', *British Journal of Medical Psychology* 9: 187–202.
Simon, B. 1978. *Mind and Madness in Ancient Greece*. Ithaca, NY: Cornell University Press.
Skura, M.A. 2008. *Tudor Autobiography: Listening for Inwardness*. Chicago, IL: University of Chicago Press.
Smith, J.Z. 1990. *Drudgery Divine: On the Comparison of Early Christianities and the Religions of Late Antiquity*. Chicago, IL: Chicago University Press.
Stewart, C. 2000. 'Evagrius Pontiarus on Prayer and Anger', in R. Valantasis (ed.), *Religions of Late Antiquity in Practice*. Princeton, NJ: Princeton University Press.
Stroumsa, G.G. 1990. 'Caro Salutis Cardo: Shaping the Person in Early Christian Thought', *History of Religions* 30: 25–50.
Tausk, V. 1948 [1919]. 'On the Origin of the "Influencing Machine" in Schizophrenia', in R. Fleiss (ed.), *The Psychoanalytic Reader*. New York: International Universities Press.
Thomas À Kempis, St. 1952. *The Imitation of Christ*. Harmondsworth, UK: Penguin.
Torrey, E.F. 1979. *Schizophrenia and Civilisation*. New York: Aronson.
Zilboorg, G. 1941. *A History of Medical Psychology*. New York: Norton.

Chapter 4

Religious Stigmata, Magnetic Fluids and Conversion Hysteria

One Survival of 'Vital Force' Theories in Scientific Medicine?

Introduction

In this chapter, we consider the nature of religious stigmata and the modes of explanation offered by psychiatry. Medical anthropology, unlike cultural psychiatry, has generally not been concerned with questions of mechanism, seeking rather to illustrate social meaning. Within psychiatry, explanations have invoked hysterical conversion, psychological processes, or factitious (self-inflicted) wounds. One cannot of course assume a single mechanism for all psycho-physiological patterns collected under the rubric of the cultural label of stigmata, especially as the Church itself seems ambivalent about the ascription of 'a miracle', preferring rather an extreme psychological identification with Jesus somehow leading to bodily changes.

An interview on the Thursday after Easter in 2003 with the noted Calabrian stigmatic Natuzza Evolo of Paravati presented certain obvious questions as to the authenticity and psycho-physiological reality of stigmata – obvious for the external student, if not for the faithful.[1]

Natuzza, as she is familiarly known, is most famous for miraculously receiving the stigmata of the Crucifixion (Jesus' wounds at his execution and finally from having his side pierced) but she has also experienced bilocation (being in two places at once) and haemographia (miraculous writing in her blood), conversations with Jesus and the Virgin Mary, and with angels and the dead, and has been also persecuted by diabolical powers (Pitaro 2003).

Natuzza was born in 1924 to an illiterate peasant family and as a young girl was sent out to domestic service. At the age of ten, when working as a servant in the house of a rich family, she started to see visions of a priest; her employers, alarmed, admitted her to a local psychiatric hospital.[2] The stigmata first appeared in 1938 after her discharge from hospital. She was then investigated by Agostino Gemelli, the psychiatrist and psychologist employed by the Holy Office to look at cases of stigmata (and later rector of the Catholic University of the Sacred Heart in Milan) (Bartocci and Littlewood 2004). Natuzza later married but, according to her husband, the couple never had a normal life together due to the frequent miraculous events. Nevertheless, they have had five children, one of them qualified in medicine. Natuzza now lives with attendants in a purpose-built building belonging to the Church with a chapel attached which contains a statue of the Virgin as seen in one of her visions. A religious foundation has been established in its name, with a regular glossy colour magazine (e.g. Barone 1996), and an Italian television programme has been made about her haemographia.

Religious stigmata of this type are most typical of Catholic southern Europe, especially Italy; few recipients, who are usually lay people, are subsequently canonized as the phenomenon is not seen as inherently guaranteeing sanctity. St Francis of Assisi in 1224 is the first well known instance; since his time there have been some 400 cases (Harrison 1998), with a female to male ratio of seven to one. There was a period of particular popularity in the thirteenth century associated with the vogue for public self-flagellation (Harrison 1995). The theological explanation is simply that the individual's identification with the suffering Christ is so great that his wounds appear on their physical bodies.

During our interview, Natuzza showed us the stigmata[3] (see Figure 4.1) and allowed us to touch them: on her left lower leg a ring pattern (the crown of thorns) and above it a rather naïve picture of Christ (reminiscent of the work of the French 'outsider artist' Aloise [Cardinal 1972]); on the right leg another circular ring and, above, letters standing for the initial Latin letters of 'Jesus, victim on our behalf'; on the dorsum of the left wrist the outline of St Peter's Dome in Rome, and another ring; on the right wrist another ring; protruberances in the centre of the right and left hand palms signifying the end of the nails; some scratches on her shoulders; and an unidentifiable mark, possibly another ring, in the centre of her cranium. The marks were purple-dark red and were quite prominent, extending some two millimetres above the skin, hard and firm, and appeared to be congealed blood or wax.[4] Natuzza showed them quite readily in spite of being surrounded by onlookers and local priests, and in a brief conversation was friendly, seemed grossly psychiatrically normal, but with a slight Parkinsonian tremor. She explained that the miraculous stigmata appear once a year in Holy Week and gradually

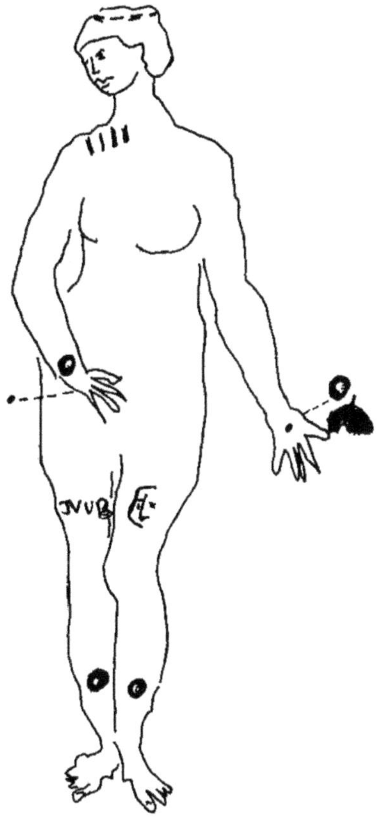

Figure 4.1. Natuzza's stigmata. © the authors.

fade away over the following weeks, and that she can see and converse with souls in Purgatory, and tell if people are ill.[5] She seemed tired and after kissing her, and she us, we departed

Given the size, form and striking three-dimensionality (thus excluding dermatographia, herpes simplex or other likely skin diseases), there appear to be three immediate mechanisms for the phenomenon: (1) a miracle; (2) an unconscious disease process (hysterical conversion); (3) a factitious symptom created by conscious or unconscious induction (known to the medical profession as dermatitis artefacta).

Stigmata and Their Medicalization

As psychiatry developed as a medical speciality in the early nineteenth century, it became common for doctors to claim that science had now liberated the descendants of the earlier victims of clerical superstition and persecution, a view that has still continued in 'Whiggish' histories of psychiatry (such as Zilboorg 1941: see his chapter in that volume on religious obscurantism, entitled 'The Great Decline'). In the nineteenth century, the student of hypnotism and hysteria, Hippolyte Bernheim, claimed that what was now recognized as hysterical conversion had been dealt with in the medieval period as demonic or other possession. The witches were revealed as merely having been hysterical women (Spanos 1975). The male psychiatrist (or more strictly the psychotherapist) became the liberator of the (usually female) hysteric: Zilboorg (1941: 365) typically declares that the neurologist and hypnotist Jean-Martin Charcot, famous for his theatrical demonstrations of hysterical patients, 'was the first to capture for psychiatry the very last part of demonological territory'. Along with demonic possession, out went states of religious ecstasy and stigmata which, while clearly valued as spiritual by the church, were often distinguished with difficulty from more demonic manifestations. (We might note that both Natuzza and the saint Padre Pio in the twentieth century were subject to demons trying to confuse them or at least cast doubt on the miracle of stigmata.) Pinel and Charcot made reference in their writings to the Devils of Loudon (demonic possession) and to religious sanctity as hysteria (Drinka 1984: 42, 88; Ellenberger 1970: 94). A patient of Charcot's identified Louise Latour, a contemporary Belgian religious stigmatic, as her 'sister', and contemporary medical photographs of this patient and another show clear resemblances to 'religious' ecstasy (Drinka 1984).

An example of the borderline between the ascription of sanctity and that of pathology might be the early nineteenth-century nun with stigmata, Katherina Emmerich of Westphalia: 'every night she had dreams that followed one another in regular sequence according to the cycle of the liturgic year' (Ellenberger 1970: 78). The psychiatrist and philosopher Pierre Janet (1925), although not claiming so dramatically as others to be the saviour of the possessed, similarly argued that medical psychotherapy provided a scientific understanding of what were previously treated as religious phenomena. Janet treated a stigmatic (who also levitated and had divine revelations) simultaneously with her priest (Ellenberger 1970: 395), but is uncertain in his conclusions about the nature of stigmata, saying they are possibly similar to dermatographism (Janet 1925: 310). By contrast, William James in his *Varieties of Religious Experience* (1964 [1902]: 291) famously criticized a 'medical materialism [which] finishes up St. Paul by calling his visions on the road to Damascus a discharging lesion of the occipital cortex, he being an epileptic. It snuffs out St. Theresa as an hysteric, St. Francis of Assisi as a hereditary degenerate.'

Hysterical Conversion

The term 'hysterical conversion' was revived and popularized by John Ferriar in 1795 in his book on 'conversion of diseases', and again by Sigmund Freud (1949 [1894]). It seems to have originated in Edward Jorden's 1603 *A Brief Discourse of a Disease Called the Suffocation of the Mother*, which was written as a response to the trial in England of a woman in 1602 accused of bewitching a young girl, causing fits and anaesthesiae (Hunter and Macalpine 1963). Jorden had unsuccessfully tried to treat the victim and subsequently gave evidence in court. The judge suggested that as the normal treatments were unavailing, and the symptoms could not be understood by medicine, the cause must therefore be supernatural. As a witness, Jorden suggested, however, that the victim might be counterfeiting her symptoms: when pressed by the judge, he withdrew this suggestion, and the witch was found guilty (although treated fairly leniently). In his subsequent book, Jorden argued that 'the mother' (womb or *matrix*) was a powerful organ which could cause related symptoms elsewhere (by 'conversion');[6] the suffocation of his title referred to the common experience of *globus hystericus* or functional blockage of the throat. He also allowed for conversion of purely mental functioning into bodily symptoms, as well as conscious simulation as in this case.

This aetiological uncertainty – 'genuine' conversion of physical symptoms or mental states into other physical symptoms, or else frank simulation – continues to bedevil the diagnosis of 'hysteria', a diagnosis often abandoned by psychiatry as unsound (Slater 1965) but then resurrected yet again (Lewis 1975). Our current manifestations might include Multiple Personality Disorder, Gulf War Syndrome and Myalgic Encephalomyelitis (Showalter 1998; Littlewood 1996, 2002). The later history of hysterical conversion, the development of the two French schools which treated it with hypnosis – Bernheim's Nancy School and Charcot's Salpetrière – and the development of Freudian psychoanalysis from the latter have been well surveyed by the historian (e.g. Zilboorg 1941; Ellenberger 1970) and need not be rehearsed in detail here. What particularly concerns us are the arguments in favour of mental representations becoming represented symbolically in the body independently of conscious motivation, how these arguments appeared at a certain historical moment, and how they served as justifications for replacing theological thinking with a more mechanistic medical science.

At the same time, Jorden's suggestion in 1602 of the deliberate induction of symptoms, or their counterfeiting, has continued as an available possibility. An instance of stigmatization in Oxford in 1222 (i.e. before St Francis) was declared self-inflicted and the man imprisoned, and a seventeenth-century Portuguese stigmatic was condemned by the Inquisition for consciously producing his wounds (Harrison 1995). In the same century as Jorden,

Kenelm Digby also argued for sympathetic contagion of religious symptoms in the case of the nuns of Loudon, and later Bernheim's idea of suggestion placed any hysterical conversion in its particular social and emotional context.[7] After Charcot's death, his disciple Babinski soon declared that all hysterical conversion was suggestion, and that therefore the key lay in normal social psychology (feigning, imitation, pretence) rather than in some mysterious mind/body interrelationship (Ellenberger 1970: 100).

The nineteenth-century technique for dismissing or inducing physical hysterical symptoms was hypnosis, a pattern whose modern manifestations may be traced back to Franz Anton Mesmer in the late eighteenth century whose treatment of a young woman with severe physical symptoms by using astronomical predictions of their severity was replaced with what came to be known as magnetism. Following some experimentation, Mesmer persuaded her to drink an iron solution, which he then directed by attaching magnets to her, upon which she felt a 'fluid' moving down her legs (Ellenberger 1970: 58–59). Mesmer then investigated individuals who had previously had a religious exorcism and argued that they had really been cured by animal magnetism. He initially conceived of this as a physical fluid (later and more ambivalently as a psychological rapport between patient and doctor) which he could convey by his hand movements. This fluid (animal magnetism) was found in everybody: indeed, it filled the whole universe – planets, earth and man. Disease, speculated Mesmer, was an unequal distribution of animal magnetism in the body, but the magnetism could be channelled or stored, with crises precipitated or treated by directing it with mirrors (Ellenberger 1970: 62). Immediate followers of Mesmer included the materialist 'fluidists' like the 'animists' who argued for an increasingly psychological idiom. The mechanistic interpretation continued during the nineteenth century at the same time as more purely psychological (largely unconscious) mechanisms were suggested: as late as the 1890s French neurologists were still attempting to transfer hysterical symptoms and even personalities from one patient to another by means of electro-magnetism, but it became increasingly accepted that the 'magnetism' of the earlier mesmerisers was just an analogy for something rather less concrete (Harrington 1987).[8]

Without wishing to put forward a general model, it seems evident that early modern science was concerned with clarifying the borderline between the personalistic and the naturalistic. Nature now has its own autonomy from human volition (except through physical actions) whilst the personalistic includes human (or para-human) cognitions and affects, memory, intention, deceit, feigning and so on (Littlewood 1996). It was agreed that there was no longer any inherent connection between the medicinal properties of a plant and that plant's shape or colour, as in the medieval doctrine of 'signatures'. No longer did each individual star have its angel keeping watch over it to ensure it appeared at its proper time and in its proper course (1 Enoch). By the seventeenth century, scientists were agreed on the 'doctrine of uniformity' – that natural laws were constant everywhere in the universe, that the universe was infinite and that a clear distinction was established between natural philosophy (i.e. science) and moral philosophy (including what is now termed social anthropology) (Singer 1941).

There was still debate as to what was a body and what was an agency which was only partially resolved in the nineteenth century. Was heat a substance, caloric, or was cold, frigorific? Such material substances without weight, the imponderables like phlogiston (the principle of inflammability which leaves a physical body when combusted), magnetic fluid (see above) or the ether (at once an agent and medium of light), were entities which had no other purpose than to explain teleologically a particular process (Toulmin and Goodfield 1965). Like the vitalist theory of human physiology or the perception through the microscope of spermatoza as little homunculi, they elided the naturalistic and the personalistic, and, by our current understanding, veered too much towards the personalistic. The point is less that they were 'wrong' than that they served to maintain some quasi-human characteristics in what came to be understood as a more purely arbitrary natural world.[9] And the persistence of conversion hysteria in contemporary psychoanalysis and psychiatry seems a persistence of this earlier 'holistic' view uniting the naturalistic and personalistic and disdaining the dualistic separation between our major disciplines (Littlewood 1996, 2002).

The historian of dynamic psychotherapy, Henri Ellenberger (1970), situated the whole debate on the materialistic versus psychological causation of conversion hysteria in the context of the development of psychodynamic (depth) psychology, in which Freud and his colleagues gradually moved away from purely naturalistic models back to the personalistic, but now through a personalistic psychology which was not immediately accessible to conscious agency. Freud (1949 [1894]: 61) argued that an unbearable idea was dealt with by the emotion being 'converted' (cf. Jorden) into a bodily symptom, 'the excitation which is directed into a wrong channel' [into somatic innovation]. Exactly how the psychological gets transferred into the physical independently of the voluntary nervous system was, and remains, mysterious.[10] It has usually been assumed fairly vaguely, as it was by the religious psychotherapist Gregory (1939: 346) discussing stigmata, as the mind 'produc[ing] through the power of the imagination extraordinary organic changes in the body.'

The rather more limited but influential theories as to the bodily specificity of psychological states were those which emerged from the psychoanalytically orientated 'psychosomatic medicine' in the 1930s (Alexander 1950). The mechanism postulated was that a particular attitude or personality trait led to adverse physiological changes which became permanent – and thus gave rise to a disease (Grace and Graham 1952). Thus, chronic diarrhoea was associated with a wish to get rid of something (and constipation the converse), vomiting followed the rejection of an undesired fantasy, and, more oddly, duodenal ulcer was associated with a wish for revenge. Though the psychoanalytical arguments were erudite, this approach fell apart not only from the lack of a clear psyche-to-soma mechanism but also for lack of empirical evidence that disease and a particular personality did indeed run together. It survives in the notion of 'Type A' personality (Helman 1987).

Given the emphasis placed by most of the later theorists on the contextual and plastic nature of conversion hysteria, there has been surprisingly little social anthropology concerned with its mechanism. The closest anthropologists come to describing how the mental and social comes to be directly represented on the physical body are perhaps the various writings on psychogenic death ('voodoo death') summarized by Marcel Mauss in 1926. A rather literary and much criticized anthropological account of shamanic healing by Lévi-Strauss in 1949 describes a woman in obstructed labour among a Central American Indian community. Resolution of the problem involves the shaman in the recitation of a myth about a quest to find the abode of the power which is responsible for the formation of the foetus. The prolonged labour implies the power has exceeded its functions and will not release the child out into the human world. The recitation is lengthy and involves the manufacture and dramatic deployment of small figures representing the protagonists whose symbolic meanings are expressed in appropriate forms, colours, textures and materials. Together, patient and healer participate in a common quest in a shared cultural idiom, linking current physiology (obstructed birth) with its cognitive representation. The healer 'rapidly oscillates between mythical and physiological themes, as if [*comme si*] to abolish in the mind of the sick woman the distinction which separates them' (Lévi-Strauss 1968 [1949]: 193). Tantalizingly vague as to the actual mind/body interactions, Lévi-Strauss returns to the Freudian idea of hysteria, or, more generally and less pejoratively, to how bodily symptoms occur in relation to popular understanding of them rather than in relation to underlying pathophysiological processes. Current psychodynamic thinking, however, like general psychiatry, rejects the idea of any standardized relationship between, say, organ and psychological complex: there is no intrinsic association between illness and disease, or at least no causal association from the former to the latter (Halligan, Bass and Marshall 2001).

Conscious (or Unconscious) Induction: A Short Conclusion

Without examining in detail the particular biography of the young Natuzza, her relations with her family, priest and employers, or looking more closely at the cultural context of stigmata in southern Italy, it is not possible to delineate a clearly satisfactory mechanism. Leaving aside the question of a miracle or of conversion hysteria, we are left with the possibility of motivated induction of the stigmata, either in a normal or restricted field of consciousness (on which see Deeley 2003). Summaries of 'secular' deliberate self-harm (including burning and 'self-mutilation') in Euro-America (Marchetto 2004) emphasize that it most commonly starts in post-pubertal single young women, usually on their legs or arms, often against a background of trauma or neglect where the biological mother fails to protect her daughter, but where the mother is overwhelming and idealized, and the person attacks herself as a substitute for attacking the mother if she is unable to otherwise verbalize her suffering; 50 to 60% have been sexually or physically abused (Favazza 1992; Favazza and Conterio 1989).[11] In psychoanalytic terms, deliberate self-harm is regarded as a way of establishing contact with a person with whom a transference relationship has been established (Walsh and Rosen 1988). According to Favazza and Conterio, 47% do it to lessen loneliness, 55% to feel 'less unreal'.

It would be quite unfair and inappropriate to speculate in detail on Natuzza's circumstances or psychological state at the time of the start of the stigmata, but we might note a young peasant girl sent away from home who in unspecified difficult circumstances develops an overwhelming attachment to the figure of the transcendent and idealized mother figure, the Madonna (Parsons 1969; Breuner 1992), and in the process gains some self-determination. It would also be inappropriate to offer a general psychosocial model for phenomena resembling stigmatization (this would have to consider all the varieties of Shi'ite, Sufi and Sinhalese Buddhist self-mutilation, for example), given the worldwide variation in patterns of bodily modification and 'mutilation'. Clearly such patterns have to be consonant with a particular culture, at the same time as the protagonist has to find a way of allowing a publicly acceptable practice to accord with deep personal motivations.

Notes

1. We are indebted to the local municipality and church for their assistance in facilitating this visit, and for their hospitality to our colleague Simon Dein and ourselves. S. Dein and G. Bartocci speak Italian and R.L. is grateful to them for translation. Interpretations are of course our own.

2. We have not been able to obtain her old medical notes, should these indeed still exist. Granone (1989: 289–91) cites Annibale Puca's original psychiatric investigation into the haemographia: the blood came from her facial skin, breast and conjunctiva. Natuzza was closely observed by two nurses and was in a dissociated state during the night, speaking in two quite different voices. Granone speculates on a 'psychokinetic' effect (*effetto psicocinetico*) but the observing psychiatrist at the time noted that when a linen handkerchief was placed under her nightdress, the writing in blood on it when seen the next day corresponded (even to mistakes in the Latin) to writing on the local church wall.
3. One curious incident: we visited Natuzza immediately after being invited to a Calabrian church conference on miracles ('Clima Culturale e Guarigioni Miraculose: Un Confronto tra Psichiatri e Antropologi': Pagnotta 2003) for which we are grateful to Dr Vittorio Infante, where Dr Dein and I both spoke from an anthropological position and apparently thus gained the approval of the local clergy (for Italian anthropology is fairly romantic, folkloric and documentatory in nature) who took us to see her after previously having expressed reservations. We were accompanied by our interpreter from the conference who had previously consulted Natuzza about her infertility ('A miracle! She said you must adopt a child and we did! All was then well'), but who on the car journey became very frightened at the idea of seeing her again, although her subsequent interview with Natuzza turned out to be fairly quiet and friendly.
4. Or very similar to freshly applied henna. The place and shape of the markings seem fairly typical of religious stigmata (with the exception of St Peter's). Simpson (1984) and Harrison (1998), summarizing the sources, say they can appear on hands, feet, side, shoulder or forehead. However, they are typically represented by bleeding or indentation (Bartocci and Littlewood 2004), not hard, raised forms. Photos of Natuzza Evola's stigmata appear on: http:// www.livingmiracles.net/Stigmata.html (accessed 21 July 2005).
5. We had the following exchange:
   Q: 'Could Dr Dein be ill?'
   Natuzza: 'No.'
   Q: 'Is Professor Littlewood ill?'
   N: 'You must pray! I can't answer these questions in public.'
   [R.L. developed intermittent claudication a few weeks later.]
6. This follows to a certain extent classical Greek ideas of the 'wandering womb'.
7. The rapport between the physical body and the local religious climate in Calabria are shown well by the *vattienti* who scourge themselves in the village streets at Easter (Ferlaino 1990). In the neighbouring towns of Nocera Teremise and Soriano Calabria, the mood on Good Friday and Easter Saturday (the day of Christ's crucifixion and of his sojourn in Hell) is mournful and subdued: the local band plays funereal music, a statue of the Pieta (the mourning Virgin cradling the dead Christ in Her arms) is slowly carried round the streets and presented in front of houses on whose balconies women weep, and the *vattienti*, grouped into informal fraternities (Mariotti, Tetui and Tripodi 1992), pass through the village, beating themselves; they bleed down the church steps and their wounds are washed down by an attendant with a pungent mixture of wine and vinegar. By contrast, Easter Sunday (the day of Christ's return from death) is characterized by circus-like brass band music, whilst another statue of the Virgin, joyful with outstretched arms, is vigorously carried along the main street of the town to meet Her resurrected Son. The two statues, together with that of the messenger to Mary, St John the Evangelist, merrily progress back up the street, the enthusiastic bearers almost tossing the figures jauntily into the air.

8. Even in the nineteenth century, the change in explanation was not always in the direction of religion to materialism, e.g. the shift from Quimby's physicalist magnetism to Mary Baker Eddy's Christian Science.
9. On the more psychotic elaborations derived from popular conceptions of the idiom of animal magnetism, see Jay (2003).
10. Freud originally attempted a mechanistic psychology based on 'psychic energy' passing through neurones (The Project for a Scientific Psychology) but it remained incomplete and unpublished in his lifetime (Littlewood 1996).
11. Five out of the six of Harrison's (1998) contemporary religious stigmatics had chronic health problems: three were anorexic and two had had severely disturbed childhoods. He notes (p. 138) that the prevailing medical explanations of wound lesions without an obvious physical cause have passed from 'autoerythrocyte sensitisation' to psychogenic purpura, and now to deliberate self-injury.

References

Alexander, F.G. 1950. *Psychosomatic Medicine, Its Principles and Applications*. New York: Norton.

Barone, P. (ed.). 1996. *Cuore Immacolato Di Maria Rifugio Delle Anime (Anno 7, Numero 25)*. Paravati di Mileto, Italy: Grafiche Abramo.

Bartocci, G. and R. Littlewood. 2004. 'Modern Techniques of the Supernatural: A Syncretism Between Miraculous Healing and the Mass Media', *Social Theory and Health* 2: 18–28.

Breuner, N.F. 1992. 'The Cult of the Virgin Mary in Southern Italy and Spain', *Ethos* 20: 66–95.

Cardinal, R. 1972. *Outsider Art*. London: Studio Vista.

Clarke, B. 1975. *Mental Disorder in Earlier Britain*. Cardiff: University of Wales Press.

Deeley, P.Q. 2003. 'Social, Cognitive and Neural Constraints on Subjectivity and Agency', *Philosophy, Psychiatry and Psychology* 10: 161–67.

Drinka, G.F. 1984. *The Birth of Neurosis*. New York: Simon and Schuster.

Ellenberger, H.F. 1970. *The Discovery of the Unconscious: The History and Evolution of Dynamic Psychiatry*. London: Allen Lane.

Favazza, A. 1992. *Bodies Under Siege: Self-Mutilation and Body Mechanism in Culture and Society*. Baltimore, MD: Johns Hopkins University Press.

Favazza, A. and K. Conterio. 1989. 'Female Habitual Self-Mutilation', *Acta Psychiatrica Scandinavica* 79: 283–84.

Ferlaino, F. 1990. *Vattienti: Osservazione e Riplasmazione Di Una Ritualità Tradizionale*. Vibo Valentia, Italy: Qualecultura.

Freud, S. 1949 [1894]. 'The Defence Neuro-Psychoses', in *Collected Papers*, Vol. 1. London: Hogarth Press, pp. 59–75.

Grace, W.G. and D.T. Graham. 1952. 'Relationship of Specific Attitudes and Emotions to Certain Bodily Diseases', *Psychosomatic Medicine* 14: 243–55.

Granone, F. 1989, *Trattato Di Ipnosi*. Turin: Utet.

Gregory, M. 1939. *Psychotherapy, Scientific, and Religious*. London: Macmillan.

Halligan, P.W., C. Bass and S.C. Marshall (eds). 2001. *Contemporary Approaches to the Study of Hysteria*. Oxford: Oxford University Press.

Harrington, A. 1987. *Medicine, Mind and the Double Brain: A Study in Nineteenth Century Thought*. Princeton, NJ: Princeton University Press.

Harrison, E.P.G. 1995. 'Medieval Phenomena in a Modern Age: A Study of Six Contemporary Cases of Stigmata and Reactions to Them', PhD thesis, University of Kent.
Helman, C. 1987. 'Heart Disease and the Cultural Construction of Time: The Type A Behaviour Pattern as a Western Culture-Bound Syndrome', *Social Science and Medicine* 25: 969–79.
Hunter, R. and I. Macalpine. 1963. *Three Hundred Years of Psychiatry 1535–1860*. London: Oxford University Press.
James, W. 1964 [1902]. *The Varieties of Religious Experience*. New York: Mentor.
Janet, P. 1925. *Psychological Healing: A Historical and Clinical Study*. London: Allen and Unwin.
Jay, M. 2003. *The Air Loom Gang: The Strange and True Story of James Tilly Mathews and His Visionary Madness*. London: Bantam.
Lévi-Strauss, C. 1968 [1949]. 'The Effectiveness of Symbols', in *Structural Anthropology*. Harmondsworth: Penguin, pp. 186–205.
Lewis, A. 1975. 'The Survival of Hysteria', *Psychological Medicine* 5: 9–20.
Littlewood, R. 1993. *Pathology and Identity*. Cambridge: Cambridge University Press.
______. 1996. *Reason and Necessity in the Specification of the Multiple Self* (Occasional Paper No. 43). London: Royal Anthropological Institute.
______. 2002. *Pathologies of the West*. London: Continuum Books.
Marchetto, M.J.A. 2004. 'Deliberate Self-Harm Subsequent to the Experience of Cumulative Trauma', PhD thesis, University College London.
Mariotti, M., V. Tetui and A. Tripodi (eds). 1992. *La Confraternite in Calabria e Nel Mezzogiorno*. Vibo Valentia, Italy: Mapograf.
Mauss, M. 1979 [1926]. 'The Physical Effect on the Individual of the Idea of Death Suggested by the Collectivity', in *Sociology and Psychology*. London: Routledge and Kegan Paul.
Pagnotta, F. 2003. 'Due Visioni Del Soprannaturale', *Il Quotidiano*, 25 April, 42.
Parsons, A. 1969. *Belief, Magic and Anomie*. New York: Free Press.
Pitaro, V. 2003. 'La Settimana Santa e la Sofferenze di Natuzza Evolo', *Gazzetta del Sud*, 24 April, 28.
Showalter, E. 1998. *Hysterias: Hysterical Epidemics and Modern Culture*. London: Picador.
Simpson, C.J. 1984. 'The Stigmata: Pathology or Miracle?', *British Medical Journal* 289: 1746–49.
Singer, C. 1941. *A Short History of Science to the Nineteenth Century*. Oxford: Clarendon Press.
Slater, E. 1965. 'Diagnosis of Hysteria', *British Medical Journal* i: 1395.
Spanos, N.P. 1975. 'Witches in the History of Psychiatry: A Critical Analysis and an Alternative Conceptualisation', *Psychological Bulletin* 85: 417–39.
Toulmin, S. and J. Goodfield. 1965. *The Architecture of Matter*. Harmondsworth, UK: Penguin.
Veith, I. 1965. *Hysteria: The History of a Disease*. Chicago: University of Chicago Press.
Walsh, B. and P. Rosen. 1988. *Self-Mutilation: Theory, Research and Treatment*. New York: Guilford.
Zilboorg, G. 1941. *A History of Medical Psychology*. New York: Norton.

Chapter 5

Jinn, Psychiatry and Contested Notions of Misfortune

Introduction

Belief in the world of the unseen (al-Ghayb) is an important part of Islamic teaching, as affirmed in various texts of the Qur'an and Sunna. All Muslims are obligated to believe in the existence of jinn (spirits). What, however, remains contentious is the degree to which they influence the human world. Over the past two years we have been conducting fieldwork among the Bangladeshi population of east London. Our particular focus has been on eliciting explanations of misfortune, more specifically sickness and the role of jinn in this process. A second focus has been to examine healing practices and the use of 'folk healers' among members of this community.

Our younger informants (more often than not born in the UK) regularly pointed out how invocation of jinn explanations was common among the elderly and relatively less educated (by Western standards) members of the community. The younger second- and third-generation Bangladeshis spoke of their parents' beliefs and those of the older generation as 'superstitious,' 'traditional' and often as 'non-Islamic.' For example, one shopkeeper, a woman born in the UK, but whose Bangladeshi parents had migrated from Sylhet thirty years earlier stated:

> It's often the older people, especially those who came from villages in Sylhet who hold these views. I think they are very superstitious. It's probably because they have had little education. They think these views are Islamic, but they are

not. They spend a lot of money visiting mullahs when they have problems, often as a last resort.

Two discourses were prevalent in the interviews. First, the younger informants typically constructed themselves as 'modern' compared with the traditional 'other,' in this case elderly members, and therefore as no longer holding to such beliefs. Much of their discourse articulated around the dichotomy 'traditional–modern.' A second discourse related to ideas of what constituted 'correct' Islam and how those beliefs of the older generation were not based upon 'proper' Islamic teachings. Despite these pejorative comments about older members of the community, almost all the informants, both young and old, were able to cite instances relating to a jinn's malevolent influence. These discourses are outlined later and are specifically contextualized in relation to beliefs about illness.

Tradition and Modernity

Tradition and modernity are terms which are commonly employed in ethnographic writing but their use is often problematic. Modernity and modernization are vague, 'taken for granted' terms that relate to a complex system of discourses, philosophies, economic trends and historical contingencies (Halliburton 2005). The terms are often deployed in a judgemental way where traditional stands for the irrational non-scientific worldview, and modern for everything which opposes that. Rippin (2005) argues that the terms are at best generalizations that do not reflect the realities of the world as is lived; they are intellectual abstractions, which can, if used reflectively, aid understanding.

Few anthropologists today would hold to the tenets of evolutionary anthropology, whereby different societies go through similar stages of development and traditional, often non-empirical, explanations are necessarily replaced by modern scientific thinking. It cannot simply be assumed that there is an evolutionary process whereby the 'modern' replaces the 'traditional.' They often abide side by side and the modern world never frees itself completely from the authority of the past: '"Traditional" does not mean rejection of the modern but the continuation in certain aspects of life in the mode authorised by the past, notably in areas of life where other people have changed to a modern view' (Rippin 2005: 177).

Although the idea of modernity appears ubiquitous and enduring, notions of modernity (and tradition) are always mediated and understood in local contexts, are historically contingent and spread through powerful political and ideological mechanisms (Pigg 1996). There is no one universal reading of modernity and it is mistaken to assume that modern equals Westernized. In some cultural contexts, the term traditional may be conflated with backwardness; Wilce (2004: 361) for example, describes communities in Bangladesh where local views on 'tradition' are often pejorative: 'Mention of anything that could be spun as a "traditional beliefs" or "traditional medicine," which find strong support in some public discourses in other Asian countries, provokes shame – at least in my presence – over "old fashioned" beliefs and practices as if the whole nation felt itself the naked object of a rational global gaze.'

Hence, we cannot take these terms as having universal meaning. They can only be understood within a cultural and historical context. Here we specifically focus upon these conceptualizations among Bangladeshis in east London.

Islam and Modernity

A second focus of this chapter is to examine how 'modernity' has impacted on the Muslim world and more specifically how this process is manifest among Bangladeshi Muslims in the UK. Rippin (2005) suggests a tripartite division of religious ways of interacting with the modern world: traditionalist, Islamist (sometimes called revivalist) and modernist. Each of these categories displays a different attitude towards the authority of the past. The traditionalist group holds that change should not and does not affect the traditions of the past. By contrast, the revivalist group is characterized by a desire to accept change in a 'controlled' fashion and uses the authoritative sources of the past to legitimize changes in the present day. It emphasizes the absolute character of the Qur'an and Sunna and results in literalism or fundamentalism. The modernist group embraces change, makes religion itself subject to change and focuses upon the differentiation of basic moral precepts from specific legal prescriptions. It is the revivalist position that is most influential for British Bangladeshi Islam and is discussed later.

By no means a new phenomenon in South Asia, Islamic revivalism or purism has erupted periodically in the face of external threats such as colonialism (Roy 1982) and as a response to political inequality (Gellner 1981). Gardner (2001 [1995]) argues that Islamic purism is inextricably linked to global processes, not least of which is migration. One effect of this globalizing process is an erosion of the social base of folk Islam, a rejection of old localized ways and a return to an emphasis on textual tradition (Abaza 1991; Gellner 1992; Robinson 1983) where the concept of a 'universal' Islam is focused on the holy texts as the only common language and Mecca as the only accepted core (Gardner 2001 [1995]). As discussed later, this process of Islamic purism is antagonistic both to folk beliefs about illness and traditional systems of healing which deploy them.

The East London Bangladeshi Community

The state of Bangladesh was established in 1972 after East Bengal seceded from Pakistan. In the 1960s and 1970s many Bangladeshis migrated to Britain, as economic migrants, particularly from rural Sylhet, with men generally emigrating several years before their wives. This community is characterized by regular travel to and from Bangladesh and it is common for young people to travel to Bangladesh for an arranged marriage.[1] These close links with Bangladesh foster continuity of beliefs and practices between Sylhet and the London communities. As Gardner (2002: 15) points out, 'many so called settlers actually participate in the economic, political and social life of both "sending" and "receiving" societies.' They are 'transnational' communities (Phillipson, Ahmed and Latimer 2003) and we would contend that traditional ideas, including those relating to illness, are maintained and reinforced through this process.

The current London Bengali population is comprised of four cohorts: the original male immigrants, their dependents, generally arriving in the 1970s and 1980s, those born in the UK, and small numbers of recently arrived adults. In the 2001 census, the Bangladeshi population represented 0.5% of the population of the UK (Office for National Statistics [ONS] 2005) and Bangladeshis and Pakistanis together constitute 36.5% of the population of Tower Hamlets in east London (ONS 2004a).

These communities have low socio-economic status with the lowest employment rates of all ethnic groups in the UK (ONS 2002). In Tower Hamlets only 30.5% of the Bangladeshi population are in employment and this situation is worsened by high levels of industrial decline (Cabinet Office 2003). There are high rates of overcrowding (23% living in overcrowded conditions; Commission for Racial Equality 2003), dependence on local authority housing and high levels of limiting long-term illness (24% of the Bangladeshi population in England and Wales in 2001; ONS 2004b). Kempson (1999) describes how one in five Bangladeshi homes are overcrowded (with more than four people sleeping in one room) compared with 1 in 200 in the general population, and many lack basic amenities. High rates of population growth, large families and increasing immigration exacerbate these problems (Eade, Peach and Vamplew 1996). Thus, deprivation and hardship are common, although there may be significant variation by region, social class, age and gender, and younger cohorts may have a more positive outlook. Bangladeshis experiencing the highest levels of social and economic deprivation are those born outside the UK, who are unable to speak fluent English. Racism, especially following 9/11, and Islamophobia (in which Islam is presented as backward and inferior) are prominent features of the lives of many people in this community.

It is not surprising that those who are subject to deprivation and racism and whose life chances are determined to a large extent by powerful, remote and capricious forces attribute their misfortunes to the operation of spiritual forces. The uncertainties surrounding the lives of members of this community and the lack of control which they encounter over earthly matters predisposes them to make such attributions and facilitate the demand for 'miracles.' It is the poor and dispossessed who often seek out miraculous transformations offered by Sufi cults in many parts of the Middle East (Gilsenan 1982) and in Bangladesh itself (Gardner 2001 [1995]) and, as discussed later, this is also the case in east London.

Islamic Revivalism in the East London Community

Bangladeshi Islam is highly influenced by Sufism and emphasizes the cult of pirs – Muslim holy men, saints who are held to have the ability to perform 'miracles' – and to whom appeal is often made at times of sickness. These pirs are familiar figures on the village scene in Bangladesh, and in some areas the shrines of saints almost outnumber the mosques. They played a key role in the early days of Islam, allowing the 'Orthodox' Sunni faith to merge with indigenous culture, which itself is highly influenced by Hindu traditions such as puja, the veneration of Hindu gods such as Lakshmi, and the use of drums and dancing, which are all elements in local Hindu rites (Ahmad 1988; Eade 1994; Murshid 1995). The popular appeal of 'miraculous healers' has not disappeared following migration. As we describe later, among the east London Bangladeshi population, resort to them is commonplace.

In Sylhet there has been a long-standing tension between the ulama (Muslim scholars) and the Sufis in relation to the 'correct' path to reaching God. Gardner (2002) has outlined how 'religious myths' – stories told by local people about pirs and their miracles – are prominent narrative genres in Sylhet. These narratives are often highly contested by those of higher status in the community and reflect an ongoing discourse about what are and what are not 'correct' Islamic beliefs. Similar processes of contestation are occurring in the UK.

East London Bangladeshis are mostly Sunni Muslims of varying degrees of orthodoxy, and many individuals, particularly young Muslims, find themselves in a conflict between secularized and strictly religious associations within Bangladeshi communities. Eade and Garbin (2002: 12) pointed out that the east London Bangladeshi community is subject to a process of Islamic revivalism, reflective of a similar movement in Bangladesh: 'As Bangladesh becomes more formally Islamicized, so Bangladeshis in London and elsewhere in the West come under pressure to conform to everyday practices, which reflect this Islamicizing development.' The religious leadership of the prominent East London Mosque is highly influential in this process. It offers literature and activities including study groups, conferences and social support to the local Bangladeshi (and Somali Muslim) population, aimed at bringing young Bangladeshis back to Islam, as an alternative to the increasingly prevalent 'gang culture' (Alexander 2000).

The leadership of the mosque emphasizes the contrast between 'authentic' Islamic beliefs and values and the inauthentic 'syncretic' cultural practices of the Indian subcontinent and actively portrays an identity linking Bangladeshis in Britain with the umma, a transnational, moral Muslim community (Werbner 2002). Glynn (2002: 970) describes how religious community leaders (from this mosque) share a 'belief in the importance of turning back to the fundamentals of religion below the cultural accretion.' For them, the Bengali traditions and culture serve 'only to obscure the real importance of Islam and divide its followers along ethnic lines' (Glynn 2002: 970). To this extent, this mosque differs from others in east London, which focus upon syncretic Bengali Islam. The East London Mosque employs three Bangladeshi imams who are held by the community to be highly educated in Islamic affairs.

The Jinn

Islam describes various classes of beings that populate the universe: jinn (spirits), *shaytaan* (satanic beings), *marrid* (demons), *bhut* (evil spirits) and *farista* (angels). The word 'jinn' derives from the Arabic root Jann which conveys the idea of protecting, shielding, concealing or veiling. They are described both in the Qur'an and Hadith (sayings of the Prophet Mohammed) as a race of intelligent beings that are normally imperceptible to the senses. Like human beings they are rational and possess a sense of agency, which is reflected in their ability to choose between right and wrong and are thus are accountable for their actions. Jinn are held to marry, produce children, eat, drink and die. However, unlike humans, they have extraordinary powers to take on different shapes, such as the ability to take on the form of birds, animals and even humans, they can move rapidly from one place to another and have the ability to move heavy objects instantly from place to place. They are said to occupy dark places, graveyards and other polluted places. Those most vulnerable to influence by jinn are those in 'transitional states' where boundaries are unclear, for example, pregnancy, menstruation or post-partum.

Most Islamic scholars accept that jinn can possess people. Some scholars disagree and assert that jinn can only influence mankind and cannot literally take up physical space within a human's body. Both, however, would agree that there are clear criteria which need to be applied before concluding that a jinn has had a role in an individual's situation, whether through possession or influence. Various passages in the Qur'an and Hadith affirm the belief that jinn can cause erratic behaviour in one's words, deeds and movements: 'Those who eat Ribaa will not stand (on the Day of Resurrection) except like the standing of a person beaten by shaytaan (Satan) leading him to insanity' (Al-Baqarah, Qur'an, 2: 275).[2]

Attribution of misfortune to malevolent forces including jinn is widely described in the anthropological literature on Islam (Boddy 1989; Kapferer 1991; Lambek 1993; Lewis 1971; Messing 1958), including disturbances of the mind, which we may liken to the Western idiom of 'mental illness,' and which are often treated by exorcism of jinn spirits (Al-Ashqar 2003; Littlewood 2004; Younis 2000). Furthermore, it can be argued that for many Islamic communities, this belief in the malevolent effects of possession is tied, particularly among South Asian migrant groups in the UK, to persistence in demand for traditional healers to resolve treatment issues associated with spirit possession and the evil eye (Aslam 1970; Dein and Sembhi 2001; Healey and Aslam 1989; Weiss et al. 1988). This close affinity between spirit possession and mental illness is not unique to Islam and similar beliefs are held in Hinduism (Halliburton 2005), Buddhism (Gaw, Ding, Levine and Gaw 1998) and Judaism (Greenberg and Witztum 2001).

To further understand the role of jinn in illness,[3] the authors conducted an ethnographic study involving interviews with 40 members of the east London Bangladeshi community. The study aimed to elicit narratives of recent misfortunes with an emphasis on sickness and informants were asked to elaborate on the role of jinn in these events.[4]

Jinn and Misfortune

All informants held jinn to exist, but there were varying views concerning the extent to which they could influence human beings and cause illness. Similarly, there was some disagreement about the sorts of illnesses caused by jinn. The possibility of jinn causing illness appeared to be held more strongly by the older informants who had lived in the UK for up to 40 years. There was great variability in the ways that jinn were implicated when 'things had gone wrong.' However, the ethnographic findings pointed to the fact that belief was a matter of degree with some informants frequently appealing to supernatural explanations while others rarely invoked them. Jinn explanations were posited by both young and old informants.

Ikram is a 40-year-old shop worker from Tower Hamlets. He was born in Sylhet and migrated to the UK 18 years previously. He pointed out that some people were 'extreme' in their beliefs about jinn or black magic, but he thought that it was quite reasonable to invoke these explanations some of the time. He went on to discuss the fact that members of the community, both here and in Bangladesh, typically differentiate dharma (religion) from shangskrite (culture).

Dharma derived from the Qur'an and was immutable, whereas culture could change over time. He emphasized that people often confused the two and believed, wrongly, that many behaviours were Qur'anic in origin when this was not the case. The problem as he saw it was that too many members of the community held jinn to cause problems, whereas this is rarely the case. Jinn do exist but it is not written in the Qur'an that they cause every illness that people complain of. He referred to those who held these beliefs as 'small minded' and 'backwards.' It was their lack of education that caused them still to hold such beliefs.

His narrative emphasized the role of education in eliminating traditional beliefs about illness. Informants often conflated western education with rationality. For them it was irrational to believe that something they could not see could harm them; a paradoxical view since they still held viruses and bacteria to be causes of illness.

The Role of Jinn in Illness

East London Bangladeshis typically divide 'illness' into three domains: illness caused by physical factors (shordi bemar), psychological illness (sintha bemar, fagol bemar) and spiritual illnesses (jinn bemar and Allah bemar, uffri bemar, batash – evil wind). Common problems where jinn were implicated included sudden changes in behaviour, a condition that resembles the western notion of 'depression' and physical symptoms where no obvious physical cause was found. Problems believed to be caused by jinn possession ranged from low mood, withdrawal, speaking 'rubbish,' a failure to observe Islamic practices, and deviant behaviour including stealing and unfaithfulness in marriage. It was the suddenness in the change of behaviour, rather than the behaviour itself, which suggested jinn possession. However, it was commonly posited that it was possible to protect oneself against jinn possession by being good and obeying Allah's words. Jinn were also held to cause physical symptoms such as pain and tiredness and were implicated where biomedical medical treatments had failed. However, not all informants believed that illness was caused by jinn possession. In cases of stroke, it might be enough to fall in the path of a jinn without being possessed. Similarly, a jinn may influence a person to varying degrees without fully possessing them. Narratives of illness are often interspersed with grander narratives in which jinn influence many aspects of a person's life. Jinn were also commonly implicated when something mysterious occurred in a house for which there was no obvious explanation.[5]

Rashida, a 56-year-old woman originally from Sylhet and living in the UK for 15 years, described the sudden onset of pain in her chest. A housewife with three children, she had received little formal education and could neither speak nor read English. She lived in a 'cold damp' two-bedroom flat with her son and his family in Tower Hamlets. Her narrative was frequently punctuated by expressions of longing for her previous life in Sylhet and her desire to return there one day. She repeatedly spoke of the fact that accessing services such as housing and health was extremely difficult, not solely on account of language problems, but due to a general lack of interest from what she referred to as 'officials,' those whom she perceived to be in a position to change things. She believed strongly that British people did not want her to be in the UK.

Despite consulting several general practitioners (GPs) and one hospital consultant, the pain did not improve. She complained that the doctors had not examined her thoroughly, showed little interest in her problem and she blamed allopathic medication for making her feel worse. Desperate, she sought the help of a local healer, a man in his fifties from Senegal, who had advertised in a Bangladeshi newspaper. Although her husband agreed with this course of action, her two sons doubted the credibility of the healer. At the first consultation the healer diagnosed jinn possession, recited a Sura from the Qur'an and also blew over her. He charged £200 for this consultation. She agreed with his diagnosis and said she had wondered if a jinn was the cause of her problem. She recovered shortly afterwards. This informant's narrative about sickness revolved around a discussion of racism and deprivation, implicitly criticized service provision and was typical of those who held a similarly marginalized status (see Gardner 2002 for similar narrative genres). The overwhelming experience expressed by many of our informants was one of total powerlessness – the inability to influence external events by their own actions.

Nirban a 40-year-old man from Sylhet had lived in the UK for 25 years and had visited relatives in Sylhet for long periods from time to time. He worked as a translator and had a master's degree from a British university. He recounted the following story. Last year, his wife's sister telephoned quite distressed and asked for help. Her family had experienced a number of difficulties, including sleep problems and a baby who would not stop crying. The doorbell would ring continuously, but when they answered there was no one there. The family thought they could see someone who disappeared in a flicker. Nirban told his wife's sister that he knew a man called Mr Choudhury, a 60-year-old Bangladeshi who specialized in working with people who have problems with jinn. He and Mr Choudhury regularly visited their local gym along with a third friend, Mohammed.

Following a phone call from his wife's sister while they were in the gym, Nirban spoke to Mr Choudhury about her problem, who agreed to help and suggested that a malevolent jinn might be causing the problem. As they were leaving the gym, Mohammed received a call from his wife to say that their 15-year-old son had collapsed in the bath. Mohammed became panic stricken and asked Mr Choudhury for help. Believing that Mohammed's son was possessed by the same jinn as had afflicted Nirban's sister-in-law, Mr Choudhury recited a passage from the Qur'an over the phone and the boy instantly revived and coughed. The three discussed the event, Mr Choudhury believing the boy's collapse to be a warning sign for him not to get involved with the treatment of Nirban's sister-in-law. However, he still felt strongly that he could help and agreed to meet her. Shortly afterwards, Nirban's sister-in-law visited Mr Choudhury in London and he explained that her problem was caused by a jinn. He recited a Sura from the Qur'an and prayed over some water. Within a short period her problems at home (sleep disturbance, the baby's crying and the ringing of the doorbell) improved considerably, but did not go away. Mr Choudhury felt that there was a problem with the house and suggested that it had been built over a graveyard. He asked Nirban's sister-in-law to enquire whether anyone had lived in the house for very long before them and she discovered that in the past people had lived in the house for less than one year and then left. This narrative underscores belief in the multifarious nature of jinn, their involvement simultaneously with several aspects of life and the dangers believed to be associated with getting involved with jinn.

While several informants warned that those who appealed to jinn for malevolent purposes (i.e. to hurt another person) should understand the possible negative consequences, more relevant to the forces of hybridization were those east London narratives about magical forces, which got woven into local descriptions of gang warfare and urban London crime. Narratives of social deprivation and jinn possession were often interwoven in a disconnected way.

Rohan a 21-year-old Bangladeshi man, born in England, lived in Tower Hamlets and had visited Sylhet on three occasions. He reported that there were problems among young Bangladeshis on different estates, which he described as 'tribal warfare' and that more young Bangladeshis are taking to drugs and crime. He saw this as resulting from the marginalized identity of young Bangladeshis who gain power through committing crimes. For him, this was a pressing issue for the community, which was more significant than discussing jinn.

Specifically in relation to jinn, he explained that people readily invoke the 'jinn' explanation for any sort of misfortune. For example, if someone suddenly changes their mood or behaviour, they might feel they are possessed by jinn. He pointed out that generally no one asks about stresses in their lives of those believed to be possessed by jinn and people do not behave in a logical way when it comes to jinn. He told me that a lady he knew had become depressed and withdrawn, but instead of asking her about the relationship with her husband, the family went to the imam for advice about getting rid of a jinn. He said that the vast majority of imams do not have the correct knowledge of Islam and therefore give people the wrong advice. He added that it is not acceptable to charge money in Islam for religious services, but if an imam comes to talk at a meeting for a couple of hours he will receive up to £200.

Bangla Traditional Healing

Episodes of sickness, which are considered more than minor, often occasion a visit to the mosque to receive prayers from an imam. Sickness of any severity is characteristically seen as being fated, Qudr, the decree of Allah, and to this extent is accepted. This, however, does not mean that the sufferer should be inactive in the face of illness, far from it. Islam teaches that the sick person should seek help for their illness first with natural medicines, then divine medicines and then a combination of the two. It is also held that there is no sickness for which Allah does not provide a cure (apart from old age).

A number of informants complained about the poor service they received from both British and Bangladeshi GPs. These complaints included long waits for appointments, being 'rushed out' by doctors and not giving them enough time. Several informants suggested that GPs did not respect the Bangladeshi population and did not understand their culture. For example, one Bangladeshi man, who was a Hindu, stated:

> "Doctors do not understand our culture. They do not listen to us and certainly do not respect us. When we come with our children, doctors do not touch them directly. They often put out their hands and touch them with a pen. They think we are dirty. The health system does not work for Bangladeshis and Bangladeshi doctors are the worst. They do not pick up illnesses and consequently people are very ill before going to see hospital specialists. It's not just a language problem. That is why we turn to other types of help when we are ill".

Sometimes people who are sick ingest olive or black seed oil or apply it to the skin and there may be recourse to folk remedies such as Zamzam water,[6] which is held to have medicinal properties. But for most health problems in east London, sick people initially seek the help of their GP.

Consistent with the literature on health-seeking behaviour in this community, it is common to consult several types of healer simultaneously (Aslam, 1970; Dein and Sembhi, 2001; Healey & Aslam, 1988). The healers most often consulted are hakims, kabiraj and mullahs (priests). Hakims were defined variously by informants as medicine men or herbalists and are consulted more often by women, often on account of marital disharmony or because a woman is afraid that her husband may be seeing another woman. None of the informants knew of a hakim in east London. Hakims visit from India or Pakistan and can cost up to £500 a consultation. Alternatively, people may travel long distances to find a reputable hakim. The term kabiraj refers to healers who use herbal medicines.

Resort to folk healers is commonplace especially when western medicine is not perceived to be effective. Healers often advertise in local Bangladeshi newspapers and claim to be devout Muslims with a thorough knowledge of the Qur'an. They often claim a long lineage with their fathers and grandfathers being healers and may trace their ancestry back to well-known pirs or mullahs. They deploy various techniques in their healing practices and often blur the boundaries between magic, herbal and Islamic healing: blowing over the patient (foo), the recitation of Qur'anic verses (mantra) and the prescription of amulets (tabiz). Healers were described as specializing in particular treatments or illnesses, for example, some claimed the ability to find lost objects or people, for instance a wife who has left the household following domestic violence. Yet others were consulted for purely malevolent purposes, such as inflicting harm on someone they did not like, or with a view to changing someone's mind, for example, to facilitate amorous feelings. Some provide a more comprehensive service and, apart from offering healing, claim that they can bring wealth to those who consult them.

An article in the Asian Times (24 September 2005) reported the case of a young Bangladeshi woman called Sureha who lived in Manchester and had become virtually mute, tearful and cut herself. Strongly believing that a jinn had possessed her, she was taken by her parents to see several healers, which cost them £3000. Her symptoms had started when her parents forced her to break up with her (Bangladeshi) boyfriend of whom they strongly disapproved and had then arranged marriage to a cousin in Bangladesh. For two months prior to her marriage, she became quiet, stopped eating and going out.

Her mood deteriorated further, and rumours started to circulate that she had become a phagal – a possessed person. Her parents felt she had been 'taken over' by a jinn and took her to a mullah in Stepney Green, who claimed to be an expert in possession. Her parents explained to him that their daughter had become withdrawn, would not eat, cried all the time and did not want to be with her husband. The mullah readily agreed that she was possessed by jinn and asked them to bring her back in one week so that he could read special prayers over her and exorcize the jinn.

Over the next year her parents spent over £3000 visiting faith healers all promising to 'bring back the old Sureha' and all of them failing. Eventually, Sureha's ex-boyfriend and his sister heard that she was ill, and went to visit her. The following day they returned with an older member of the community who insisted that Sureha should be taken to a doctor as soon as possible. According to Sureha, 'my ex and his sister are very educated and don't believe in jinn possession. I think they could see straight away that I was ill and not "possessed." Nobody realized I was suffering from depression as these faith healers were so convincing.' This case history is typical of many accounts provided by east London Bangladeshi families about their visits to local traditional healers. All were characterized by a number of themes: healers who claimed descent from Islamic saints, exorbitant fees, forceful treatment, exorcism of jinn spirits and guarantees that their treatment would be successful. Anecdotally, from discussion with several informants in east London, it appears that resorting to these healers is commonplace, a fact confirmed by the large number of newspaper advertisements and reports devoted to this phenomenon in South Asian newspapers.

The Views of Local Imams Concerning the Jinn and Their Role in Illness

During a meeting held in east London in 2003 by a local Bangladeshi health education group in collaboration with the East London Mosque, a local imam decried the fact that members of the local Bangladeshi community frequently sought help from traditional healers, often at great cost to themselves, in the mistaken belief that their problem was caused by a jinn or black magic. The imam described these healers as non-Islamic on account of the fact that their healing occurred through magic or jinn not through the direct influence of Allah. According to him only forms of healing that deployed the Qur'an or other Islamic texts (either orally or in written form) and involved Muslim prayer and evoked Allah as being in control of all events, were true Islamic healing.[7] This imam's major bone of contention was that members of this community readily resorted to these supernatural explanations instead of seeking the help of doctors. This was especially the case with 'mental illness,' which east London Bangladeshis readily attributed to jinn possession. Although the meeting was held to educate the community about biomedical causes of illness and treatment of mental illness, the imam's underlying motivation went far deeper than this and involved a discussion of the authenticity of Muslim beliefs concerning jinn possession and witchcraft. The imam repeatedly asserted that the practices of lay healers were often not Islamic and that most of them, 'could not call themselves Muslims.' He readily resorted to textual justification for his arguments and provided the text of Qur'anic passages, which he claimed expressed 'orthodox' views on jinn and their involvement in human affairs. For him, any statement that was not taken from the Qur'an, Sunna or Hadith was not acceptable in Islam. Another local imam reported that: There are many spiritual healers in this area. They advertise in the newspapers. They are from Africa, India or Pakistan. They call themselves spiritual healers. People often go to them when doctors can't help. They explain people's problems in terms of black magic or jinn. My impression is that people never feel better after going to the spiritual healers. The population here are very under-educated both in general education and also in terms of religion. They believe that the spiritual healers are following Islamic beliefs, which they are not. They charge a lot of money. Many have little knowledge of Islam although some claim to have descended from Muslim saints and to be holy in this respect.

These imams are sometimes consulted by members of the community who consider their problems to be related to jinn. Some of these people are advised to consult a doctor if the imam considers the problem to be 'medical' or 'psychiatric.' Those whom the imams consider possibly to be possessed by a jinn (usually on the basis of rapid changes in character or failure to respond to biomedical treatment) are referred to a local expert who is able to deal with such problems. One well-known person is Abdul, a 50-year-old man who works part-time in an office. Born in Syhlet, he moved to the UK at the age of 5 but has spent short periods back in Syhlet over the past 20 years. He is married with three children. He explained how he himself had been a victim of jinn possession, which was cured by exorcism. Following this possession experience, Abdul himself 'trained' to become an 'exorcist.' His friend taught him the relevant Qur'anic verses and the 'signs' of jinn possession and imams at several London mosques refer patients to him. He sees on average one 'patient' a week. He explained that each exorcism can take up to two hours and said he does not charge for his services although many people offer him money. He will often visit patients in their homes. Abdul said that the consultation starts with a number of questions relating to symptoms, mood, sleep and life stresses. Patients are asked if they have been to a doctor to establish what treatment they have had and whether or not it was effective. These questions are followed by recitation of different verses of the Qur'an.

He elaborated: "If a jinn is present, the patient will react in a number of ways. First, he or she will complain of a rushing feeling in the body and might feel hot. This rushing feeling is caused by a jinn moving up and down the body. The person starts to shake. This shaking might be in one part of the body where the jinn is hiding. If these symptoms occur, I know a jinn is definitely present. I will then read several more chapters from the Qur'an such as the Sura Fatiha. The person will then become unconscious, and the jinn will start to speak to me. It often shouts, screams or swears. They sometimes foam at the mouth and the mouth becomes a strange shape. I tell the jinn to leave. By this time the jinn is in a lot of pain and has to leave. The jinn can be male or female. Occasionally a jinn will tell me about someone performing magic. By reading the Qur'an I can break the spell. Sometimes if the magician has used a talisman the jinn will tell me where it is and I will burn it. Generally, jinn will leave after all this. If they do not I will read more verses from the Qur'an. I will also read the verses over water and give the patient this water to drink or wash with. If the jinn is very stubborn I say they must leave or they will die. Rarely, I have to hit the jinn. The person does not remember this when they wake up. Following this exorcism people are better and their symptoms disappear".

"People come to me with many types of problem: anger, poor sleep and nightmares. Some have physical symptoms such as weakness in one limb. If this is the case I give them olive oil to rub on the site. The weakness is caused by a jinn in that part of the body. The response to reading the Qur'an determines whether or not they are possessed. If there is a jinn present the patient will react in this way. Sometimes the patient feels calmer after reading the Qur'an but does not show any other symptoms I have described. This suggests that the patient is depressed."

Hence, the jinn specialist is able to discern whether the person is possessed by a jinn depending on their response to reading passages of the Qur'an. Religious and biomedical themes run closely together. Those who feel calmer during this recitation are held to be 'depressed.'

Discussion

This article has examined a micro-politics of belief in the east London Bangladeshi community. As discussed earlier Bangladeshis in the UK are subject to a process of increasing revivalism and purification, a process propagated by local imams, especially those from the East London Mosque. There is an attempt to divest religious practices from their cultural accretions, to replace 'low' or folk Islam (based upon magic rather than rule learning) with 'high' Islam, which is oriented towards scripturalism and puritanism, to deploy Gellner's (1992) terms. This is reflected in efforts by religious authorities to arbitrate on what constitutes 'genuine' jinn influence. Despite these attempts, belief in the malevolent influence of jinn runs high in this community.

Although the younger members of the community speak about traditional explanations of misfortune in a disparaging and often critical way, this study suggests that members of the Bangladeshi community in east London still commonly employ 'traditional' explanations for illness, although there is marked variability in the ways that these explanations were deployed in specific cases of illness. Of course, it is impossible to know whether our younger informants were reluctant to admit to believing in the malevolent influence of jinn. As we pointed out earlier, Wilce (2004) noted that some Bangladeshis hold pejorative views concerning tradition and this is born out by the narrative of Ikram.

Specifically in relation to jinn, all the informants believed in their existence, which is consistent with orthodox Islamic belief. What differed between informants was the degree to which jinn were perceived to have agency in the human world. In general, elderly and less 'educated' informants were more likely to invoke jinn at times of misfortune. It appears that western education with its emphasis on 'rationality' has to some extent moderated belief in jinn among younger members of the community. The imams held that jinn possession was consistent with Islamic beliefs but overrated by the community as a cause of illness. They not only attempted to decree what constituted 'orthodox' Islamic belief but made themselves the arbiters of who was and who was not genuinely possessed, and in this sense played a seminal role in constituting the discourse about possession. This discourse is informed by ideas about what constitutes 'correct' Islamic beliefs.

The experience of 'modernity' does not necessarily erode 'traditional' conceptualizations. This is increasingly born out by anthropological research, which suggests that traditional ideas adapt to new environments and often become incorporated into modernist ways of thinking. Relations between traditional beliefs and modernity are complex. For example, Pigg (1996) in her study of Nepalese shamanism points out that it is all too easy to assume that the educated urban elite have abandoned shamanism in favour of 'modern medicine.' Far from this being the case, ritual healing survives alongside the country's best and readily available biomedical services. These ritual healers 'step in' where 'modern medicine falls short.' She contends that discussion about belief is informed by an ambivalence to 'modernity,' which the elite see as partial or second rate compared to that of the developed world. Halliburton (2005) found a decline in the incidence of spirit possession as well as a homogenization of the identities of spirits in his study of possessed and mentally ill patients in the state of Kerala, India. However, the idiom of spirit possession was still found to be common in the psychological advice columns in the popular media. As Stewart and Strathern (2004) state in relation to African witchcraft, 'Witchcraft ideas in contemporary Africa have become a prominent way of conceptualizing, coping with and criticizing the very "modernity" that was supposed to have done away with them.'

Migration leads some people to adhere more strongly to their traditional cultural practices (Knott, 1986), in order to reinforce their identity, especially during times of serious illness (Blackwell, 2005), and the decision to invoke culture in sometimes novel ways, tells us something about what is salient to the values they migrate with. So, how can the persistence of these beliefs be explained?

As described earlier, this community is one of the most deprived in the UK with high indices of social disadvantage and high levels of discrimination. The overwhelming experience of our informants was one of powerlessness – the inability to change their lives through their own actions. This is exemplified in the narrative of Rashida who reported that she could do very little to change her life. In this community, fate is largely perceived to be influenced by external factors outside their control. Jinn represent forces external to them, which control their lives. They are metaphors for powerlessness. Just like the British authority figures of which some of them speak and which ultimately control their fate, so to do these supernatural phenomena.

Gilsenan (1982) has argued that belief in 'miracles' is related to perceptions of powerlessness and lack of control, and it is those who are marginalized and lack power who often seek out these 'miraculous' transformations. This fact provides some insight into why those who lack power in their community commonly resort to pirs who are attributed with the ability to affect miraculous transformation, often manipulating these very phenomena over which ordinary people have little control. It is not surprising that those with little autonomy and personal control have faith in the supernatural powers of pirs to affect worldly change. This is not solely in cases of sickness, but is of note that many of these pirs claim to bring wealth to those who consult them.

We must also take into account the transnational character of this community. As pointed out earlier, despite living in the UK, members of this community regularly travel to and from Sylhet. In fact, several of our younger informants' lives were characterized by spending long periods in Bangladesh where they lived in rural environments and were exposed to traditional ideas about jinn.

These phenomena provide culturally plausible explanations for misfortune – in Evan's Pritchard's terms the why rather than the how of misfortune. A great deal of religious activity is driven by the need to deal with adversity, whether it is experienced personally or to one's family. At one level, Islam provides such an explanation for adversity in terms of Allah's will. As Ballard (2006) points out, these explanations are supplemented by a host of 'additional visions of the potential source of personal distress, as well as remedies which are available to cause such afflictions to lift.' These specific traditional explanations might function to further explain the cause of misfortune.

However, there is a third explanation involving disillusionment with biomedicine. Several informants expressed dissatisfaction with primary care services and rationalized from their experiences in the UK that poor medical services resulted from pervasive racism and inequality (in terms of health, unemployment and poor housing). Problems in communication, a perception of not being respected and cultural misunderstandings might also disparage east London Bangladeshis from using these services and even if they can overcome these barriers, many aspects of services offered appear tangential to their needs. Established forms of health service delivery are often incapable of diagnosing, let alone providing any kind of meaningful response to some causes of distress. They lack the capacity to locate explanations for illness within an appropriate cultural context leading to disillusionment and contributing to the rationale used to justify consulting traditional healers. This point has been argued by Sharma (1990) in her study of the use of complementary therapies in the UK.

The 'Modern' and 'Traditional' in Healing

A second finding from this study is that local imams hold both 'traditional' and 'modern' beliefs about illness concurrently, which they often deploy in the same narrative. As Stewart and Strathern (2004) point out, people feed their ideas into new circumstances. The imams speak of 'depression' as a biomedical diagnosis, which requires psychiatric intervention, but at the same time accept the fact that 'depression' which does not respond to this treatment might really be caused by jinn possession necessitating exorcism. The exorcist deploys the response of their patient to the recitation of Qur'anic verses to help in the differentiation of depression from possession. Unlike other forms of healing deployed by the 'folk' healers described earlier, the imams were generally favourable toward local exorcists and sometimes referred people to them. Parkin (2007) describes the complex interweaving of medical and religious themes in Islam, and more specifically in the Qur'an. There are many stories of healing in the Qur'an and the book itself is held by many Muslims to have healing properties. It is therefore not surprising that reading verses from it is seen as a potent mode of healing and that some Muslims believe that many biomedical discoveries were predicted by the Qur'an. Thus it is also no surprise that biomedical and religious themes occur often in the same narrative. What the imams express opposition to is any form of healing that does not invoke Allah as controlling all events. Islamic methods of healing insist that there is only one route to well-being: the rigorous assertion of Allah's authority. Folk healing in east London which does not invoke the power of Allah (such as kabiraj which invokes magic and witchcraft) is seen by the imams as anti-Islamic.

What is remarkable about this hybridized discourse on ill-health is the extent to which a medical and psychological idiom is imported into modes of explanation that would, in other settings, stand alone as modes of explanation. To attribute ill-health to 'depression' or 'anxiety' in the context of religious healing is both an acknowledgment and an appropriation of the otherwise hegemonic relationship between local and global systems of meaning. At times, these systems appear to be entirely independent (as say when Islamic texts are given canonical and absolute interpretations), while at other times global ('western') categories are imported in the interests of adjusting more rigid, canonical values to local circumstance. Indeed, it may be within this very ambiguity that the adaptability and power of religious values is evidenced; for otherwise, the denouncement of exorcism as a mode of praxis would not be accepted in the framework of prescribing such exorcisms to those who find them meaningful.

Conclusion

This study examined understandings of the role of jinn among Bangladeshis in east London, an economically deprived community that experiences racism, poor health service provision and cultural misunderstanding in relation to contacts with statutory services. The ethnographic findings suggest that traditional explanations of misfortune are prevalent in this community and are deployed especially as a way of coping with distress, psychological disturbance and unexplained physical symptoms. The popular appeal of 'miraculous healers' has not disappeared following migration and resort to them is commonplace to resolve treatment issues associated with spirit possession and evil eye. Exorcism was accepted both within the community and by local imams as a healing tool in certain defined clinical situations. Acceptability of this practice was found to be associated with the degree to which the Qur'an and appeals to Allah were part of the healing process. An important finding was the role of imams and the lay exorcist in 'triaging' their patients in terms of the distinction between illnesses and conditions that needed a biomedical or spiritual intervention. This was especially interesting in relation to mental illness and the willingness of imams and the exorcist to refer patients to each other and to local doctors.

The experience of 'modernity' does not appear to erode 'traditional' conceptualizations of the cause of illness, nor for deprived communities does it bring social empowerment. Rather, in our cohort, the lack of autonomy and the dependence on poor, culturally inappropriate medical services, may increase faith in supernatural explanations of illness. In terms of modernity, we argue that education may not transform beliefs associated with causation of illness and healing in a globalized world. Wider economic, social and cultural factors have a highly significant impact on these beliefs. These beliefs may disappear as this community becomes more integrated into mainstream society, but the degree to which the community benefits from economic development is likely to be a key fact in this process. A key question in this research is whether the acquisition of wealth will enable people to gain a sense of power to act in the world and abolish the need for jinn to do this for them. We intend to address this issue in future research in this community.

Acknowledgements

We are grateful to Dr Gerard Leavey for his comments on an earlier draft of this paper.

Notes

1. Bose (1997) describes how families are often housed in close proximity to their male and female kin, which facilitates the continuation of social organization familiar in Bangladesh. Entire families sometimes make trips to Bangladesh during which children attend school there and become acquainted with the way of life.
2. The Islamic faith decrees that Muslims should not pay interest (ribaa) on a loan. It is held that those who do this will be punished on the Day of Resurrection. Those who consume food bought from this interest will be beaten by Satan which renders them insane. Thus there is a close association between jinn and madness.
3. Gardner (2002) and Pollen (2002) have briefly examined understandings of illness in this community. For a good discussion on madness in this community see Bose (1997) who presents two case studies outlining the relationship between psychosis and jinn possession in adolescence.
4. The research involved detailed focused ethnographic interviews over one year with 40 east London Bangladeshis (mean age 42 years; 22 male, 18 female). Using a snowballing technique, a wide range of informants was recruited from the east London community including elderly Bangladeshis attending a local community centre, imams from the East London Mosque, businessmen, restaurant workers and health professionals. Narratives were elicited concerning recent misfortune, specifically related to episodes of sickness and its perceived causes (Mattingley, 1998). In most cases, the interviews were conducted in English, but where informants did not speak English, a Sylheti-speaking researcher con-

ducted the interview. Interviews were conducted at the informants' homes, but for the elderly informants they were conducted in a local day centre. To facilitate discussion of folk ideas about misfortune, informants were shown an advert from a Bengali newspaper concerning a mullah who was also a traditional healer. Because some of the informants objected to the interviews being audiotaped, the responses were recorded by hand.

5. Informants frequently mentioned Sihr (black magic) and nozoor (evil eye, literally 'sight,' 'vision') as causes of illness. Sihr is performed for a fee by 'specialists,' known in the community as jhadu kor. Informants commonly held that Sihr was practised by members of their community, as a way of forcing someone else to be compliant to their wishes, for example, engaging in a relationship contrary to their will. It was commonly held that hair from the victim was needed to perform Sihr. Women particularly feared Sihr because of its use in inducing them to go to Bangladesh to marry someone against their will. Sihr was also cited as a means of inducing illness but was not implicated as often as jinn possession. Many informants also spoke of the evil eye. This refers to the malevolent influence of one person's envious glance on another. Those who give the evil eye are often said to be unaware that they are doing it. Envy and the evil eye are potentially harmful to the thing that is liked or envied. Sometimes a person comments on how pretty fruit looks, only to find the following day that the fruit is rotten. A compliment might turn out to be destructive. Everyone in the community is vulnerable to nozoor, but some are held to be more vulnerable, for example, babies. To avert the effects of the evil eye, a black mark is often painted on the head of a baby, or the baby might be covered. Nozoor is often implicated in cases of weakness, especially in children who fail to thrive or lose their appetite.
6. Zamzam is the well within the sanctuary of Mecca that sprang up to provide Hagar with water in the wilderness.
7. Eade (1997) has documented a similar phenomenon among imams in Tower Hamlets and reports on a conference in 1992 organized by a community mental health team, where the majority of the participants were Bangladeshis. An article by a local imam contrasted the low level of Islamic knowledge and superstitious beliefs of the local Bangladeshis, with what he held to be 'correct' Islamic beliefs and practices concerning health and illness.

References

Abaza, M. 1991 'The Discourse on Islamic Fundamentalism' In *The Middle East And South East Asia: A Critical Perspective*. Sojourn, 6(2): 203–239.

Ahmad, R. 1988 'Conflict and Contradictions in Bengali Islam: Problems of Change and Adjustment'. In K. P. Ewing (Ed.), *Shari'at snd Ambiguity in South Asian Islam*. Berkeley: University of California Press.

al-Ashqar, U. S. 2003. *The World of the Jinn & Devils in the Light of the Qur'an and Sunnah*. Islamic Creed Series, Volume 3. Columbia, NC: International Islamic Publishing House.

Alexander, C. 2000. *The Asian Gang: Ethnicity, Identity and Masculinity*. Oxford: Berg.

Aslam, M. 1970. The Practice of Asian Medicine in the United Kingdom. PhD thesis, University of Nottingham, UK.

Ballard, R. 2006. 'Popular Islam in Northern Pakistan and Its Reconstruction in Urban Britain'. in J. Malik & J. Hinnells (Eds.), *Sufism in the West* (pp. 160–187). London: Routledge.

Blackwell, D. 2005. *Counselling and Psychotherapy with Refugees*. London: Jessica Kingsley.

Boddy, J. 1989. *Wombs and Alien Spirits: Women, Men and the Zar Cult in Northern Sudan*. Madison: University of Wisconsin Press.

Bose, R. 1997. 'Psychiatry and the Popular Conception of Possession among the Bangladeshis in London'. *International Journal of Social Psychiatry*, 43(1): 1–15.

Cabinet Office. 2003. *Ethnic Minorities and the Labour Market (Chap. 7).* London: Cabinet Office. Available: http://www.strategy.gov.uk/work_areas/ethnic_minorities/index.asp.2003Survey of English housing. Provisional results: 2002–2003, based on 1999–2000 data (Table 2). London: Commission for Racial Equality. Available: www.cre.gov.uk/duty/reia/statistics_ housing.html.

Dein, S., & Sembhi, S. 2001. 'The Use of Traditional Healers in South Asian Psychiatric Patients in the Uk: Interactions between Professional and Folk Remedies'. *Transcultural Psychiatry*, 38(2): 243–257.

Eade, J. 1994. 'Identity, Nation and Religion: Educated Young Bangladeshi Muslims in London's 'East End.' *International Sociology*, 9: 377–394.

Eade, J. 1997. 'The Power of the Experts: the Plurality of Beliefs and Practices Concerning Health and Illness among Bangladeshis in Contemporary Tower Hamlets, London'. In M.Warboys & L. Marks (Eds.), *Migrants, Minorities and Health: Historical and Contemporary Studies* (pp. 250–271). London: Routledge.

Eade, J., & Garbin, D. 2002 'Changing Narratives of Violence, Struggle and Resistance: Bangladeshis and the Competition for Resources in the Global City'. *Oxford Development Studies*, 30(2): 137–149.

Eade, J., Peach, C., & Vamplew, T. 1996. *Bangladeshis in Britain: The Encapsulated Community.* in C. Peach (Ed.), *Ethnicity in the 1991 Census* (Vol. 2, pp. 150–160). London: HMSO (Office National Statistics).

Gardner, K. 2001. *Global Migrants, Local Lives: Migration and Transformation in Rural Bangladesh.* Oxford: Oxford University Press.

Gardner, K. 2002. *Narrative, Age and Migration: Life History and the Life Course Amongst Bengali Elders in London.* Oxford: Berg.

Gaw, A. C., Ding, Q.-Z., Levine, R. E., & Gaw, H.-F. 1998. 'The Clinical Characteristics of Possession Disorder among 20 Chinese Patients in the Hebei Province of China'. *Psychiatric Services*, 49: 360–365.

Gellner, E. 1992. *Postmodernism, Reason and Religion.* London: Routledge.

Gilsenan, M. 1982. *Recognising Islam: An Anthropologist's Introduction.* London: Croon Helm.

Glynn, S. 2002. 'Bengali Muslims: The New East End Radicals'. *Ethnic And Racial Studies*, 25(6): 969–988.

Greenberg, D., & Witztum, E. 2001. *Sanity and Sanctity.* New Haven, CT: Yale University Press.

Halliburton, M. 2005 'Just Some Spirits: the Erosion of Spirit Possession and the Rise of 'Tension' in South India'. *Medical Anthropology*, 24: 111–144.

Healy, M. A., & Aslam, M. 1989. *The Asian Community: Medicines and Traditions.* Huddersfield, UK: Amadeus Press.

Kapferer, B. 1991. *A Celebration of Demons: Exorcism and the Aesthetics of Healing in Sri Lanka.* Oxford: Berg.

Kempson, E. 1999. *Overcrowding in Bangladeshi Households: A Case Study of Tower Hamlets.* London: Policy Studies Institute.

Knott, K. 1986. *Religion and Identity, and the Study of Ethnic Minority Religions in Britain.* Community Relations Project Research Papers No 3. Leeds, UK: Department of Theology and Religious Studies (University of Leeds).

Lambek, M. 1993. *Knowledge and Practice in Mayotte: Local Discourses of Islam, Sorcery, and Spirit Possession.* Toronto, ON: University of Toronto Press.

Lewis, I. M. 1971. *Ecstatic Religion: An Anthropological Study of Spirit Possession and Shamanism.* Harmondsworth, UK: Penguin.

Littlewood, R. 2004. 'Possession States'. *Psychiatry,* 3: 8–10.

Mattingley, C. 1998. *Healing Dramas and Clinical Plots: The Narrative Structure of Experience.* Cambridge: Cambridge University Press.

Messing, S. D. 1958. 'Group Therapy and Social Status in the Zar Cult of Ethiopia'. *American Anthropologist,* 60: 1120–1126.

Murshid, T. 1995. *The Sacred and the Secular: Bengal Muslim Discourses, 1871–1977.* Calcutta, India: Oxford University Press.

Office for National Statistics. 2002. *Annual Labour Workforce Survey, Working-Age Employment Rate By Ethnic Group, 2002/03* (Table 3.1). London: HMSO. Available: www.statistics.gov.uk/downloads/theme_labour/ethnicity/Wkage_Employ.xls.

Office for National Statistics. 2004a. *Local Market Data for Local Areas by Ethnicity,* Keith Brook, *Labour Market Trends* (Vol. 112). Available: www.statistics.gov.uk/downloads/theme_labour/ethnicity/Wkage_Pop.xls.

Office for National Statistics. 2004b. *Focus on Social Inequalities: Health* (Table 6.14). London: HMSO. Available: www.statistics.gov.uk/downloads/theme_compendia/fosi2004/Health.pdf.

Office for National Statistics. 2005. *Focus on Ethnicity and Identity* (2001 census data). London: HMSO. Available: http://www.statistics.gov.uk/downloads/theme_compendia/foe2004/Ethnicity.pdf.

Parkin, D. 2007. *In Touch without Touching: Islam and Healing.* in R. Littlewood (Ed.), *the Importance of Knowing about Not Knowing* (pp. 127–139). Walnut Creek, CA: Left Coast Press.

Phillipson, C., Ahmed, N., & Latimer, J. 2003. *Women in Transition: a Study of the Experiences of Bangladeshi Women Living in Tower Hamlets* (Chap. 5). Bristol, UK: Policy Press.

Pigg, S. 1996. 'The Credible and the Credulous: The Question of Villagers' Beliefs in Their Fall'. *Cultural Anthropology,* 11(2): 160–201.

Pollen, R. 2002. *Bangladeshi Family Life in Bethnal Green.* Unpublished thesis, University of London, UK.

Rippin, A. 2005. *Muslims: Their Religious Behaviour and Practices.* Routledge.

Robinson, F. 1983. 'Islam and Muslim Society in South Asia'. *Contributions to Indian Sociology,* 17(2): 185–203.

Roy, a. 1982. *The Pir Tradition: A Case Study in Islamic Syncretism in Traditional Bengal.* in F. Clothey (Ed.), *Images of Man: Religious and Historical Process in South Asia.* Madras, India: New Era.

Sharma, U. 1990. *Using Alternative Therapies: Marginal Medicine and Central Concerns.* In P. Abbott.

G. Payne (Eds.), *New Directions in the Sociology of Health* (pp. 127–139). London: Falmer Press.

Stewart, P., & Strathern, A. 2004. *Witchcraft, Sorcery, Rumours and Gossip.* Cambridge: Cambridge University Press.

Weiss, M., Desai, A., Jadhav, S., Gupta, L., Channabasavanna, S., Doongaji, D., & Behere, P. 1988. 'Humoral Concepts of Mental Illness in India'. *Social Science & Medicine,* 27(5): 471–477.

Werbner, P. 2002. *Imagined Diasporas Amongst Manchester Muslims.* James Currey.

Wilce, J. 2004. 'Madness, Fear, and Control in Bangladesh: Clashing Bodies of Knowledge Power'. *Medical Anthropology Quarterly,* 18(3): 357–375.

Chapter 6

The Use of Traditional Healing in South Asian Psychiatric Patients in the UK

Interactions between Professional and Folk Psychiatries

Anthropological studies in developing countries suggest that patients with mental health problems often resort to both professional and folk systems simultaneously (Hohmann et al. 1990; Sandoval 1979, 1983; C.I. Weiss 1992). Relatively little is known, however, about the use of traditional healing in populations who have migrated from the developing world to the West. Migrants bring with them their traditional beliefs and values but undergo a degree of acculturation. Once the migrant community has become established, the important question is whether subsequent generations consult traditional healers. Although there has been some work looking at the use of traditional healing for physical disorders in the UK, there is very little examining their use in mental health care (Bhui and Strathdee 1993).

Aslam (1979) and Healey and Aslam (1990) found that traditional healing was frequently used by Asian patients in Bradford, where there is a large Muslim population, particularly from the rural region around Mirpur in Pakistan. Appeal to hakims was common,[1] comprising an un-official health service. Some were full time and held recognized qualifications from their home countries. The majority, however, were unqualified. The consultation with the hakim lasted about twenty minutes and physical examination was restricted to feeling the pulse. Aslam (1979) points out that the majority of consultations were for a psychiatric problem often related to sexual anxiety.[2] Of seventy-nine patients treated over a four-week period, 30% had a psychosexual problem, 13% had excessive fatigue, which Aslam diagnosed as depression, and the others suffered from physical disorders.

A diagnosis of a supernatural illness led to referral to a mullah (religious leader). This would occur if the patient had broken a religious ordinance or appeared to be in a state of possession as implied by altered level of consciousness. Aslam noted a frequent belief in the evil eye (*nazar*) according to which illness was held to result from the jealous glance of another person (Spooner 1970). The *taveez*, consisting of holy words from the Qur'an incorporated into an amulet, was frequently deployed. About two-thirds of the sample were satisfied with the hakim's treatment. The majority had visited their general practitioner (GP) first and would consult a hakim if they were dissatisfied with the GP's treatment because the family were excluded from the consultation, or the treatment was ineffective. Often hakims were visiting for short periods from India or Pakistan, and these were especially popular. They were consulted most frequently for psychiatric and psychosexual problems, such as *dhat*, along with anxiety, sorrow and *fikr* (fright illness). Illness was understood in terms of a humoral theory of excess hot or cold (Leslie 1976) and frequently necessitated dietary manipulation. Consultation usually resulted in the prescription of a herbal preparation, and in fact some of these preparations had serious interactions with biomedical drugs (for example, the vegetable karela could interact with hypoglycaemic agents prescribed by doctors; see Aslam and Stockley 1979). A nosebleed was held to occur because the body was too hot and required treatment with a cold mixture such as honey and water.

Aslam points out that there may be problems of compliance when a Western medicine (most of which are considered to be hot) is used to treat a hot condition such as dysentery or kidney problems (see Dein and Lipsedge 1998: 149, in relation to the management of mental illness among Vietnamese clients). Aslam suggests that Asian patients may prefer to see a traditional healer because there is no language barrier, they have more time, are more holistic and include the whole family. GPs are often ignorant of the use of hakims and traditional remedies. Although Aslam found that hakims were often consulted for psychiatric problems, he did not examine the relationship between professional psychiatry and traditional healing among patients with mental health problems.

Other studies indicate, however, that resort to traditional healers is uncommon among Asian patients in the UK, although the use of traditional remedies is commonplace. In her community sample of 388 Sikhs in Southall, West London, Karmi (1985) found that 46% used traditional medicine. There was no difference in education, marital status, employment or place of birth between those who used traditional medicine and those who did not. Those using traditional medicines manufactured them at home. Advertisements about hakims were frequently found in local newspapers. A minority of her sample (22%) had visited a hakim, sometimes from abroad, before seeing a GP. Resort to traditional healing was most common for digestive and respiratory problems. Two GPs were interviewed, one of whom did not think that hakims were used by patients. Bhopal (1986) looked at the use of folk remedies in Glasgow in a community sample of sixty-five patients taken from a general practice register. This was chosen for its high proportion of Asian patients. A high proportion of patients had an awareness of traditional remedies, of which 48% were culinary ingredients. Few people preferred traditional medicine to Western medicine and there was some disagreement about safety. It was impossible to identify any traditional healers in Glasgow, but two people had consulted them in England and a number had returned to India to do so. However, they derived little benefit from consultation. Asian remedies were used concurrently with Western remedies, but GPs were unaware of their use.

A study by Donaldson (1986) of 726 Asian patients in Leicester over sixty-year years of age found that only 6% had consulted a traditional healer. He noted the increased rate of GP consultation of these elderly patients above that of the indigenous population (see Blakemore 1982; Johnson, Cross and Cardew 1983). He speculated that this might relate to cultural differences in illness behaviour and attitudes to medical services. Elderly patients suffer not only from socio-economic disadvantage, but also from anxiety, stress, loneliness and cultural dislocation to a greater extent than the indigenous population. Johnson et al.'s (1983) large-scale household survey of primary care use and provision in Asians, Afro-Caribbean and white groups in inner city areas in the West Midlands reported very little use of traditional remedies or practitioners by Asian patients. However, 51% of Afro-Caribbean, 33% of white and 24% of Asian respondents expressed the opinion that there are many conditions for which traditional remedies are better than conventional medicines, for example, chronic fatigue.

Understanding the use of traditional remedies and consultation of traditional healers is important for Western-trained health professionals as it improves the provision of culturally appropriate service to patients. It is also important to understand ethnic minority clients' explanatory models of illness in an attempt to negotiate between different treatment modalities and enhance compliance. Asian patients may appear to differ from non-Asian patients in their utilization of state health services, which may be a reflection of their experience in their country of origin (Raschid and Jagger 1992). These issues may be of importance for health planning (Karmi 1985). While there has been some research looking at the use of traditional healers among ethnic minority patients in the UK, there has been little work examining their use among those with psychiatric problems.

The aims of this study were to examine how traditional healing is used in collaboration with professional psychiatry and the factors responsible for the choice of treatment modalities. Specifically, the following questions were addressed:

I. How common is resort to traditional healing (healers) while attending professional psychiatrists?
II. What factors result in the use of traditional healing or traditional healers?
III. How does their use of treatment modality relate to their underlying explanatory models?
IV. How do South Asian patients view professional psychiatry?

Method

Setting

This study was carried out among patients attending a mental health service in the Waltham Forest area of north-east London. The London Borough of Waltham Forest has a large South Asian population (15%) and the highest Pakistani population in London (8%) (London Borough of Waltham Forest 1996). Asian patients in London suffer from high rates of unemployment and poor quality, overcrowded housing (Peach 1996) and are frequently subjected to racial abuse. In the UK the term 'Asian' refers to subjects born in the Indian subcontinent and also to children whose parents were born in the same region (in accord with the Office of Population Census Survey definition).

Participants

All eligible participants were either born in South Asia (India, Bangladesh, Pakistan or Sri Lanka) or, for the minority who were not born there, their parents had been born there and were under sixty-five years old. The mean age was forty-two years (range twenty-five to sixty-four years old). Patients had the following ICD-10 diagnoses: schizophrenia, 12; depression, 12; bipolar affective illness, 1. Eleven were born in Pakistan, three in the UK, two in India, two in Sri Lanka and seven in East Africa (although their parents derived from India). The group comprised fourteen Muslim, two Christian, four Sikh and four Hindu patients; religion was unrecorded for one patient. Some of the participants had been brought up within a Western medical system although at times had consulted traditional healers for various complaints. All defined their ethnicity in terms of country of descent or religious affiliation. Twenty-five patients were interviewed (9 men, 16 women).

Procedure

All Asian patients who were cared for by community psychiatric nurses (CPN) or attending the day hospital were asked whether they would participate in a one-hour open-ended interview. Of the forty patients approached, twenty-five (63%) agreed to be interviewed by a psychiatrist, with the presence of an interpreter where required. The interpreter spoke both Hindi and Urdu. The aim was to elicit the patient's experience of healing. Questions were asked about current and past health problems. The interviews were guided by the use of a theme list using an explanatory model framework (Kleinman 1980). Questions focused on lifestyle, religious beliefs and practices, symptomatology, understandings of symptoms, use of and satisfaction with Western psychiatric treatments, resort to traditional remedies and healers (including foods, herbs, penance, use of religious objects and astrology) and their perceived efficacy both for psychiatric and physical illness (this distinction was made by the interviewer).

Results

Among the twenty-five patients, six reported using home remedies, generally folk medicines or herbs, three used home remedies for psychiatric illness, five used traditional healers for non-psychiatric illness, and seven (28%) had consulted a traditional healer at some time during the course of their psychiatric illness. Although not examined in detail, several of those who did not use traditional healers stated that they did not know of healers in the UK, or they believed that they were very expensive. However, they stated that they would consult them if they were available.

Use of a traditional healer was significantly related to age, with patients younger than forty years old being more likely to consult a traditional healer (chi-squared = 4.4, df = 1, p = 0.046). There was no significant association of use of a healer with gender, country of origin or religious affiliation.

Case Studies

Case 1

Mr D. is a thirty-five-year-old mechanic.[3] He was born in the UK and is a practising Muslim although he did not become religious until fairly recently. Both his parents were born in Bangladesh and are devout Muslims. They came to the UK forty years ago. He had a traditional upbringing and as a young child went regularly to the mosque with his family and regularly fasted at Ramadan. Although he had never made Haj, he reiterated several times how much he would like to do this. He has been diagnosed as having a depressive illness by his psychiatrist. He has been depressed for many years and has low self-confidence, poor memory and is unable to work. His depression started when he was about twenty years old on account of work problems and was characterized by tearfulness and extreme tiredness. At times it was so severe that he spent days in bed, much to the dismay of his parents. After being treated by a doctor in his local casualty department, he saw several psychiatrists and has attended the out-patients department for several years. He regularly takes an antidepressant medication, which helps a little, but he believes that it does not really get to the cause: 'Tablets can only help a little, I need something else to help me feel better.' On account of this he later sought the help of a Muslim healer. He now wears two *taveez*. One contains holy scriptures (sura) from the Qur'an given to him by the healer for his depression. The second protects him against jealousy and the evil eye in his marriage. He has also received special prayers from the healer. The sura were selected specifically for his problem. He was unable to explain exactly how these *taveez* worked.

He found the healer by 'word of mouth' and was told that this healer will give 'relief not a cure.' He met up with the healer in his house and initially emphasized that he hoped he would completely cure him very quickly since several years of tablets had only helped a little and he had been waiting a long time. After his first visit to the healer, the latter visited him at home. He received the prayers at the first meeting and only later received the *taveez*. The consultations were free, and Mr D. was told that the prayers could exorcise black magic. Mr D. reports that the *taveez* and prayers are particularly helpful for his panic attacks. However, he was keen to point out that *taveez* can only help 'if you believe, otherwise it is just two black strings and two little bags around your neck.'

He had wanted to visit a hakim but was unable to do this due to the high cost involved (£100). He was concerned that some were untrained: 'I don't trust people who say they are a hakim and give you any mixture.'

Case 2

Mr S. is a forty-one-year-old Muslim man who suffers from schizophrenia. He was born in Pakistan and came to England aged thirteen years in order for his father to find work. After completing a period of college education, he has worked mainly in factories. He has two younger sisters who do not suffer from mental illness. He lives with his elderly parents and generally has a good relationship with them. He spends his days reading the Qur'an and sleeping. He was careful to tell the interviewer that, although he was ill, he still kept up his religious responsibilities, such as regular prayer, and this in itself made him feel better. He has regular injections of a long-acting antipsychotic, fluphenazine decanoate.

He believes that he suffers from schizophrenia as a result of injuring his face in an accident as a child after falling down the stairs. Following this, his nose was very swollen and children at school mocked him causing him to become withdrawn. He described himself as a 'zombie': 'I would just stay in my room and not go out and I became afraid of everything.' Of particular significance, he believes, is the fact he neglected his religious obligations, which played a large part in making him ill. In 1976, he started to believe that the wall plugs had microphones in them and people were spying on him. He was diagnosed with schizophrenia by a psychiatrist who put many of his problems down to puberty and told him to go to Pakistan for a visit. The psychiatrist also started him on a regular injection of depot antipsychotic medication. While visiting some members of his family in Pakistan, his grandfather suggested he visit a herbal doctor for treatment of his condition. The doctor told him that this injury he had sustained as a child had caused blood to clot in the small arteries of his brain and he should shave his head and rub medicine onto it to draw the clotted blood out. He did not do this as his father advised him to continue with his regular injection of depot antipsychotic and not to do as the hakim recommended since he had no faith in him. He did, however, visit an Unani doctor suggested by his grandfather who told him he had constipation and prescribed a mixture of crushed spices and herbs to be taken for this. He also gave him a herbal preparation called *Atrifal astkhudes* for his mind which he said would not interfere with Western medicine. It came as a semi-solid in a bottle and was taken in warm milk. Mr S. found that it helped him overcome his feelings of paranoia.

Following a visit to Pakistan three years earlier Mr S. has worn a *taveez* given to him by a mullah. It contains a sura 'for the mind' and he wears it constantly. This protects against bad *gini* (spirits) and helps to fight off depression by stopping bad things happening to him. He was also given a ring containing an agate gemstone, used to ensure good health. The mullah also dissolved passages of the Qur'an in saffron water and asked him to drink this again to protect him against evil forces. He finds the ring and *taveez* helpful and feels they protect him. He also finds that his regular prayer and reading of the Qur'an helps his mood. When visiting Pakistan Mr S. says he would visit a hakim 'without hesitation'. However, in his experience, it is expensive to see a hakim in the UK as they import their medicines from Pakistan. This deters him from visiting one and he sees his GP. He stressed the need for a personal recommendation of a doctor in Pakistan and hakim in the UK to ensure that they are qualified. He is now keen to see a sufi

(Islamic mystic) but is concerned that some sufis 'deal in evil and are wizards' and cannot be trusted.

Overall, he held that his depot injection was helpful and 'changed the complexity of his brain', whereas herbal medicines could also cure schizophrenia by 'clearing out the brain.' He himself now did not use herbs because he believed they were not available in the UK. He stated that for a Muslim spiritual healing could be helpful and could in some cases cure schizophrenia.

Case 3

Mr M. is a sixty-six-year-old married man who was born in Sri Lanka. He came to the UK aged eighteen years but became ill while studying. He is a practising Hindu and regularly attends a Shivaic temple in London. He is a retired clerk and has been diagnosed with schizophrenia on account of long-standing persecutory delusions and intermittent voices shouting and swearing at him. He himself did not describe his illness as schizophrenia but said that family worries and anxiety had caused excess bile to rise to his head. As a result, he was 'unable to concentrate and heard voices'. This condition was severe and interfered with everything in his life.

He explained that his view of his illness was based on Ayurvedic principles. He uses lime juice and sugar to treat excess bile. This was recommended to him by a family friend. Citrus fruit is a cold food that restores balance when suffering from a hot condition, in this case increased bile. Taking lime and sugar generally keeps him in balance from day to day and controls his voices. However, if he becomes very unwell, he has crossed a threshold beyond which this treatment can no longer keep him in balance and he knows that he requires Western medicine, which he takes. He said that 'Western medicine only treats symptoms and not disease – if you are high, it brings you down and if you have a cyst, they take it off but not away.' He believes that Western medicine does not treat the underlying cause, while Ayurvedic medicine does.

As a child in Sri Lanka, his mother would take him to a biomedical doctor if he had a cut, bruise or broken arm but to an Ayurvedic practitioner for something 'inside' the body. He does not know of any Aryuvedic doctors in the UK and so did not have the choice to visit one when he became unwell. He finds alternative medicine too expensive to use.

Case 4

Mrs Z.H. is a fifty-three-year-old Muslim woman from Pakistan who has been living in the UK since the age of eighteen. She is married and has three children. She has never worked. Her illness started when she was about eighteen years old at which time she 'thought too much' and developed 'useless thoughts'. She became preoccupied by the colour and faces of people and at times would hear 'bad voices' talking to her. At times she has been aggressive, and the police have taken her to hospital. She holds that these experiences were brought on by the fact that her aunt continuously told her to marry a rich man, which upset her. As a young woman she was diagnosed as suffering from a schizophrenic illness and treated with a depot antipsychotic medication. Since then, she has had many admissions to hospital with restlessness, excitability and confused speech. She rarely takes medication for longer than a few weeks and held that it was of no use as she felt the same on and off it. She believes that her main problem is anxiety caused by her past and medicine cannot change this. Only God can heal her.

In an attempt to cure her, her husband took her to two local Asian homeopathic doctors in London who both prescribed herbs. They asked her very little and did not examine her. One of the homeopathic doctors told her to stop her depot injection. Although the herbal preparations cost about £100 (US $170), they did not help her. One herbal doctor told her to stop her injection, which she did for some weeks but became very ill. She also approached a lady in a shop who acted as an agent for a herbalist. The lady obtained tablets for her to help with her weight (she was apparently told that being overweight was part of her problem). Both she and her husband felt these herbs were expensive and did nothing to help her. While taking these herbal preparations, she continued with her antipsychotic medication when her community nurse could persuade her to take it.

Nine years ago, she returned to Pakistan to see a reputable homeopathic doctor in Lahore. She told him she thought too much, was restless and could not sleep. After a brief examination (feeling her pulse), he prescribed a bottle of liquid containing herbs and 60% alcohol. Her mood lifted for some weeks after taking this. However, both she and her husband believed that it was the social support she received from her extended family which helped. Overall, she feels that both professional psychiatric treatments and traditional remedies have not helped her. She remains a difficult management problem, and her husband has given up work to look after her full time. She has also consulted a number of both Muslim and Hindu priests. One priest told her there was no problem, she simply needed to go out more. Another told her she was possessed by jinn spirits, but she did not believe him and did nothing more about this.

Case 5

Mrs B. is a fifty-two-year-old married Muslim woman. She is a housewife and mother. She was born in Pakistan but has lived in London for most of her life. She emphasized that her life was one of 'great religion' and she has been on a pilgrimage to Mecca with her family several times. She has been diagnosed as having a depressive illness. She herself does not have a term for her illness but says it is caused by marital problems.

She treats ill health with home remedies handed down through family generations or learned from her friends. She herself has never consulted a traditional healer, but several of her family have done so, for various health problems such as tiredness and diarrhoea. These remedies are based on a humoral theory of disease balancing hot and cold states. She also judges her body from day to day and varies her diet accordingly. She does not find Western medicines of any benefit at all. Initially, she took an antidepressant for her illness but it made her feel very tired and so she stopped it and took a herbal remedy. This helped her and she uses 'hot' foods, such as green peppers, with every meal to protect against depression. This helped her with depression, which she believes was a cold illness. She explained that depression could be caused by too much cold in the body, although on further questioning she could not elaborate further in terms of humoral theories, nor was she aware of classical teachings about madness in Ayurveda.[4] When her daughter was unwell, she stopped the Western treatment and manipulated her foods and her daughter improved. When she heard her mother was ill with pneumonia in Pakistan, she sent her almond oil, which cured her. She says there is no specific treatment for depression. She suggests that people will improve by keeping themselves occupied, meeting up with others to discuss things, and looking after the home. Overall, she felt that these hot foods effectively helped her cope with her moods.

Discussion

The study has a number of limitations. First, the numbers are small, and the population is heterogeneous in terms of country of origin, length of time in the UK, psychiatric diagnosis and religious affiliation. Future studies need to concentrate on specific populations such as Muslims from India. Second, all patients were already attending Western psychiatric services. Future studies should examine clients of traditional healers, some of whom may not have seen psychiatrists. Lastly, the analyses are based on self-reports which are subject to reporting biases.

In discussions about traditional healing several themes recurred: patients used traditional remedies concurrently with professional psychiatric treatments. Often several types of treatment were used at one time.

Although some of the patients understood how traditional remedies worked, others did not understand, nor were they particularly interested as long as they got better quickly. Aslam (1979) comments on the idea of the 'quick fix' held by some Asian patients. Hot and cold imbalances were cited by two informants and food was used as a remedy, while other informants used herbs.[5] These remedies led to increased feelings of wellbeing. Although, in general, Western medication helped a little, the patients believed that it did not get to the root of the problem and could never cure the problem in itself. Religious practices were held to be as important as medical treatments in healing illness. Traditional healers were thought to be effective but were considered expensive and at times were mistrusted.

Interestingly, choice of healer was not determined by religious affiliation, with both Muslims and Hindus consulting both types of healers. This is contrary to the findings of Schiller and Levin (1988) who observed that religious affiliation was an important factor in health-seeking behaviour. Traditional healers usually did not dissuade patients from using professional psychiatric treatments (except in one case). The use of traditional healers did not appear to be directly related to the underlying explanatory model of illness. In this study, only the age of the subjects showed a significant relation to the use of traditional healers, with younger patients being more likely to consult a traditional healer. This finding is contrary to expectation and requires further replication. Economic factors may play a part. Older patients may not have the necessary financial resources to pay for traditional healing, which, as the study indicates, can be expensive. Attending a healer may be a way for younger patients to reassert a cultural identity that is already strong in older patients.

The choice of treatment adopted by members of a particular society is not only a reflection of their view of ill health, but also what is available to them (Young and Garro 1982) and financial constraints (Madan 1969). Health-seeking behaviour may be more constrained by objective social and material conditions than by the patients' rational beliefs (Good 1994). It may have less to do with agency and more to do with power relations, whether located in the family (Wilce 1998) or within wider social structures (Morsy 1990; Myntti 1988). Individuals do not simply choose from a pre-existing range of therapies but constitute, reproduce and destabilize therapies through their health-seeking practices (Brodwin 1996).

Conclusion: Globalization and Biomedical Hegemony

The evidence presented suggests that traditional healers are used in conjunction with professional psychiatry by South Asian psychiatric patients. Asian immigrants are subject to the forces of modernization and globalization. However, despite the global hegemony of Western biomedicine, itself replacing religion as a legitimating and charismatic ideology (Littlewood and

Lipsedge 1987), local healing practices survive in many parts of the world. Perhaps this is because local healing succeeds where biomedicine fails by recognizing the links between disease and social, moral and religious events (Ayora-Diaz 1998), or because traditional beliefs and healing systems are anchors of security for people undergoing the stresses of uprooting, translocation and adaptation to a new society (Lefley, Sandoval and Charles 1998). We can only speculate what will happen in the future to traditional systems of healing among Asian patients. Will they be replaced by biomedicine or will traditional systems themselves appropriate biomedical symbols and therapies without accepting biomedicine's naturalistic ideology (Brodwin 1996)? Will exposure to the market forces of capitalism change the ways in which traditional healers practise, leading to new opportunities for mercenaries and charlatans as Lefley et al. (1998) suggest? These questions remain to be empirically examined.

Notes

1. The term 'hakim' refers to healers in the Unani tradition deriving from the Arabic word meaning wise or learned. The term is often used to describe Asian healers in general, including Ayurvedic healers who are strictly called Vaids. Both types of healers undergo rigorous training in India and Pakistan and can only practise after taking and passing a number of examinations. However, in the UK anyone can call himself or herself a hakim, irrespective of whether they are qualified. For a good discussion of theories of mental illness in the Ayurvedic tradition, see M.G. Weiss et al. (1986; see also M.G. Weiss, Desai, Jadhav and Gupta 1988). Weiss outlines contemporary humoral theories of *unmada* (severe mental disorder) in India. Ayurveda acknowledges various causes of *unmada* including possession, violation of taboos, stressors along with imbalances of the three *dosas* (humours). Illness results from humoral imbalance. Foods play a large part in treatment. There are 'hot' and 'cold' foods which address humoral imbalances. Hot foods cause excess bile and must be treated with a diet of cold foods and other cold medications. Ayurveda also includes a theory of temperament. A patient whose temperament results from excess bile is prone to illness caused by excesses of this humour and should avoid heat-producing foods. Unani (lit. Ionian) medicine is not an intrinsic part of Indian culture but extended from its origins in the Mediterranean with the spread of Islam. Deriving from Galenic medicine, it similarly emphasizes humoral imbalances, and treatment is based on the principles of *contraria contrariis*. All food and medicines are classified as hot or cold. Siddha medicine is practiced among the Tamils of Southern India and Sri Lanka and although closely related to Ayurveda, it places greater emphasis on drugs and minerals to treat illness.
2. In the UK, many male Asian patients present to their general practitioners complaining of weakness deriving from loss of semen, a syndrome called *dhat*. These ideas derive from Ayurvedic teachings of the derivation of blood from semen.
3. A modified version of Case study 1 appeared in Sembhi and Dein (1998).
4. In his study of psychiatric clinics in Bombay, M.G. Weiss et al. (1988) found patients commonly resorted to humoral explanations of mental illness even though they were generally unfamiliar with the classical treatises of Ayurveda.

5. Aslam (1979) presents evidence that some of the herbs prescribed by hakims have metabolic effects. For instance, M. charantia lowers blood sugar. The medicine Kushta Surb containing bamboo reed is used as an aphrodisiac. The effects on the central nervous system await empirical research.

References

Aslam, M. 1979. 'The Practice of Asian Medicine in the United Kingdom', PhD thesis, University of Nottingham, UK.

Aslam, M. and L. Stockley. 1979. 'Interaction Between Curry Ingredient (Karela) and Drug (Chlorpropamide)', *Lancet* 1: 607.

Ayora-Diaz, S. 1998. 'Globalisation, Rationality and Medicine: Local Medicine's Struggle for Recognition in Highland Chipias, Mexico', *Urban Anthropology* 27: 165–95.

Bhopal, R.S. 1986. 'The Inter-Relationship of Folk, Traditional and Western Medicine Within an Asian Community in Britain', *Social Science and Medicine* 22: 99–105.

Bhui, K. and G. Strathdee. 1993. 'Asian Inpatients in a Psychiatric Unit: An Examination of Presenting Features and Routes into Care', *International Journal of Social Psychiatry* 39: 208–20.

Blakemore, K. 1982. 'Health And Illness Among the Elderly of Minority Ethnic Groups Living in Birmingham: Some New Findings', *Health Trends* 14: 69–72.

Brodwin, P. 1996. *Medicine and Morality in Haiti*. Cambridge: Cambridge University Press.

Dein, S. and M. Lipsedge. 1998. 'Negotiating Across Class, Culture and Religion: Psychiatry in the English Inner City', in S. Okpaku (ed.), *Clinical Methods in Transcultural Psychiatry*. Washington, DC: American Psychiatric Press, pp. 137–55.

Donaldson, L.J. 1986. 'Health and Social Status of Elderly Asians: A Community Survey', *British Medical Journal* 293: 1079–82.

Good, B. 1994. *Medicine, Rationality and Experience*. Cambridge: Cambridge University Press.

Healy, M. and M. Aslam. 1990. *The Asian Community: Medicines and Traditions*. Huddersfield, UK: Amadeus Press.

Hohmann, A., M. Richeport, B.M. Marriott, G.J. Canino, M. Rubio-Stipec and H. Bird. 1990. 'Spiritism in Puerto Rico: Results of an Island-Wide Community Study', *British Journal of Psychiatry* 156: 328–35.

Johnson, M.R., M. Cross and S.A. Cardew. 1983. 'Inner-City Residents, Ethnic Minorities' Health Care', *Postgraduate Medical Journal* 59: 664–67.

Karmi, G. 1985. *Traditional Asian Medicine in Britain*. Wisbeck, UK: Menas Press.

Kleinman, A. 1980. *Patients and Healers in The Context of Culture*. Berkeley: University of California Press.

Lefley, H., M. Sandoval and C. Charles. 1998. 'Traditional Healing Systems in a Multicultural Setting', in S. Okpaku (ed.), *Clinical Methods in Transcultural Psychiatry*. Washington, DC: American Psychiatric Press, pp. 88–110.

Leslie, C. 1976. *Asian Medical Systems: A Comparative Study*. Berkeley: University of California Press.

Littlewood, R. and M. Lipsedge. 1987. 'The Butterfly and the Serpent: Culture Psychopathology and Biomedicine', *Culture Medicine and Psychiatry* 11: 289–335.

London Borough of Waltham Forest. 1996. *Borough Profile*. London: Borough Of Waltham Forest Policy Analysis Unit.

Madan, T.N. 1969. 'Who Chooses Modern Medicine and Why?', in G.R. Gupta (ed.), *Main Currents in Indian Sociology*. New Delhi: Vikas, pp. 1475–84.

Morsy, S. 1990. 'Political Economy in Medical Anthropology', in T. Johnson and C. Sargent (eds), *Medical Anthropology: A Handbook of Theory and Method*. Westport, CT: Greenwood Press, pp. 26–46.

Myntti, C. 1988. 'Hegemony and Healing in Rural North Yemen', *Social Science and Medicine* 27: 515–20.

Peach, C. 1996. *The Ethnic Minority Population of Britain: Ethnicity in the 1991 Census*. London: HMSO.

Raschid, A. and C. Jagger. 1992. 'Attitudes to and Perceived Use of Health Care Services Among Asian and Non-Asian Patients in Leicester', *British Journal of General Practice* 42: 197–201.

Sandoval, M. 1979. 'Santeria as a Mental Health Care System: An Historical Overview', *Social Science and Medicine* 13B: 137–51.

______. 1983. 'Santeria', *Journal of Florida Medical Association* 70: 620–28.

Schiller, P.L. and J.S. Levin. 1988. 'Is There a Religious Factor in Health Care Utilisation? A Review', *Social Science and Medicine* 27: 1369–79.

Sembhi, S. and S. Dein. 1998. 'The Use of Traditional Healers by Asian Psychiatric Patients in the UK: A Pilot Study', *Mental Health, Religion and Culture* 1(2): 127–33.

Spooner, B. 1970. 'The Evil Eye in the Middle East', in M. Douglas (ed.), *Witchcraft Confessions and Accusations*. London: Tavistock, pp. 311–19.

Weiss, C.I. 1992. 'Controlling Domestic Life and Mental Illness: Spiritual and Aftercare Resources Used by Dominican New Yorkers', *Culture, Medicine and Psychiatry* 16: 237–71.

Weiss, M.G., A. Desai, S. Jadhav and L. Gupta. 1988. 'Humoral Concepts of Mental Illness in India', *Social Science and Medicine* 27(5): 471–77.

Weiss, M.G., S.D. Sharma, R.K. Gaur, J.S. Sharma, A. Desai and D.R. Doongaji. 1986. 'Traditional Concepts of Mental Disorder Among Indian Psychiatric Patients: Preliminary Report of Work in Progress', *Social Science and Medicine* 23(4): 379–86.

Wilce, J.M. Jr. 1998. 'The Pragmatics of "Madness": Performance Analysis of a Bangladeshi Woman's "Aberrant" Lament', *Culture, Medicine and Psychiatry* 22(1): 1–54.

Young, J. and L. Garro. 1982. 'Variation in the Choice of Treatment in Two Mexican Communities', *Social Science and Medicine* 16: 1453–65.

Chapter 7

TRAUMA AND THE KANUN

Two Responses to Loss in Albania and Kosova

Therapy and Social Ritual

Psychology and social anthropology have differed as to whether societies can be compared under equivalent institutions that reflect approximately similar spheres of interest – very generally, the psychological and personal, or the moral and social – or whether, as many anthropologists argue, the scale of each particular institution is different in different cultures. And thus they cannot easily be mapped onto each other. In the most extreme case, anthropologists have argued that Euro-American ('Western') societies are particularly ego-centred and hence psychological, whilst 'traditional' societies have a more extended moral and social domain in which actions which would be seen as individually motivated in the West are merely customary procedures, participation in which is presumed for all members of that culture (for example Needham 1962; Shweder and Bourne 1982). If personal experience of one's own self and agency may sometimes follow the social ascription, as anthropologists argue, then emotion and suffering must follow different models and involve us in rather different types of understanding (Lutz 1988); or, to put it another way, the master discipline for non-Western societies will be anthropology, for Western societies psychology.

Social anthropologists have thence long argued for non-industrialized societies a relationship between what initially appear as social institutions represented in individuals, and responses more easily interpreted by us as essentially personal and psychological (Littlewood 1992). At the most accessible, standardized social ritual or other practices may serve as a 'therapy' for a whole community where the putative patient, identified as such by the observer, is only one among many people whose psychological state is altered by collective action (Turner 1964). (Indeed, similar ideas deriving from Gregory Bateson and Victor Turner have proved influential in our structural theories of group and family therapy.) Certain 'ritual' institutions have been interpreted as subserving a clearly psychological function for the individual. The decay of a Zulu rite of symbolic inversion (Needham 1973) which annually adjusted relations between men and women was found to be later associated with a more evidently personal and arguably 'decultured' psychological response by the women who then demonstrated individual anxiety. And conversely, the women's health movement in the United States has attempted to prevent or heal personal psychopathologies arising from gender antagonisms through the elaboration of new types of ritual action (Teish 1985). At a certain level of generality then, therapy and social ritual may be seen as alternative routes to the same psychosocial end, or even as transformations of each other, as the etymology of 'therapy' itself might indicate: from hypothesized proto-Indo-European *ar* ('way of being, orderly and harmonious arrangement of the part of whole'), and hence Hittite *tarpan-alli* ('ritual substitute') (Tyler 1986).

It is particularly in the response to the sudden loss of one's immediate kin that standardized social action may be seen as alleviating or preventing an individual grief reaction. The traditional Haitian family's response to the unexpected death of a young person may be that they have been zombified: in other words kidnapped and killed but in a way in which their individual personality will continue in a not so remote form (Littlewood and Douyon 1997), not so different from the Druze family's concept of immediate and recognized reincarnation of the dead relative (Littlewood 2001), or the Omani idea of *mu ghayeb* in which the dead person is only regarded as ensorcelled, to eventually return alive and well in their usual form (Al-Adawi, Burjarjee and Al-Issa 1997). A problem for considering the therapeutic value of such standardized social systems for analogues of grieving is that we cannot start from any 'natural' baseline uncontaminated with culture. As Phillips (1999: 6) notes, 'It is possible that we have no idea what secular grief is: what grief unsanctioned by an apparently coherent social system would feel like'. The modern clinical assumption that the experience of loss first passes through the three fixed stages of acceptance, working through and detachment (Parkes 1972) is closely tied to a Western and modern moral economics, with its particular concepts of an individual and individual finality, the ties between persons, and of justice, retribution and reconciliation. Nor can we assume that there is an inevitable global process of psychologization and interiorization going on, towards the Euro-American perspective with its own characteristically psychological notions of an individual: Good and Good (1988) demonstrate how Iranian patterns of mourning after the Islamic revolution moved from a previously new Westernizing response back to a more 'traditional' contextual and socially embedded response emphasizing shared values of moral justice and retribution rather than the more individualized character of personal grief.

Rather than argue then for or against some general process of globalization in a psychological direction, as many psychotherapists have been tempted to do (e.g. Hiev 1964), we can more modestly consider situations in which the two perspectives, the psychological and the moral (or social) may come into opposition and conflict. The case considered here is the type of response now available to Albanian Kosovars after the Serbian intervention and massacres of 1999: blood vengeance or psychological trauma.[1]

The Historical Setting

Albanian speakers have been settled in what is now Kosova since at least the early medieval period (Malcolm 1999; Vickers 1999) and now comprise around a third of Balkan Albanians (Judah 2000). Coming under the control of the Ottomans, Albanians were then among the last to seek a national identity separate from Ottoman Turkey in the late nineteenth century. In spite of Kosova having been a centre of resistance to the Ottomans (for instance, the League of Prizren in 1878), when Albania achieved independence from Turkey in 1912, the area east of the Accursed (Prokletije) Mountains, Kosova, was occupied by Serbia in 1913, and has remained part of Serbia and thence Yugoslavia. During the First World War, the Kosova area was the seat of fighting by various groups of Serbs, Greeks, Turks, Macedonians, Italians and Britons, but the pre-war settlement was re-affirmed by the League of Nations; the boundaries between Kosova and the rest of Albania have remained the same in spite of the recent collapse of Yugoslavia into (among others) Macedonia, Bosnia, Serbia and Montenegro. By the early 1990s, relations between Serbs and Albanians in Kosova had become tense: Kosova's status as an autonomous unit within Serbia was revoked in 1989, and resistance grew to the Belgrade administration and Serbian education system during the 1990s, at the same time as many ethnic Serbs left Kosova for Serbia proper. The attempt at reconciliation at Rambouillet in 1999 failed as Serbia refused to grant autonomy with international inspection, and Kosova was first bombed and then occupied later that year by Nato forces – the current situation. Relationships between Albanians and the remaining Serbs in Kosova are still extremely confrontational.

Albania proper, on the Adriatic coast, has remained independent, first as a republic then as a monarchy under King Zog, was occupied by the Italians and then the Germans in the Second World War, with a period of extreme isolation under the communist Enver Hoxha and his successor which ended with elections in 1992, and now a return to a nominal parliamentary system but with frequent and widespread civil disturbances often approaching civil war and a vacuum of power at the political centre.

The Kanun: Death and the Customary Law

During the twentieth century, Kosova and Albania had remained the poorest part of Europe (Economist Intelligence Unit 1998–1999), isolated from the rest of the continent by geography and politics. Despite attempts at centralization from Belgrade or Tirana, rural life was dominated by a network of exogamous patrilineal clans or tribes (*fis*, or at the village level *bajraks* or Banners) especially among the Ghegs of northern Albania and Kosova. Without a nationally enforced system of justice, customary law prevailed among the transhumant peasants living in wooded multi-generational family settlements (*shtëpi* or *zadrugas*). The majority of Albanians are Muslim, with a Catholic majority in the north and an Orthodox majority in the south. In spite of the Hoxha regime's opposition to the traditional social order and to religion (Albania was the world's first 'atheist state'), notions of the customary law remain to adjust personal relations in what is once again a clan-based society with limited central authority. The most influential of the codifications of this law is the medieval Kanun (Canon) of Lekë Dukagjini collected together with twentieth-century revisions by a Kosovar priest in the 1920s (Gjecov 1989), presumably in an attempt to standardize and attenuate more inchoate forms of immediate revenge (Black-Michaud 1975). 'The importance of the kanun to the ordinary life of the Albanians of Kosova and the Matësi [mountainous northern Albania] can hardly be exaggerated', says the Balkanist historian Noel Malcolm (1999: 17). 'It still influences life in the entire area' (Senechal 1997: 5), and traditionally took precedence over state or church law (Gjecov 1989).[2]

Striking similarities have been noted between the Kanun of Lekë and North Caucasian customary law and, indeed, the Indian Laws of Manu (Gjecov 1989). Whilst much of the Kanun is taken up with marriage, hospitality and the resolution of rights in livestock and property, it is most well-known in Western Europe for its regulation of homicide and blood feud (*gjakmarrje*) of the type associated with other Mediterranean societies such as Sicily or Corsica (Peristiany 1965): particularly since the translation of the Albanian novelist Ismail Kadare's famous *Broken April* (1991). One of the most striking aspects of this ethnographic novel and the Kanun which it illustrates is the location of experience and revenge within the standardized setting of the Kanun itself: as if individual perception and experience are of no real significance in the working out of the process of the local moral economy. However it starts (quarrels over boundaries or grazing rights, insults to guests or women), its continuation has an almost inexorable public form. On the death of a man in feud, his blood-stained shirt was hung up: when the dried blood turned yellow, it was then time to avenge the death. One of the aspects noted by commentators on the blood feud (Durham 1909; Hasluck 1954; Kadare 1991; Senechal 1997) is how little individual motivation to continue the feud is actually determined by feelings of loss or personal revenge: all the commentators note that it is the expected public response to an insult to the 'law of blood' (Durham 1909; Hasluck 1954): 'Till you had taken blood everyone would talk about you. You could not live like that' (ibid.: 112); 'strangely impersonal, abstract, the blood feud is a collective concept involving the whole community' (Senechal 1997: 29, 30). An individual engages in return assassination because he must, as part of the accepted order: he goes into ambush, shoots a male member of the opposing family, carefully turns him on his back and places his gun by his head (as the Kanun specifies: §3846; Gjecov 1989), goes back to his own family stronghold (*kulla*) and sends a neutral messenger to the opposing family (or tribe in the case of inter-tribal feud) stating what he has done and claiming a period of *besa* or pledged truce, during which he attends the funeral and wake of his victim in the latter's house, pays a monetary compensation to the ritual authorities and then awaits his own death (or that of another male family member) on completion of the truce: 'For a moment he felt as if he were trapped in bird-lime by the bloody part of the kanun' (Kadare 1991: 30).

Hutton (1954) terms Albanians 'head hunters' and compares them with the Pathans and Nagas. It appears that formerly the assassinated corpse was decapitated and the head carried by the extended tuft of hair that Albanian male hairdressing once afforded (Hasluck 1954). The display of expected and permitted grief after a death is clearly specified by the Kanun: '§1235: The men who bewail the dead scratch their faces and beat their clothes. §1236: The women lament, but do not scratch their faces. §1239: Men do not lament over women, except in the case of a son over his mother or a brother over a sister' (Gjecov 1989).

With the frequency of male deaths, women can elect to become honorary males and, declining marriage altogether, inherit and act as heads of households – as 'sworn virgins' (*virgjinesha*: Durham 1909) – and take part in blood feuds (Young 2000). In both Catholic and Muslim Albanian communities, the levirate (here additional common law marriage to the deceased brother's widow) was formerly practised.

Women had little voice in the Kanun: they could not be the target of a blood feud, could not inherit, nor refuse their arranged marriage, were assumed to be virgins on marriage, and must 'submit to the husband's domination' (Kanun: §33, §57): 'a woman is a sack made to endure' (Gjecov 1989) – in other words, perform an essentially child-bearing role as the property of her husband (Whitaker 1981). At her marriage, a wife's parents formerly gave their son-in-law a cartridge to kill their daughter should she be adulterous or 'betray hospitality' (Hasluck 1954). The association of men with the blood feud is exemplified by the expression for tracing relationships agnatically (recognized descent, through men) 'by blood'; through women (uterine relationships) 'by milk'. The almost erotic symbolism of the man's gun is commented on by Edith Durham (1909: 176): 'His "well-beloved" had cost twelve napoleons, the price of an ordinary wife, and he spent eight guilders a year – exactly half his income – "feeding" it [buying cartridges]'. Durham describes how everyday interest and occupation are monopolized by the 'law of blood', and how sardonically but light-heartedly men pursue its course. She says little of women's interest: they are (like priests) not legitimate targets of the blood feud. The idiom of 'blood' thus variously connotes Albanian kinship and thus identity, social position and honour, custom and communal acceptance, masculinity and, as we shall see, certain psychological notions of both anger and anxiety. 'Blood' rather than 'honour' appears to be the persistent idiom (Black-Michaud 1975).[3]

The Kanun's regulation of homicide is concerned with individual acts, carefully tallied, often in an interminable sequence of reprisal, which is difficult to break: 'At the end of the Ottoman period it was estimated that 19 percent of all adult male deaths in the Matësi were blood feud murders, and that in the area of Western Kosova with 50,000 inhabitants, 600 died in these feuds every year' (Malcolm 1999: 20). Feuds can be theoretically commuted by paying blood money but this, although allowed by the Kanun, is regarded as dishonourable, and many a feud previously settled by mediation is opened up again by a young man seeking to restore family honour. Mediation by outsiders, a common occurrence in Arab blood feuds, was relatively unusual in Albania, although sometimes a local priest, mullah or elder could carry this out. Resolved blood feuds may result in 'blood brotherhood' and fictive kin links between the adversaries: thus, their families cannot intermarry.

It might be expected that the Kanun refers to a now disappeared past yet since the early 1990s, with the decline in communist authority, blood feuds in Albania and Kosova have proliferated with the privatization of communal land (Malcolm 1999; Schwandner-Sievers 1999; Young 2000) 'at a remarkable rate' (Hing 2000), shading into new urban and rural criminality and now 'without order' (Hrasztev 2000). Schwandner-Sievers (1999) discusses the survival of various Kanuns after communism; their modifications and exploitation, particularly by Sali Berisha (President, 1992–1997); and newer 'national' attempts at offering processes for reconciliation (see also Miller 1999). A recent study found that over a hundred young boys in northern Albania were in protective hiding, fearing to go out of their *kulla* because of an ongoing feud (Hing 2000). Perhaps a hundred families in Shkodra, a town of some 80,000, are 'in blood' at the moment (Hrasztev 2000). A recent case involves two members of the parliament (ibid.).

Trauma

During this same modern period, Albanian communities have also been subject to external war, civil war based on political affiliation, and massacre by the Serbs and others. Here, the social intelligibility and, in a sense containability, of the feud type of deaths is no longer possible. And it might seem that the notion of 'trauma' as advanced by Western psychology is more appropriate. Since 1999, no less than six international intervention agencies have been involved in projects dealing with 'traumatization' in Albanian Kosova (International Organisation For Migration 2000).

Yet the notion of something which may be considered 'trauma', and particularly the notion of 'post-traumatic stress disorder', has been questioned as a universal human response (Marsella et al. 1996; Bracken and Petty 1998; Summerfield 1999). Like the blood feud, it may in fact be culturally limited. Allan Young (1995) and Ruth Leys (2000) propose that trauma, as a psychological response, is a nineteenth-century extrapolation from physical trauma. With various putative psychophysiological mechanisms, post-traumatic stress disorder (PTSD) entered the American Diagnostic and Statistical Manual of Mental Disorders in 1980 as a successor to earlier Vietnam War concepts of 'delayed massive trauma' with symptoms of guilt, rage, psychological numbing, alienation and the sense of being scapegoated by others: the last not so unlikely given that, as Young argues, PTSD provided medical exculpation for soldiers who had committed atrocities in Vietnam. Since then, treatment for PTSD in the form of cognitive behavioural therapy (CBT) has been used for a large number of civil and military disasters (including accidents and earthquakes), and 'trauma' has become a major new paradigm for psychopathology and culture (Farrell 1998; Leys 2000). Central to both nineteenth-century and more recent ideas is the notion of a 'hidden memory' of the trauma, those apparently most at risk of PTSD being individuals who in a psychodynamic sense 'repress' their memories of extreme violence or atrocity (Young 1995: 289). And now the newer international aid agencies promote the related idea of a whole 'culture of silence' preventing traumatized local communities from processing their memories (e.g. Boyder and

Gibbs 1996). Antze and Lambek (1997) suggest that our current emphasis on memory goes along with a new interest in individual and group identity, identity being inevitably dependent on memory.

According to the International Organisation for Migration's working party on Kosova (IOM 2000), all six agencies working there on post-intervention psychological response privilege the notion of PTSD as the diagnosis most useful with individually focused CBT as the therapy. (This conflicts with earlier notions that war was good for individual mental health presumably because of enhanced social cohesion and purpose.) By contrast, the IOM project in Kosova has attempted to translate individual diagnosis into collective experience, with the use of role play, theatre, workshops, video, open-ended fieldwork and the compilation of an 'archives of memory' historical and experiential project (Zur 1996; IOM 2000).

Is PTSD a universal human response? Both Bracken (1998) and Summerfield (1999), who have worked therapeutically post-atrocity, suggest it derives from highly individualized and psychological notions of the individual (e.g. Horowitz 1986; Janoff-Bulman 1992), and while it may make some sense of severe experiences in the industrialized West, it cannot be automatically presumed for other societies. The IOM (2000) found it difficult to provide an Albanian gloss for trauma: local responses from their trained personnel in Kosova elicited notions such as 'deep spiritual disorder' (or 'wound' or 'pain') when the concept was more directly introduced. Many Kosovars saw the killings of their family by Serbs as fate determined by God (IOM 2000), yet some who had been raped committed suicide (ibid.). Bracken (1998) notes that as industrialized countries reduced their total overseas aid budget in the 1990s, 'trauma' and 'trauma counselling' became popular idioms in supposedly more focused and targeted interventions which could be quantitatively evaluated. Summerfield (1998) comments that as civilians have represented a higher proportion of war casualties (5% in the First World War, 40% in the Second, 90% in current wars), trauma has become the prevailing international idiom. He summarizes critical objections to the interventionist projects' use of PTSD: trauma is used inconsistently as a description of external events impinging on the individual; the Western idea of 'ventilating' difficulties is precisely that, Western; human response is not uniformly the same; we cannot assume that in periods of war large numbers of people inevitably require professional help, particularly those identified by outsiders as vulnerable – children or rape victims; nor that rapid intervention is necessary to prevent a mental health disaster or that local workers cannot assist because they are traumatized themselves (Summerfield 1999). To which we might add that 'trauma' like 'stress' (both attempts to link the individualized biomedical subject to the social environment) confusingly refers to both the external traumatizing events as well as the presumed internal psychological response to them.

Trauma and the Kanun

The psychological idiom of PTSD and the prescriptive social code of the Kanun are not immediately comparable. We cannot easily match them one to the other. Clearly the Kanun does not pretend to be a psychological theory. It is concerned with considerations of gender and kinship, and with an affirmation of normative behaviour, rather than being an empirical account of psychological process. 'The individual was almost completely submerged in his family' (Hasluck 1954: 219). Indeed Durham (1928) speculates that the ultimate meaning of the feud is that of a sacrifice to the souls of the dead rather than a type of vengeance, and we can certainly adduce the social accretions which appear to have grown up around it: the black ribbon marking the arm of the killers and now potential targets (Hadare 1991), the extension of the *besa* (truce) to include protected highways (ibid.; Durham 1909), and the almost phasic movements of the feuds so that the population whose turn it is to take vengeance (the 'owners of the blood' with 'blood to redeem') can irrigate their fields and till their crops with impunity, whilst those awaiting vengeance to be dealt to them ('incurring blood') neglect their agriculture and retreat into their *kulla*; or, now, the 'Blood Quarter' of Shkrodra. Durham (1909: 146–47) even describes the effects noticeable on the local agricultural landscape from which the current state of social relations may be deduced. There is a complex economics of blood vengeance when mediated so that monetary compensation for a wound is equivalent to half that for a death and wounds in different parts of the body may be compensated differently (Hasluck 1954; Gjecov 1989; Kadare 1991). While the Kanun provides expectations of experience and for action, it clearly does not offer a full account of psychological responses to loss by killing (certainly not for women).

And yet a more nuanced questioning about personal experience is itself likely to produce a more psychologized response, if not to generate a now indigenous psychology of something recalling trauma (cf. Lutz 1988; Young 1995). In a converse way, emphasis on PTSD as a solely internal process ignores the historical circumstances under which this psychology has been elaborated (Young 1995), just as PTSD checklists, presumed to be universal, ignore the contextual meanings of the particular external trauma itself (Bracken 1998) from which, indeed, indigenous ways of coping may be elaborated. What we can do is to start from the social (the Kanun) or the psychological (PTSD), and move towards the other position (Littlewood

1993). Customary law and psychological theory both contain elements of social relationships and psychological experience, cultural order as well as personal therapy.

Each is clearly culturally and historically embedded, PTSD in late twentieth-century notions of accountability and the private self, the Kanun in what we may take as a pre-modern 'traditional' (Littlewood 1995) clan-based society. They are dealing with different types of violence and personal loss: the Kanun with the shared legitimacy of a practice within a society itself, PTSD with external and almost arbitrary violence, of here a 'meaningless' intercommunity war (cf. Loizos 1988). The blood feud already contains two recognized psychological responses. First, does the Kanun derive from, and still contain as a codification, an individual tendency to revenge or 'natural justice' (cf. Rivers 1916)? It appears very different, indeed impersonal, but the impulse to immediate retaliation is already recognized by the Kanun as a state of boiling blood: the first twenty-four hours *besa* prevents sudden retaliation and thus any interruption of the accepted process – if a person is killed in revenge immediately, 'that person is simply avenging blood and does not incur blood' (§871, 873 of the Hanun), i.e. they do not incur a continuation of the blood feud. Secondly, a state of blood sickness is also recognized in the killer; often a man's 'blood seized him' (Hasluck 1954: 228) with somatic anxiety symptoms and he could not run from the corpse until he had bitten the used cartridge or performed a similar action.

There is clearly some relationship between the matched vengeance of the Kanun and the equivalence of matching insult with insult, atrocity with atrocity, of the recent war (Judah 2000). The Kosova Liberation Army (KLA) developed as an extension of the older *kacak* (informal guerilla) band, based on the kin mobilized in a blood feud (Judah 2000: 147). A difference is that war involves escalation, feud reciprocity. Though some impulse to retaliation appears common to both PTSD and the feud, revenge is relatively neglected by academic psychology except in certain studies of 'natural justice' or 'equalization' – the impulse which the semi-legendary Lekë Dukagjini codified as the Kanun. Blood feuds could only be conducted properly within the Albanian speaking community itself; although variants could be practised against neighbouring families of a fairly similar background (Montenegrins, Serbs), on the whole the conflict then became an inter-community one, more of a war than a feud (cf. the Nuer: Evans-Pritchard 1940; or Cypriots: Loizos 1988). As this occurred, women and children became legitimate targets for reciprocal violence, often sexual (Littlewood 1997), as representatives of the opposing collectivity, in a way they could not in the course of the feud. While the inter-communal war thus contains some elements of the feud, and inter-communal atrocities have continued in Kosova for most of the twentieth century and thus have some claim to be institutionalized, we cannot easily assume that war generates similar sentiments to feud on a larger scale (Loizos 1988). Nor do we have any account of such 'standarized' responses to earlier wars as psychological experiences. And increasing anti-Serbian feeling in Kosova was associated with a diminution in intra-Albanian feuds and increased attempts at reconciliation (Young 2000).

A common feature though of both Kanun and trauma is how perpetrators and victims gradually become interchangeable in a web from which there is no escape: blood feuds continue as an obligation for years, those 'owing blood' becoming those with 'blood to redeem', and with PTSD the perpetrator of atrocities becomes in turn the traumatized victim (Young 1995). In both, we have a vicious circle into which external attempts at reconciliation – mediation or therapy – appear only imperfectly to enter.

Notes

1. My grateful thanks to Lucia Nixon for advice, and to the International Organisation For Migration (IOM) project on trauma response in Kosova, particularly Natale Losi and Monica Goracci; for conversations with Patrick Bracken, Derek Summerfield and various Kosovar therapists from the IOM; for discussions with mediators Alexander Hola and Father Dionis Maka, and with various (unnamed) families 'in blood'; and for comments on an earlier draft of this chapter from Stephanie Schwander-Sievers, Charles Stewart and participants at LSE, Oxford and UCL seminars.
2. Pauli Qesku, a former Albanian ambassador to London, has produced an Internet book (The Albanian Implosion, http://www.albania.memail.com/author.html) which argues that the various Kanuns have provided a central national identity for Albanians in opposition to external powers.
3. Black-Michaud (1975), following Anatol Rapaport, comments that a feud approximates to our notion of a rule-governed 'game', albeit one which is deadly and taken as such by the participants. Arguably the same is true of early modern 'chess board' war (Littlewood 1997).

References

Al-Adawi, S., R. Burjarjee and I. Al-Issa. 1997. 'Mu-Ghayeb: A Culture-Specific Response to Bereavement in Oman', *International Journal of Social Psychiatry* 43: 144–51.

Antze, P. and M. Lambek. 1997. 'Introduction: Forecasting Memory', in P. Antze and M. Lambek (eds), *Tense Past: Cultural Essays in Trauma and Memory*. New York: Routledge.

Black-Michaud, J. 1975. *Cohesive Feud: Feud in the Mediterranean and the Middle East*. Oxford: Blackwell.

Bracken, P.J. 1998. 'Hidden Agendas: Deconstructing Post-Traumatic Stress Disorder', in P.J. Bracken and C.I. Petty (eds), *Rethinking the Trauma of War*. London: Free Associations.

Bracken, P.J. and C.I. Petty (eds). 1998. *Rethinking the Trauma of War*. London: Free Associations.

Boyder, J. and S. Gibbs. 1996. *Vulnerability and Resilience: Perceptions and Responses to Psycho-Social Distress in Cambodia*. Oxford: INTRAC.
Durham, E. 1928. *Some Tribal Origins, Laws and Customs of the Balkans*. London: Allen and Unwin.
______. 1985 [1909]. *High Albania*. London: Virago.
Economic Intelligence Unit. 1998–1999. *Albanian Country Profile*. London: Economist.
Evans-Pritchard, E.E. 1940. *The Nuer*. Oxford: Oxford University Press.
Farrell, H. 1998. *Post-Traumatic Culture*. Baltimore, MD: Johns Hopkins University Press.
Gjecov, S. 1989. *Kanuni I Lekë Dukagjini (The Code of Lekë Dukagjini)*. Orig. collect. 1933. Trans. L. Fox. New York: Gjonlekaj.
Good, M.-J. and B. Good. 1988. 'Ritual, the State and the Transformation of Emotional Discourse in Iranian Society', *Culture, Medicine and Psychiatry* 8: 315–43.
Hasluck, M. 1954. *The Unwritten Law in Albania*. Cambridge: Cambridge University Press.
Horowitz, M. 1986. *Stress Response Syndromes*. New Jersey: Jason Aronson.
Hutton, J. 1954. 'Introduction', in M. Hasluck, *The Unwritten Law in Albania*. Cambridge: Cambridge University Press.
International Organisation for Migration. 2000. *First Seminar on Psychosocial and Trauma Response in Kosovo: Working Documents*. Geneva: I.O.M.
Janoff-Bulman, R. 1992. *Shattered Assumptions: Towards a New Psychology of Trauma*. New York: Free Press.
Judah, T. 2000. *Kosovo: War and Revenge*. New Haven, CT: Yale University Press.
Kadare, I. 1991. *Broken April*. London: HarperCollins.
Kiev, A. (ed.). 1964. *Magic, Faith and Healing*. New York: Free Press.
Hing, C. 2000. 'Singular Oaths', *Times Literary Supplement*, 7 July: 27.
Hrasztev, P. 2000. 'Back to the Torn-Out Roots: Reflections on Vendetta in Contemporary Albania', Conference on 'Intersecting Times: The Work of Memory in South East Europe', Swansea University.
Leys, R. 2000. *Trauma: A Genealogy*. Chicago: Chicago University Press.
Littlewood, R. 1992. 'How Universal Is Something We Can Call Therapy?', in J. Kareem and R. Littlewood (eds), *Intercultural Therapy*. Oxford: Blackwell.
______. 1993. *Pathology and Identity: The Work of Mother Earth in Trinidad*. Cambridge: Cambridge University Press.
______. 1995. 'Psychopathology and Personal Agency: Modernity, Culture Change and Eating Disorders in South Asian Societies', *British Journal of Medical Psychology* 68: 45–63.
______. 1997. 'Military Rape', *Anthropology Today* 13: 7–16.
______. 2001. 'Social Institutions and Psychological Explanations: Druze Reincarnation as a Therapeutic Resource', *British Journal of Medical Psychology* 74: 213–22.
Littlewood, R. and C. Douyon. 1997. 'Clinical Findings in Three Cases of Zombification', *Lancet* 350: 1094–96.
Loizos, P. 1988. 'Inter-Communal Killings in Cyprus', *Man (N.S.)* 23: 639–53.
Lutz, C. 1988. *Unnatural Emotions: Everyday Sentiments on a Micronesian Atoll and Their Challenge to Western Theory*. Chicago: University of Chicago Press.
Malcolm, N. 1999. *Kosovo: A Short History*, 2nd ed. London: Macmillan.
Marsella, A.J., M.T. Friedman, T. Gerrity and M. Schonfield (eds). 1996. *Ethnocultural Aspects of PTSD*. Washington, DC: American Psychological Association.
Miller, M. 1999. 'Family Feuds Are No Game in Albania', *Los Angeles Times*, 12 July.
Needham, R. 1962. *Structure and Sentiment*. Chicago: University of Chicago Press.
______. (ed.). 1973. *Right and Left: Essays on Dual Symbolic Classification*. Chicago: University of Chicago Press.

Parkes, C.M. 1972. *Bereavement: Studies of Grief in Adult Life*. Harmondsworth: Penguin.
Peristiany, J.G. (ed.). 1965. *Honour and Shame*. London: Weidenfeld and Nicolson.
Phillips, A. 1999. 'Commanded to Mourn', *London Review of Books*, 18 February: 3–6.
Rivers, W.H.R. 1916. 'Sociology and Psychology', *Sociological Review* 9: 1–13.
Schwandner-Sievers, S. 1999. 'Humiliation and Reconciliation in Northern Albania: The Logics of Feuding in Symbolic and Diachronic Perspective', in G. Elwert, S. Feuchtwang and D. Neubert (eds), *Dynamics of Violence: Processes of Escalation and De-Escalation in Violent Group Conflicts*. Berlin: Duncker and Humblot.
Senechal, M. 1997. *Long Life to Your Children: A Portrait of High Albania*. Amherst: University of Massachusetts Press.
Shweder, R.A. and J. Bourne. 1982. 'Does the Concept of the Person Vary Cross-Culturally?', in A.J. Marsella and G.M. White (eds), *Cultural Conceptions of Mental Health and Therapy*. Dordrecht: Reidel.
Summerfield, D. 1998. 'The Social Experiences of War and Some Issues for the Humanitarian Field', in P.J. Bracken and C.I. Petty (eds), *Rethinking the Trauma of War*. London: Free Associations.
______. 1999. 'A Critique of Seven Assumptions Behind Psychological Trauma Programmes in War-Affected Areas', *Social Science and Medicine* 48: 1449–62.
Teish, L. 1985. *Jambalaya*. San Francisco: Harper and Row.
Turner, V. 1964. 'An Ndembu Doctor in Practice', in A. Kiev (ed.), *Magic, Faith and Healing*. New York: Free Press.
Tyler, S.A. 1986. 'Post-Modern Ethnography', in J. Clifford and G.E. Marcus (eds), *Writing Culture*. Berkeley: University of California Press.
Vickers, M. 1999. *The Albanians: A Modern History*, Rev. ed. London: Tauris.
Whitaker, I. 1981. 'A Sack for Carrying Things: The Traditional Role of Women in Northern Albanian Society', *Anthropological Quarterly* 54: 146–56.
Young, A. 1995. *The Harmony of Illusions: Inventing Post-Traumatic Stress Disorder*. Princeton, NJ: Princeton University Press.
Young, Antonia. 2000. *Women Who Become Men: Albanian Sworn Virgins*. Oxford: Berg.
Zur, J. 1996. 'From PTSD to Voices in Context: From an "Experience-Far" to an "Experience-Near" Understanding of Responses to War and Atrocity Across Cultures', *International Journal of Social Psychiatry* 42: 305–17.

Chapter 8

DRUZE REINCARNATION AS A THERAPEUTIC RESOURCE

The relations between the social and psychological sciences have never resulted in an agreed use of individual (psychological) interpretation in explaining or understanding social institutions, including standardized beliefs. Generally, social anthropologists have not followed Weber in employing interpretation of individual motivations and emotions as a possible social or historical datum. Emile Durkheim famously declared that social facts are independent of individual psychology: 'there is between psychology and sociology the same break in continuity as there is between biology and the physical and chemical sciences. Consequently, every time a social phenomenon is directly explained by a psychological phenomena, we may rest assured that the explanation is false' (Durkheim 1982: 129). In particular, he emphasized that no widespread social phenomenon such as 'religion' or 'culture' (or, in his words, 'collective representations') could be attributed to the psychology of the individual, notably in his well-known study of suicide, whose methodology still influences social science (Durkheim 1952). Social institutions, he suggests, consist of 'certain ways of acting . . . imposed or at least suggested *from outside* the individual and . . . added on to his own nature' (Durkheim 1982: 248, emphasis in the original). One must look for the social in the social.

Despite his later use of what are essentially socio-physiological hypotheses (Durkheim 1915), he did not alter his opinion, and his methodological emphasis continues as fairly normative in the social sciences, despite a recent interest in questions of individual agency and subjectivity, hermeneutics and pragmatic relativism in relation to the 'facts' of social life (Littlewood 1995;

Obeyesekere 1981). Outside the minor disciplines of psychohistory and psychobiography – both heavily influenced by Freud, who was apparently not familiar with Durkheim – it is generally considered unacceptable to relate a shared culture back to individual cognitions, affect and experience (Littlewood 1993). This remains generally true of medical anthropology and medical sociology where, although obviously local health related practices may be expressly set up to serve certain recognized psychological or medical needs, more widespread social institutions such as religious or marriage systems are not directly related to particular individual psychological experience.

If social scientists have sometimes assumed that for times of rapid social change they might justifiably have resort to psychological explanations more than for more settled periods (ibid.), there remained a more general problem of the role of psychology in seeking to understand culture. Durkheim's pupil, Mauss, followed him in 1934 to describe 'psychological facts as connecting cogs and not as causes, except in moments of creation or reform' (Mauss 1979: 121). Whilst the social anthropologist Malinowski (1944) argued that any culture must satisfy certain 'basic [physiological] needs', he gave a minor place to the possibility of psychological needs. Turner (1967), by contrast, proposed that the components of any successful culture must have both a 'public' (Durkheimian, social) utility at the same time as they are psychologically meaningful and satisfying to the individual: indeed, for the psychologist it is difficult to see how they could not. Social anthropologists and sociologists, however, have always been vague about individual motivation and the communication of cultural knowledge, simplistically assuming that something called 'socialization' makes all individuals in a society think and behave in the same way (Boyer 1994). A more recent solution argues that individual agency and experience just seem to act in a different 'direction' to social structuring (Bourdieu 1977) and that we continually have to place one against the other in particular situations (Littlewood 1993, 1998).

By contrast, the idea that institutions, including religion, exist for a specific collective purpose – solidarity or cohesion – is today regarded as frankly banal. That social institutions subserve particular social needs is regarded as self-evident – and thus not requiring particular comment. But when the reasons given by the people themselves are couched in such socially functional terms, they are generally regarded as irrelevant and as self-serving.

Despite Durkheim's strictures, it is commonplace for cultural psychiatrists and psychologists to maintain a psychological function for religious doctrine: i.e. that certain 'collective representations' exist essentially to subserve individual psychological needs (e.g. Kiev 1972; Murphy 1982; Tseng and McDermott 1981). Certain shared religious practices – confession, shamanism, possession, glossolalia, and certain types of religious 'consolation' – are seen as 'intended' to satisfy a person's distress or existential doubt. Indeed, religious practice in general is seen as 'therapeutic', whilst allowing that certain religious practices may be taken as 'pathological'. This has occurred within a context of widespread interest in the mental health advantages of religious practice: advantages intended or otherwise. The instance considered here is a set of explanations about reincarnation after death among the followers of the Druze religion in the Lebanon which might seem to have an obvious psychological value, a point which is maintained by the people themselves.

The Druze

The Druze are a heterodox movement in Ishmaeli ('Sevener') Shia Islam, originating during the Fatimid caliphate in Cairo (Abu-Izzeddin 1984; Betts 1988; Firro 1992). The capricious and antinomian Caliph al-Hakim bi amr-Allah, said by some followers to be the Mahdi or even God, disappeared suddenly in the year 1021 CE after which his followers entered a period of proselytization. In a period of persecution by normative Islam, the sect's major religious books were written and the faithful departed north for the relative isolation of, first Syria, and then the Shuf mountains of what is now South Lebanon, coming under Ottoman rule in the sixteenth century and a French mandate in the twentieth (Salibi 1988). Both polygamy and slavery had been abolished by the Druze in the eleventh century, but their universalist and millennial aspirations seemed to have declined by the time of European intervention in the Lebanon and are currently not prominent (Abu-Izzeddin 1984).

The call to convert (*da'wa*) into the group ended in 1042, and membership since then has been hereditary: no new members are accepted or can marry in. The Druze now number about 900,000 Arabic speakers in the Lebanon, Syria, Jordan and Israel, with a considerable diaspora in Europe, South America and the USA. Under the Lebanese National Pact of the 1940s, they are recognized as a permanent political and religious constituency in the country with guaranteed governmental representation: an agreement which has survived the recent civil war and Syrian intervention.

The community divide themselves into the uninitiated majority (*juhhal*) and the enlightened (*uqqal* or sheikhs) who have access to the six holy books: the latter, both men and women, comprise about 10% of the community and have somewhat stricter obligations (no alcohol, no tobacco, strictly no adultery) and a traditional costume of white fez, dark gown and knee-breeches for men, and they meet regularly on Thursday evenings in the *khalwa* (religious meetings) to discuss the religious texts and matters of welfare and social interest to the community. Initiation into sheikh-hood typically takes place in one's fifties but may be earlier among the more earnest members. Druze religious beliefs have traditionally been regarded as esoteric if not secret, but in conversations with both *juhhal* and *uqqal* I found no evidence of evasive answers:[1] Druze are nominally monotheistic (*tawhid*) although not Islamic, with a long history of protective dissimulation (*taqiyya*), and have collected together a set of ideas which can loosely be termed neo-Platonic (and which in the past have led them to being confused with Masonic and other Hermetic Christian philosophies; e.g. De Nerval 1984), without a clear notion of a judgment to come or of predestination, no practice of ritual circumcision nor adherence to the five fundamental tenets of Islam and, in their newer forms, sympathy for what might be called 'New Age' beliefs common in the contemporary West.[2] Druze now have monogamous extended households which still place emphasis on female sexual honour (*ird*) but with considerably more female autonomy than in most Muslim societies, with preferential parallel cousin marriage, and their social organization is very similar to that of rural Maronite Christians, Sunni and Shia Muslims in the Lebanon (Salibi 1988): local residence in kin-related villages with loyalty to a feudal chief (*bey*) (see Gilsenan 1996, for a Sunni example).

Whilst it was difficult to regard the average adult as especially 'religious' in the sense of referring everyday events to religious dogma, all Druze agree that acceptance of reincarnation (*tanasukh*) is crucial to Druze identity. All Druze I spoke with – doctors, businessmen and peasants – accepted reincarnation. This idea seems to have been present from their formation in the eleventh century (Makarem 1974). At the moment of death, one is automatically reincarnated as a new-born baby: 'You breathe your last, then the second breath is the first breath of the baby'. All souls were created at the beginning of time, and the individual soul enters the body at birth, the body being compared to a shirt which you discard. Unlike Hindu or Buddhist ideas, subsequent lives are not seen as so dependent on action in past lives or as going in a particular direction (cf. Daie, Witzum, Mark and Rabinowitz 1992). The soul matures by experience quite variously as a rich person and as a poor person, as healthy and as sick. The main purpose seems to be for it to gain the full range of human experience; where it all ends is now none too certain: most say in full unity with the deity. Male Druze reincarnate as male Druze, female as female. Generally, Druze do not reincarnate as non-Druze (but some say they might appear in Christians), although Druze souls may be present in those who are apparently non-Druze.[3] There is according to local ideas a Druze community in India and China, although its members may be unaware of being Druze; the soul cannot be split and the 'numbers problem' (an increasing population needs more souls) is solved by this unknown number of 'surplus' Druze souls (and also non-observant Druze in the diaspora). Non-Druze souls are similarly reincarnated among non-Druze, say some, generally also in a gender-specific way. Druze teaching on reincarnation is echoed among the Alawites of Syria, although these are closer to orthodox Islam. Western advocates of reincarnation have recorded various instances in the Lebanon (Stevenson 1980), and Daie et al. (1992) cite a clinical instance among the Druze in Israel.

Memories of a past life are usually triggered by some partial reminder. Four-year-old Naseem saw his father cut a sheep's throat and, bursting into tears, recalled that he himself had been a soldier who had attacked a Christian village with sixteen others, all of whom were captured and had their throats cut three days later. (In this case he was later found to have been born three months before the actual raid and was not able to recognize anybody in his previous life village, so he is not generally regarded as being that particular reincarnation.) Hareem's father Faris (Case 3 below) tells of how he had gone to a local well with his own father as a boy, and then recalled how in a previous life as his father's boss he had drowned in the well: his last memory was lying in the water with a rescue ladder on top of him. Faris' father had then taken him to the presumptive past-life family where he recognized photographs of his past-life wife and her relatives. He was recognized by his past-life daughter who still visits him, but not by his past-life uncle who is the head of the household (apparently because he then tried to help the daughter claim some property in Beirut).

Knowledge of past lives is normally limited to the one immediately before the current life. Generally, human souls have no such knowledge of a past life unless they die violently: the reason given being that the 'person' is not easily reconciled to a sudden death and is taken protesting from their previous body. This memory possessed by the soul is especially significant in the surge of reincarnation beliefs in the aftermath of the Lebanese civil war of the 1980s, of which I shall give some illustrations. Most Druze, like other Lebanese, are currently engaged in reconstruction after the war: few families have been left untouched by the war killings, massacres of civilians and other atrocities of that period (see Fisk 1992, for a detailed account).

Reincarnation Narratives

Case 1

Alaa S. is now twelve years old, the son of a plumber. At the age of two years, he demonstrated a familiarity with both car engines and guns, including habitually lying under a favourite car exhaust, which his family could not readily explain. As he learned to talk, he used phrases usually only spoken by old people and sheikhs. At six years old he led his father to a shop some miles away where in a previous life he used to run a car-exhaust business. People working there told me he knows the details of the business and can describe work-people and incidents in the workplace which he could not have known about by general conversation. He asked about holes in the garage floor which were filled in seven years before. His death in an earlier life is recalled by people in the car exhaust business: he was a sheikh, one of six Druze militiamen in a car who were taking another soldier to hospital when a rocket hit the car, and all were killed. In his current life he does indeed seem very familiar with car engines and trade details of replaceable parts such as tyres and exhausts for which he does not seem to have had any special training: 'I look at a car and what's in it; it's knowledge that came with me. Nobody taught me'. The boy does not seem to have gained financially by being identified as a reincarnation of the dead man, but his family regularly visits his past-life relatives, and a friendship has grown up between them.

Case 2

Abeer S. is now twenty-one years old, the daughter of a life insurance salesman. When she was about the age of four or five years, her parents became concerned about her because she spent a large part of the day by herself moping and crying. She had one older brother who was handicapped, whom she had to look after and who died when he was eighteen: there are no other siblings. A couple of years later, her grandfather saw her crying again and asked her why. She told him she missed her previous-life family and he insisted that her parents located them. She went with her father in his car and turned up at a village some twenty miles away (familiar to him from his work, apparently not to her in this life) and she recognized the house of a previous-life aunt and the neighbourhood. Her past-life father told me she had not hesitated in the recognition; and he himself had known at once that she was the reincarnation of his daughter who had died some years previously at the age of fourteen after a mortar shell hit the car in which she was travelling (when shopping with her cousin who had also died). He told me that since his daughter's death he had kept an eye open for her reincarnation, for he missed her. When Abeer appeared at the age of ten, he knew immediately that she was the reincarnation of his daughter. His wife backed him up but other daughters of his had agreed somewhat more slowly and (reluctantly?) that she was their sister. Relations between the two families are now very close, involving mutual exchanges of gifts and regular visiting, although Abeer's pre-reincarnation family is much wealthier and is considering putting her through college which she could not otherwise afford. Her present-life parents express no doubts about the relationship, pointing out that her 'new' parents have an equal share in her. Relations between the two families appear very cordial. Abeer was only born two months after the death of her previous life incarnation, but Druze allow for a short 'detour' between lives. I took her to the site of her earlier death where she recalled standing by the side of the car when the shell hit. She met again the men who had retrieved her body, one of whom she said she had known in her earlier life.

Case 3

Haneen A. is a ten-year-old schoolchild in Eghmid who recalls a past life as a school teacher and mother of five, Safa, who was killed in her back garden in Bchamoun (ten miles away) by a shell from the US battleship New Jersey.[4] In 1984 it was shelling the Shuf mountain villages at a point in the civil war when the Druze were opposed to the Maronite Christians who then had American support (Fisk 1992). Her elderly husband, Ajaj, was in the garden putting out a fire caused by the shelling and as she went to call him to come in out of danger, she was struck by a shell splinter in her neck and was killed. She recalls her body being licked after death by the household dog, of which she is still frightened because he had 'eaten' her. She then remembers being carried away by some soldiers but nothing more. Haneen now recalls the names of her two pre-reincarnation sons, Riyadh and Nedr, and her three daughters Shahira, Adla and Nebila, after whom she had spontaneously named her dolls, and details of the house. Her present-life parents report that at the age of 2 ½ years she had talked of having a son named Riyadh and of living in a village, Bchamoun, about ten miles away. Haneen's 'this-life' father, Faris, had also been reincarnated and told her stories about it. She was identified by the now grown-up daughter from her past life, Shahira, who had visited her after hearing rumours of a reincarnation, and recognized her because of her immediate familiarity with the names of the family. Haneen was immediately taken back to visit her past-life family where they say she successfully found her way around the home and identified objects and people, although being frightened of the garden where the shell had landed. Her past-life son, Riyadh, immediately recognized her as his mother and hugged her. Relations between the two families are cordial, although her current-life father is a bus driver whilst her past-life son is a wealthy currency dealer. She expresses sadness at the recent illness of her past-life husband, Ajaj, who is now an old man, attends like a wife to his plate at mealtimes and calls him by his first name, and as a young girl once slapped the face of her adult 'grandson' for talking rudely to his 'grandmother'. When Adla, one of her past-life daughters, appeared wearing her own mother's (Safa's) clothes, Haneen asked if they were her (Adla's) own, and Adla said 'yes': Haneen then called her a liar. Riyadh told me that Haneen talks like an adult and to outsiders appears a strange mixture of adult and child. She appears very confident in her role as an elderly woman, taking on the gestures and mannerisms of an adult. Riyadh confirms that she has the same personality as the dead woman, proud and moral, and that she worries about Riyadh and Shahira as if they were her children. Her present-life father, Faris, says she is now more settled having discovered her original family.

Bereavement: The Local View and Psychological Interpretation

Less than 10% of Druze seem to have firmly accepted memories of a past life, although all assume that they have been reincarnated.[5] They reluctantly admit that the rediscovered past-life family is often wealthier than the present-life family but say that this is no motive for asserting a particular reincarnation. Recognition as a reincarnated person confers no accepted special status (inheritance, etc.) and appears to operate socially through affective bonds and gifts alone. In many instances, the bereaved family had searched for the reincarnated soul of the dead person and met the claimant to reincarnation 'half-way', the criteria for authenticity in such cases being fairly low, generally being an apparent ability to recognize relatives. Evidence for and against the reincarnation of a lost relative is debated vigorously and I came across various 'failed claimants' (who are regarded as innocently mistaken), such as Naseem above. Hussan, a ten-year-old boy from a broken home, remembers that in a past life he was a soldier called Raja who was shot in the ear and died. But Raja (who lived in a neighbouring village) was actually still alive and it was his brother Murfa who died. A friend of Murfa also died at the same time and had already been accepted as having been reincarnated in Hussan's village. Hussan is now recognized as having been mistaken but nobody attributes mercenary motives to him (Raja's family again were relatively wealthy compared with Hussan's, whose father had no job).

What actually constitutes a 'soul' and its continuation across different lives is uncertain. Some argue for common features of personality (such as courage, nurturance or generosity), particularly in socially acknowledged instances, but many say the soul has no recognizable human characteristics at all. Most reincarnations are instantaneous, but the Druze were skilled at avoiding questions about the correlation of battle deaths and new pregnancies (which would be necessary to make available new human bodies).

In relation to the personalities of the children who claim (or are recognized) to be specific reincarnations, there appear to be no abnormal features, except for a slight sense of dissatisfaction; but we cannot exclude this from the normative expectations of everybody being reincarnated. This would agree with Daie et al. (1992). It may be significant that the period of volunteering reincarnation narratives – typically between three and six years of age – corresponds to the 'family romance' period identified by psychoanalysts, when the child is apparently prone to fantasize that they are really the children of more glamorous or famous parents. In one case reported by Stedman (1998), a three-year-old Druze village boy claimed he was the reincarnation of a well-known footballer and singer, whose own family accepted the relationship. It is not too difficult to realize how general expectations, reinforced by grieving relatives, confirm the child in their identification. In some cases, such as Haneen (Case 3), the identification is primarily made by the bereaved relative. As Stevenson (1980: 13) comments: 'Druze parents nearly always encourage their children to tell them whatever they can remember of their previous lives'.

When asked directly about any personal value for the belief, Druze unanimously agree it has had a validity in having bound together as a single community people who were dispersed over four different countries with diverse public policies of their governments. Druze in Israel have been at war with those in Syria (Israeli Druze join the Israeli armed forces).[6] To acknowledge some function for customary ideas in no way questions the belief itself and I met no Druze who doubted the likelihood of reincarnation. Many mentioned that the idea usefully led to fearlessness in battle and quoted a Druze battle cry 'Tonight my mother's womb' (I'll be killed in battle today, but I shall be instantly reincarnated), which may go some way to explain the ferociousness of the Druze in war (Fisk 1992).

The most evident locally stated utility of the belief in reincarnation (given that bereaved relatives tend to seek out the soul of the one who has died) appears as part of a process of bereavement. Druze spoke of reincarnation beliefs as a support for the bereaved person. Though few of the personal characteristics of the dead person are believed to continue in their soul, enough survives to mitigate the loss of a person's identity. The social recognition of what constitutes death differs widely (Eisenbruch 1984b; Hertz 1960) whilst the actual type of mourning in Islamic societies may change fairly fast depending on political and cultural changes (Good and Good 1988). A problem for considering the therapeutic value of cultural systems for grieving is that we cannot start from any 'natural baseline' uncontaminated by culture (Eisenbruch 1984a, 1984b). As Phillips (1999: 6) notes, 'It is possible that we have no idea what secular grief is; what grief unsanctioned by an apparently coherent symbolic system would feel like' (see Wieseltier 1998). Psychological theory, deriving from Euro-American experience, argues that first the reality of the loss has to be accepted, then the emotional pain is 'worked through', with an eventual detachment from the deceased (Parkes 1972; Pincus 1976). Druze ideas would seem to contradict the first stage. The cross-cultural evidence however argues that denial of the actual death, if supported by a systematized set of values, may be adaptive for the individual.

Al-Adawi, Burjorjee and Al-Issa (1997) describe the *mu ghayeb* concept in (Arab) Oman in which an assumption that the dead is only ensorcelled and will return alive usefully seems to deny the loss altogether, in a similar way to zombification ideas in Haiti (Littlewood and Douyon 1997). Assumptions of reincarnation, though equally contrary to Islamic tradition, are not such a radical denial of the death itself. The individual has died in a real physical sense and yet the notion of death itself is attenuated compared with other societies in which death is the immediate end of the individual.

Mourning among the Druze is restricted to a short period and overt grieving discouraged, as I witnessed at funerals (also see Firro 1992; Stevenson 1980). Thus, the psychological substitution of the dead relative by the hypothetical reincarnee takes place at a fairly early stage in the grieving process. The obvious sort of psychological interpretation would be that having reincarnation beliefs to account for violent deaths in the civil war usefully diminishes socially wasteful mourning in the context of a central religious tenet which already provides solidarity and unity for a community under immediate threat.

That Druze give psychologically functional reasons of this sort for their reincarnation beliefs – that it serves to alleviate grieving – in no way alters the validity of the belief itself. But nor does it necessarily provide a model for us to decide the origin and individual articulation of the phenomenon: Durkheim (1982: 171) expressly ruled out agents' explanations for their own actions, a view with which 'structural' anthropologists and sociologists concur. We are enmeshed in a web of culture which we can never comprehend objectively. If we do follow the local informants, however, and argue for some sort of psychological purpose for reincarnation beliefs, where does this leave Durkheim's view that religious institutions cannot be explained by individual psychology? Various possibilities include:

(1) The Druze tradition of reincarnation has only become 'psychological' in response to a modern worldview (individualization and psychologization) and, particularly, the immediate context of my investigation and its reception by the Druze.
(2) Satisfying psychological needs is not primarily related to an institution but it may later serve to maintain it by some process of social selection.
(3) Psychological need satisfaction is an occasional and insignificant by-product of social institutions.
(4) We are unduly influenced by the explicit local views as to what constitutes a psychological explanation.
(5) Durkheim is mistaken when he maintains of a person that 'beliefs and practices of his religious life [,] if they existed before he did, it follows that they exist outside him' (Durkheim 1982: 50–51).

The evidence offered here does not easily help us to answer this difficult epistemological question one way or another, but I would support (2) as the most promising. It does, however, call attention to a too-easy assumption that social institutions are to be explained through their satisfying individual psychological needs.

Notes

1. On a brief fieldtrip in 1997/98 to make a film on Druze religion. Interviews were carried out in homes and workplaces, at funerals and during religious meetings (*khalwa*) in the Shuf mountains south of Beirut. I owe a particular debt to Jad Al Younis for local Druze knowledge and for interpreting from the Arabic, and especially to Chris Ledger, without whose preparatory work this study would have been impossible.
2. I talked with the son of the paramount Druze religious figure (sheikh al-aql), Sheikh Bahjat, who publishes a religious magazine which combines Druze religion with an interest in pyramidology, flying saucers and Teutonic mythology. His father maintained to me that there is no esoteric Druze religious doctrine at all, for all religions aim at the same truth, yet one should not seek for a Creator outside oneself. This set of 'liberal' and near-pantheistic ideas is somewhat at variance with the past Druze tradition of not sharing their religious ideology with outsiders (De Nerval 1984), and the fierce solidarity of the Druze community during the recent civil war in the Lebanon (Fisk 1992). I was openly invited to attend the regular meetings of the *uqqal* with my interpreters (a Druze man and later a Sunni woman). It is likely that the Druze tradition of dissimulating their beliefs in the past was to avoid orthodox (Sunni and Shia) persecution: as they put it, 'a Muslim outside and Druze "at home"' (Daie et al. 1992).
3. The possibility was often raised that I myself was a Druze 'inside' because of my interest in the community, and after I became ill Sheikh Bahjat's son wondered whether if I had died my soul would have become incarnated in a recognized Druze. It might be noteworthy that, in the nineteenth century, the Druze accorded a special religious status to the English (Inchbold 1906: 83), perhaps a consequence of the 1830 Druze–British alliance against the French-backed Maronite Christians. There have been various speculative theories for Druze origin, giving them an English or Frankish (French) crusader ancestry.
4. My companion Roy Stonman has reported this incident at greater length (1998).
5. On going to a local school and asking an assembled class of twelve–fourteen-year-olds, about 10% agreed they had accepted memories of a previous reincarnation.
6. In another example, Adham B. at the age of three years reported a past life as Ràad Ismail (the same name as a schoolfriend of his). In this past life Ràad was apparently the pilot of a Syrian air force plane which crashed in the Barouk Mountains in 1984, together with Ràad's father as navigator. Plans to visit Syria with Adham were prevented by the refusal of a visa from the Syrian authorities.

References

Abu-Izzeddin, N.M. 1984. *The Druzes: A New Study of Their History, Faith and Society*. Leiden: E.J. Brill.

Al-Adawi, S., R. Burjorjee and I. Al-Issa. 1997. 'Mu-Ghayeb: A Culture-Specific Response to Bereavement in Oman', *International Journal of Social Psychiatry* 43: 144–51.

Betts, R.B. 1988. *The Druze*. New Haven, CT: Yale University Press.

Bourdieu, P. 1977 [1972]. *Outline of a Theory of Practice*. Cambridge: Cambridge University Press.

Boyer, P. 1994. *The Naturalness of Religious Ideas: A Cognitive Theory of Religion*. Berkeley: University of California Press.

Daie, N., E. Witztum, M. Mark and S. Rabinowitz. 1992. 'The Belief in the Transmigration of Souls: Psychotherapy of a Druze Patient with Severe Anxiety Reaction', *British Journal of Medical Psychology* 65: 119–30.

De Nerval, G. 1984 [1853]. *Journey to the Orient*. London: Owen.

Durkheim, E. 1915 [1912]. *The Elementary Forms of the Religious Life*. London: Allen and Unwin.

______. 1952 [1897]. *Suicide*. London: Routledge and Kegan Paul.

______. 1982 [1895]. *The Rules of Sociological Method and Selected Texts on Sociology and Its Method*. London: Macmillan.

Eisenbruch, M. 1984a. 'Cross-Cultural Aspects of Bereavement: 1. A Conceptual Framework for Comparative Analysis', *Culture, Medicine and Psychiatry* 8: 283–309.

______. 1984b. 'Cross-Cultural Aspects of Bereavement: 2. Ethnic and Cultural Variations in the Development of Bereavement Practices', *Culture, Medicine and Psychiatry* 8: 315–47.

Firro, K.M. 1992. *A History of the Druzes*. Leiden: E.J. Brill.

Fisk, R. 1992. *Pity the Nation: Lebanon at War*. Oxford: Oxford University Press.

Gilsenan, M. 1996. *Lords of the Lebanese Marches: Violence and Narrative in an Arab Society*. London: Tauris.

Good, M.-J. and B. Good. 1988. 'Ritual, the State and the Transformation of Emotional Discourse in Iranian Society', *Culture, Medicine and Psychiatry* 12: 43–63.

Hertz, R. 1960 [1907]. *Death and the Right Hand*. London: Cohen and West.

Inchbold, A.C. 1906. *Under the Syrian Sun*. London: Hutchinson.

Kiev, A. 1972. *Transcultural Psychiatry*. Harmondsworth: Penguin.

Littlewood, R. 1993. *Pathology and Identity*. Cambridge: Cambridge University Press.

______. 1995. 'Psychopathology and Personal Agency: Modernity, Culture Change and Eating Disorders in South Asian Societies', *British Journal of Medical Psychology* 68: 45–63.

______. 1998. *Reason and Necessity in the Specification of the Multiple Self*. Royal Anthropological Institute, Occasional Paper No. 43. London: RAI.

Littlewood, R. and C. Douyon. 1997. 'Clinical Findings in Three Cases of Zombification', *Lancet* 350: 1094–96.

Makarem, S.N. 1974. *The Druze Faith*. New York: Caravan.

Malinowski, B. 1944. *A Scientific Theory of Culture*. Chapel Hill, NC: North Carolina University Press.

Mauss, M. 1979 [1934]. 'Body Techniques', in M. Mauss, *Sociology and Psychology*. London: Routledge and Kegan Paul.

Murphy, H.B.M. 1982. *Comparative Psychiatry*. Berlin: Springer.

Obeyesekere, G. 1981. *Medusa's Hair: An Essay on Personal Symbols and Religious Experience*. Chicago: University of Chicago Press.

Parkes, C.M. 1972. *Bereavement: Studies of Grief in Adult Life*. Harmondsworth: Penguin.

Phillips, A. 1999. 'Commanded to Mourn', *London Review of Books*, 18 February: 3–6.
Pincus, L. 1976. *Death and the Family: The Importance of Mourning*. London: Faber and Faber.
Salibi, K. 1988. *A House of Many Mansions: The History of the Lebanon Reconsidered*. Berkeley: University of California Press.
Stenman, R. 1998. 'Lebanese Research among the Druze', *Reincarnation International* 15: 11–21.
Stevenson, I. 1980. *Cases of the Reincarnation Type: 3. Lebanon and Turkey*. New York: Alloh.
Tseng, W.-S. and J.F. McDermott. 1981. *Culture, Mind and Therapy*. New York: Brunner/Mazel.
Turner, V. 1967. *The Forest of Symbols: Aspects of Ndembu Ritual*. Ithaca, NY: Cornell University Press.
Wieseltier, L. 1998. *Kaddish*. New York: Knopf.

Chapter 9

Apocalyptic Suicide

> . . .this heaven and this earth shall cease, and a new world shall begin . . . Then shall the world's corruptible qualities be burnt away, and all those that held correspondence with our corruption shall be made fit for immortality, that the world, being so substantially renewed, may be fitly adopted unto the men whose substances are renewed also.
>
> —Augustine, *The City of God*, Book 20, ch. 14, 16

Introduction

Research into individual suicide is commonplace, but little work has been done in relation to group suicide. It cannot be assumed that the dynamics of group suicide mimic those of individual suicide, nor that each person in the group has exactly the same motive (or indeed intention) for committing suicide. The individual may be conforming to what for shorthand we may refer to as 'social pressures' deriving from the group dynamic. Here we concentrate on one particular form of group suicide: apocalyptic suicide – suicide amongst a group who hold that the world will end imminently. The issue has been briefly reported on by Dein and Littlewood (2000) who have discussed the psychological circumstances in which apocalyptic suicide occurs. It is well recognized that religious or religio-political groups can be violent either to themselves or to others, reminding us of the proximity of violence to the sacred (Girard 1977; Grotanelli 1988).

Mass suicide among religious groups has been recorded among the Jews of Masada during the Roman war of the first century CE, among the heterodox Christian group of Montanists (Cohn 1993), the Jews of medieval York (Alexander 1984), and among the sect of Old Believers in Russia (Robson 1995). We might note affinities with suicide in other circumscribed small-scale societies, such as the practice in Rajasthan of *jauhar* where a group of women carried out self-immolation to avoid capture and subsequent dishonour (Harlan 1992; Adityanjee 1994). Such group suicide may be understood analytically as a form of resistance or even rebellion, which expresses discontent, or in a limited attempt to disrupt or modify the wider social order (Grottanelli 1985).

Over the past thirty years there have been a number of reports of mass suicide among the newer religious groups in Western societies. In 1978 mass self-poisoning occurred among nearly all members of Jim Jones's Peoples Temple in Jonestown in Guyana, a group uniting contemporary Pentecostal healing with left-wing American political activism (Hall 1987; McCoy 1988). In the course of an investigatory visit by a United States Congressman, he and four companions were shot, and immediately afterwards Jones and his followers committed suicide by drinking cyanide-laced Fla-Vor-Aid (a soft drink). In 1993, near Waco, Texas, the US Bureau of Alcohol, Tobacco and Firearms (BATF) carried out a raid on the Branch Davidians, a breakaway group of the Seventh Day Adventists led by one David Koresh. After a siege of more than a month, almost all Branch Davidians who remained in the compound died after it was set alight by Koresh's followers (or perhaps by the BATF: the question of who, precisely, remains controversial) (Lewis 1994; Tabor and Gallagher 1995; Wright 1999).

In the Solar Temple episode of 1994, a 'New Age' homeopathic doctor Luc Jouret and fifty-two of his associates killed themselves simultaneously in Canada and Switzerland in order to bring about 'transit' to the star of Sirius. Fourteen months later, sixteen of their colleagues died in a related incident in France, and five more committed 'ritual suicide' at the time of the spring equinox in 1995 (Introvigne 1995). In the Heaven's Gate suicide in 1997, thirty-nine followers of a Californian 'flying saucer cult' died from auto-asphyxiation apparently in the assumption that after bodily death, they would join a spaceship that awaited them behind the Hale-Bopp comet. Other less well publicized incidents include the suicide among seven members of the Friends of the Truth Church in Japan following their leader's death in 1989 (Takahashi 1989), and the threats of the Concerned Christians, a group led by Monte Kim Miller in 1999, who promised suicide and violence in order to 'force the end' (as Martin Buber put it) – the return of Jesus at the end of the last millennium. Although all similar in that they committed or planned to commit suicide, the internal ideologies of the groups clearly differed widely:

Christian millennialism, science fiction themes. All however were similar in that they were isolated from the outside world, and members appear to have been firmly monitored by the leaders (Galanter 1999). Certainly not all of them were 'millennial' in the strict definition: that is, concerned with the Second Coming of Christ or the arrival of the year 2000. The term 'apocalyptic', though still derived from Christian tradition, is perhaps more appropriate in generally signalling the eruption of a transcendent catastrophe into our mundane world.

What factors result in acts that to non-members appear totally irrational? Theories have ranged from focusing on the characteristics of the members before joining, the authority of the leader and on influences from outside the group. An adequate theory presumably must be able to discriminate between those apocalyptic movements that are violent and the vast majority, which have never been, nor are likely to become, violent. One of us has recorded a Jewish apocalyptic group who anticipated an imminent and radical change in the world order but have never been violent (Dein 2001).

Psychological Theories of Apocalyptic Suicide

In terms of personality, we have little evidence that the members who participated in these suicidal groups were radically different in any way from others in their society (Hall and Schuyler 2000). There are few empirical psychological studies of the members for obvious reasons, but one interpretation suggests that some possess 'borderline personality' traits and in psychodynamic terms are prone to splitting, idealization and projective identification (Zee 1980). Survivors' accounts are biased to the extent that there is a need to justify post hoc their attraction toward and conversion to the movement (Littlewood 1993), but studies of new religious members suggest that their members are not conspicuously deviant. Similarly, an approach that focuses on the personalities of the leaders has little discriminative value. Storr (1996) speculatively points out that leaders of many new religious movements share some similar characteristics: an absent father from a young age, solitude in childhood, intolerance of criticism, a personal revelation, and narcissistic and paranoid personality traits. Storr's examples include Jim Jones, David Koresh and Shree Rajneesh (the founder of the Hindu Rajneeshi sect). All three possessed narcissistic and paranoid personality traits and were intolerant of criticism, with a background of childhoods marked by distant fathers.

Charisma and Pathology

The notion of charisma is commonly invoked as a reason 'why' cult members perform the actions they do and is appealing to psychiatric and psychological commentators because of an easy assumption of psychopathology in the leader. The term is employed by sociologists to refer to a group characterized by special personal qualities or powers claimed by and for the individual leader and was introduced into social sciences by the sociologist Max Weber. In his discussion of types of authority, Lifton (quoted in Lamberg 1997), a psychiatrist with an interest in authoritarianism, uses the term to argue that the leader has 'total control' over the group on account of his perceived exemplary qualities. It has, however, been argued by sociologists and anthropologists that charisma has no explanatory value in itself and is merely the description of a type of society (Worsley 1973; Littlewood 1993). However, this type of leadership might seem relevant to mass suicide because it seems sometimes to be associated with group fragility precisely because it is inherently precarious (Weber 1946): clearly the leader may at times become ill, elderly or even die.

If millennial or revitalist leadership often seems consequent on some intense personal experience, the model most applicable to the relation between prophet and follower – the reception of the message and its amplification and reworking – would appear to be that of charisma. As elaborated by Max Weber and his successors, charismatic authority derives not from the occupation of an already structured status but in the development of a highly personalized relationship between leader and follower which involves 'the social recognition of certain extrasocially sanctioned qualities imputed to the person of the leader' (Weber 1947). This seems particularly relevant to millennial movements for, as the student of 'the religions of the oppressed', Vittorio Lanternari (1963: 304), argues, 'there is probably no known religious phenomenon in which the dialectical interpretation of relationships between personality (the individual personality of the prophet) and culture (the social personality of the group) becomes more convincing than it does in regard to messianic cults'. Given psychiatry's presumptions of pathology (and thus idiosyncrasy) in millennial leaders, how did it envisage their influence over their followers? This is largely through the postulated mechanism of 'suggestion' (later to reverse its object and become 'transference'), which derives from Gustave Le Bon's studies of the crowd. Paradoxically, this argued for a loss of unique and 'higher' qualities in each individual participant to reduce the self to the lowest common denominator of the existing culture, where a single emotional tone could resonate spontaneously with that of the others; and thus we might suppose a situation of little innovation. Conceptualized primarily as a psychological mechanism, suggestion presumes a disengagement of the cognitive in favour of the affective. Freud has argued that the critical passivity of the crowd was a return to archaic patterns by a leader who took the place of the developed 'superego' (parental values internalized in childhood) of each follower, but Roheim (1940) emphasizes the attempt by all participants to rediscover a state of childhood bliss, a state which Devereux (1955: 156) restricts to the 'infantilised leader' alone.

Devereux and La Barre, however, agree with Freud that the charismatic leader, devoid of moral scruples, infects his entranced followers: 'All mobs forget their inhibitions, their critical judgement and their superego controls, and borrow for a time the superego of their leader. . . . The psychopathology of the mob leader that propels him to antinomian leadership in crisis now releases and mobilizes the hidden psychopathology in each mob member' (La Barre 1970: 14). La Barre identifies charisma as a contagious pathology: 'a folie a to a geometric power [in which] an authentic schizoid component in the prophet or the temporary schizophrenia of his dream speaks to passive fantasy in his faithful communicants' (La Barre 1970: 307). Devereux suggests that this sickness is already located in the prophetic moment: the charismatic leader takes power during a crisis when the usual adaptations to stress are inadequate, and society is in a 'schizophrenia-like disorientation' with individuals engaging in 'catastrophic behaviour'. But the solution then adopted is frankly irrational and can only lead to a vicious circle in which the actual situation gets increasingly out of control (Devereux 1955).

Lifton and Erikson have brought a greater epistemological sophistication to bear on these 'tenuous boundaries between identity crisis, psychosis, theological innovation and individual and historical revitalization' (Lifton 1974). Erikson (1965) argues that 'the great man of history' is less a psychopathic mesmerist than one who shares and anticipates the personal dilemmas of his contemporaries and, by solving them for himself by external action in society, solves them for others; leaders then are healers who have a 'grim willingness to do the dirty work of their ages'.

The objections to the type of unitary psychological closure offered by Devereux and La Barre are those which we offer against the nineteenth-century social theorists: an oversimplified unitary hypothesis based on second-hand comparative data that assumes a unilinear mode of cultural evolution and hence an inherent racism, together with ignorance of the specific contexts in which the particular institution has developed. We might add that unitary theories always have problems with anomalies, and historical 'survivals' are simply equated with pathologies, not surprisingly given the identity in psychoanalysis of the archaic, the primitive and the sick. While the analytic tradition appears superficially attractive in its claim not to split mechanism from meaning, thus promising a fruitful dialectic between psychopathology and society, the priority it gives to culture-bound and unitary biosocial categories reduces society itself to sickness, couched in the popular idiom of psychiatric denigration.

Given its clinical interests, for psychoanalysis there may be some slight justification for perceiving history through an idiom of pathology. Yet contemporary sociologists, who might be alarmed at the suggestion of any explicit affinity between themselves and psychoanalysts, share the assumption that the developments of millennial groups can be explained in terms of psychology, more specifically in the satisfaction of psychological needs through the generation of certain emotional states. In his account of the sociology of the Jehovah's Witnesses, James Beckford offers three explanations, two of which are pure psychology – frustration/ compensation and social solidarity, plus worldview construction. Beckford cites Lofland, whose sociological studies of a chiliastic sect led him to comment: 'It would seem that no model of human conduct entirely escapes some concept of tension, strain, frustration, deprivation or the like, as a factor in accounting for action' (Beckford 1975: 126). Barkun actually characterizes millennial movements as a 'regression from the social to the psychological' (Barkun 1974: 7). It may be that sociologists ignore individual (psychological) choices in established societies as apparently redundant but invariably introduce them when considering social movements, particularly those which appear dramatic and chiliastic. Those inclined to functionalism were concerned with social order in 'steady-state' systems for which there could be no ultimate cause and effect in linear time; psychological states, taken as autonomous and biological, seeking 'release', then had to be introduced to explain the rare change.

Millennial groups certainly engage frequently in antinomian actions – deliberate contraventions of conventional morality – but why should this be seen as primarily emotional? The particularly 'affective' idiom of such groups seems deployed to qualify them as undesirable, maladaptive and regressive – as not 'rational' in either the Weberian or the everyday sense. As with the evolutionary schema of psychoanalysis, the regression is both to hypothetical infantile and to archaic patterns. Devereux had stated that such groups have little hope of lasting success because of 'the health, maturity and potentiality of the [wider] public' (Devereux 1955: 156). In his textbook on social movements, Toch argues that 'fringe groups' must fail because they are specifically orientated to the emotional needs of their participants rather than to any wider intellectual or political concerns (Toch 1971, ch. 2). Wilson states that millennial groups are a 'deviant religious response', doomed to impotence by their affectivity and the contradictory doctrines of their disordered leaders (Wilson 1970: 37). Groups initiated by the mentally ill are considered particularly short-lived as Cohn (1957: 248) suggests in his account of the seventeenth-century British Ranters. Wilson (1975: vii) adds that these 'spontaneous' and 'non-rational' mechanisms are usually religious, for 'The only claim that could hope to stand against constituted authority . . . was a claim to power from a transcendent source great enough to be set over against existing power structures'.

Even apparently sympathetic observers are inclined to emphasize affectivity. George Woodcock, defending the Canadian Doukhobors who set light to their homesteads in protest at conscription and compulsory state schooling, cites: 'their irresistible excitement [for] Fire had become its own end, a passion that excited some of the arsonists to the point of orgasm as they watched the deadly splendour of their handiwork burst out against the night sky' (Woodstock and Avakumovic 1968: 347).

The argument of the sociologists approaches that of Freudian massenpsychologie. Some social groups, sects and rabble, have regressed from, or not evolved into, rational civil society, and remain dependent for their perverse ideology and degenerate actions on the authority of certain powerful others. They 'abdicated the responsibility they would have as individuals' (Robert Waelder, cited in Wolman 1973: 12); their primitive mental mechanisms have burst through the existing constraints by which society is properly constituted. Down there lies something nasty:

> a subterranean world, where pathological fantasies disguised as ideas are churned out by crooks and half-educated fanatics . . . There are times when that underworld emerges from the depths and suddenly fascinates, captures and dominates multitudes of usually sane and reasonable people . . . And it occasionally happens that this underworld becomes a political power and changes the course of history. (Cohn 1981: 14)

By relying solely on the overt normative values of the bounded society, this sentiment precludes the possibility that a society already contains dominant and subdominant sectors, out of whose conflicts and oppositions, contradictions and latent variants are always being generated, neutralized, accommodated or at times becoming central; for the 'present' has always to be recreated in our actions. The reason for change is seen then simply through those elements which do change as a distorting impulse external to proper society (as 'stress' or 'pressure'), as is the arbitrary mechanism ('affectivity' or even 'pathology'), and the immediate consequences are regarded as maladaptive. If the movement is 'established' and its motive returns to ends-means pragmatism, then emotion is said to ebb and we return to steady-state theories of social cohesion, recruitment, management of deviance and the like. We might note that even if an influential novel doctrine and practice must resonate with personal emotional experiences – what we may term 'affect' – such affects are themselves always socially constrained and are not independent of existing personal and social cognitions.

Societies have a culture no more than sects, sects a psychology no more than societies. Dominant ideologies, however, represent their dominance, to themselves and others, as a state of things independent of human choices: deviants and dissidents are relegated to an arbitrary under-world of personal pathology and emotion which alone can explain their futile actions. The subdominant live their lives through this ascription and thus there is more 'psychology' around at periods of revolt, in the experience of participants at least. And this experience becomes taken up into social theory as an explanation for how a given society (whose continued 'stability' is unproblematic and in which individual motivations and choices are apparently redundant) transforms itself: a dramatic leap into purely psychological if not psychopathological explanations to explain 'change', and then a return to the previous perspective. Sects (and societies) however continue to change, for, as Godfrey Lienhardt argues: 'their coherence is not that of a logically thought out, rational scheme of ideas produced by one mind only. After the initial appeal others make their contribution to ritual and doctrine. The "vision" of one man then becomes accepted by his followers as a source of their own distinctive collective experience' (Lienhardt 1974: 135–36).

Social scientists, anthropologists as well as sociologists, have shown little interest in examining how the fortuitous experiences of individuals may become formalized in an ideology, where tenets and actions are now tacit, less able to be negotiated; in which the random becomes transformed into the customary as the frame to which successive events and experiences themselves come to be referred, and in which individuals come to see themselves in a new way. The notion of 'charisma' is not unhelpful as a typological category for certain social institutions: as a general explanation it explains nothing. An adequate sociology of the genesis of new formations must demonstrate the relationship of the existing social order and its symbolic representations to the individual experiences through which are generated both customary understandings and any novel understandings on the part of the visionary, and how these experiences are taken up and revised, employed by others and structured through active social appropriation and transformation.

Sociological Theories of Apocalyptic Suicide

Emile Durkheim's claim that social institutions and values exist independently of particular individuals, are outside and above them and exert a constraining effect on them, shaping their lives, is taken as axiomatic by most sociologists: 'Insofar as he belongs to society the individual transcends himself, both when he thinks and when he acts' (Durkheim 1965: 29). It is not simply that human beings are driven both by internal (psychological) and external (social) factors but society functions to shape individual agency, socializing the individual into accepting that certain ends or goals rather than others should be pursued. Durkheim is well known for his functionalism whereby any social phenomena are explained by their interrelationship with other social institutions and serve to maintain overall coherence.

In his classic text, *Suicide*, he argues against the common sense nineteenth-century view that suicide is the most individual of actions. We cannot understand why people in these groups commit suicide by studying individual cases; while not totally denying that individual motivations may play some part in suicide, for him this act is enacted by the social collectivity. He attempted to demonstrate how suicide rates vary between different societies whilst for any given society the suicide rate remained constant over many years.

To explain this internal constancy and external variation he appealed to the two concepts of social integration and moral regulation. The former refers to the sharing of values, attitudes and beliefs among individuals. The latter refers to the fact that society functions to provide constraints over individual desires. Durkheim postulated a relationship between suicide rates and degree of social integration. He differentiates between four types of suicide: egoistic, altruistic, anomic and fatalistic, all of which are related to the cohesion and integration of the social group.[1] However, we would comment that concepts such as regulation and integration which are used to operationalize Durkheim's distinctions are not easy to define nor examine empirically.

Black (1990) deploys these concepts in his analysis of the Jonestown suicides using audio-tapes made by Jones and his followers prior to suicide. He argues that two typologies of suicides are relevant: altruistic and fatalistic. Some of the residents of Jonestown died because they put the group above the self and committed altruistic suicide:

> I would just like to thank Dad [i.e. Jones] and say that he has given us life and also death and I appreciate the fact of the way our children are going, because like the way I see it, when they come, what they are going to do to our children – they are going to massacre our children and also the ones that they take, they are going to just let them go out and be dummies like they want them to be and not grow up to be persons like the one and only Jim Jones. (Tape recording by follower prior to suicide)

The majority died for fatalistic reasons, according to Black, having lost hope in a demeaning and antagonistic external environment.

One member of Heaven's Gate, interviewed before the deaths, simply said she was bored with life and wanted to die (Hall 2000). What Durkheim does usefully suggest is that our idea of 'suicide' may cover a variety of different situations of self-killing: 'assisted suicide', sought martyrdom, a belief in 'translation'. We cannot assume that the internal thoughts of all members were identical at the time of death (any more than we can with individual suicide); they may include boredom, hope, or hopelessness, revenge or escape, or even an accentuation of a group's ideology of 'self-harm' (Old Believers barricaded themselves and their families in a church, which they set alight; the Skoptsi castrated themselves, as did Origen, some Montanists and members of Heaven's Gate), often in an attempt to shame the external world (the Doukhobors stripped off their clothes in the Canadian winter in front of the police and dynamited their villages). The Black Panthers' idea of 'revolutionary suicide' (better than the slow suicide of ghetto life) influenced the People's Temple (Hall 2000).

Apocalyptic Suicide as a Result of Perceived or Actual Outside Hostility

Perhaps a more useful approach is that which looks at a particular group's ideology in the context of the whole society. This argues that violence is precipitated through the actual or perceived interaction of the apocalyptic group with the host community. It emphasizes the ways in which members of the group recognize outside hostility and persecution (which they can often expect to experience on account of their deviant perspectives). This may be exacerbated by negative media reporting of the groups. In terms of their own apocalyptic scripts, outsiders embody the forces of evil which must be overcome at any cost in a great cosmic battle, and if this is not possible the group must escape from their influence even if it means suicide. Lindholm (1990: 155) writes in relation to Jonestown:

> Because Jim Jones had brought them together, because they had lost themselves and been reborn in the Temple, because they could not imagine any alternative to their unity, because they believed themselves to be under attack, the members were ready and willing to give up their lives rather than lose their community or the leader who crystallized it.

Similarly at Waco the federal agents represented an evil government system which had been referred to in the Book of Revelation as 'Babylon'. The idea of surrendering to 'proper authority', as the government agents demanded, was totally out of the question since these were in opposition to both God and his anointed prophet David Koresh.

In these two instances (Jonestown and Waco) there appeared to be real persecutors (the American Congress and BATF respectively). By contrast, for the Order of the Solar Temple the apparent threat was one of an imminent ecological catastrophe for the planet Earth, in other words a purely 'internal' view. But there was also a real threat from 'evil' authorities who tried to prevent what in internal terms was the expected transit to another planet.

Eschatological Dualism

'Evil' can be perceived as moral, located as a predisposition in humans, or as natural – as events in an external world (Neiman 2003): it is particularly in the former sense that we find it in religious and religio-political groups. Given the significance of a dualist eschatology in these groups, it may be helpful to trace this notion in the, particularly, Western religious tradition (Judaism, Christianity and Islam). In all three 'Abrahamic' faiths we find an idiom of the 'last days' in which the world will revert to a pure uncompromised state.[2]

Normal Cohn (1993), in his book on apocalyptic faith, argues that the Eurasian moral order before Zoroaster was primarily cyclical, immutable but constantly threatened by chaos – disease, witchcraft, famine, inundation, war. Chaos was kept at bay by everyday rituals or by a number of divine or semi-divine mythological heroes quite separate from the creator who fought with the chaos-threatening demons. The procession of time was essentially endless but with minor cyclical events such as the seasons as part of it. The rightful world order was identified with the intentions of the creator and might be glossed as righteousness, justice or the good (*ma'at* in Egypt, *rita* in Vedic Sanskrit, *kettu* in Akhadian, *asha* in Iranian Avestan, *tredeq* among the Hebrews). The rather minor role of the disparate demonic forces[3] took on in Iran, under the influence of the Zoroastrian reforms, a more severe and total form (*druj*), a single entity and power opposed to the order of *asha*; there is a constant battle between *asha* and *druj* which are now beginning to take the form of absolute good and evil, to end in the complete and total defeat of *druj*. Individual humans by their free choice have a part in the cosmic drama; by their seeking (or otherwise) for purity, they are constantly involved in this. In other words, a rather heterogeneous collection of ills and misfortunes are placed together as a cosmic evil, and the afterlife is transformed from a hazy Homeric afterworld into a radical dichotomy of heaven and hell.[4] This is now democratized: all people by their choice and actions will proceed to one or the other place in an end time when the world will be purified in a final cosmic battle after a period of tribulation, with a resurrection of the good dead to an eternal changeless bliss.

We have moved away from a series of rituals to protect the fertility of the crops to a cosmic drama which entered Jewish apocalyptic literature such as Daniel and the apochryphal 1st Book of Enoch, says Cohn, from Iran during the Achaemenian post-exile period, and thence to various Jewish sects including the Essenes and Christianity. The Judaeo-Christian Book of

Revelation proposes that transfigured human beings will be immune from disease, ageing and death: that time and history will have an end: and that the non-believers will be cast into the abyss.

The Relationship Between Apocalyptic Suicide and Suicide Terrorism

There has been an escalation of religious violence over the past ten years and at present reports of suicide bombing in the Middle East are commonplace. The events at the World Trade Centre on 11 September 2001 emphasize the close connection between religion and violence. What motivates young people to take their own lives in the name of religion? We would argue that a similar motive of overcoming the forces of evil underlies this form of religious violence. In a similar way to apocalyptic suicide, perpetrators of the attacks on America appeal to the notion of a cosmic war to provide the script being played out by militant religious activists. As Bin Laden proclaimed in a *fatwa* in 1998, months before the bombing of the American embassies in Kenya and Tanzania, the actions of the Americans had constituted 'a clear declaration of war on God, His messenger and Muslims'.

Whatever the rationale for suicide bombing, be it retaliation, martyrdom, economic rewards for one's surviving dependents or the promise of eternal happiness, it occurs against the background of a perceived state of war between Islam and the secular West, a situation generated in the gradual erosion of Islamic moral and family values by Western (especially American) globalization (Juergensmeyer 2000). The presumed attackers involved in the September 11 events derived from the Sunni tradition and were atypical to the extent that they were products of the Westernized middle and upper classes and led secular lives. There is little evidence that suicide bombers suffer from any formal mental illness: a recent attempt to account for suicide bombing in terms of *folie à deux* (or *folie à plusieurs*: Salib 2003) does not further our understanding of this phenomenon.

The cult of martyrdom is a predominantly Shi'ite phenomenon and generally not recognized in the Sunni *ulama,* and suicide bombing may be a new phenomenon with hardly anyone in a Muslim country having a notion of the suicide attacker until two decades ago (Kermani 2002). The first contemporary suicide bombers seem to have been Hindu Tamils in Sri Lanka fighting a Sinhalese-dominated government, and Hinduism is not generally perceived as immediately apocalyptic (see Note 2). Suicide is strongly forbidden by the Qur'an as is violence beyond that required for defending the faith. The idea of violence to root out moral and social injustice is not a Qur'anic principle. The terrorists' intellectual universe seems a deeply syncretic worldview involving Shi'ite traditions of martyrdom and novel Islamic notions of war, which put the protagonists into the position of victims who had every right to defend themselves. Makiya and Mneimeh (2002) discuss how the terrorists were informed by a manual containing Qur'anic notions of a 'holy raid' (*ghazwah*) condoning the slaughter of 'prisoners of war' (the airline passengers), hence justifying their actions. Both apocalyptic suicide and religious suicide bombing use the rhetoric of a final cosmic war in their justification of violence to rid the world of evil forces.

Conclusion

Apocalyptic suicide is a rare but significant event. A full understanding involves an examination of the complex interplay between the individual and the social. How do the individual motivations of the leader become incorporated into the social formation? How do the leader's aspirations articulate the group's concerns? By what processes do the members lose their sense of individuality to the collective self of the group? How does the ideology of the group develop into one whereby death is seen as transcendence? Ultimately, the question of apocalyptic suicide relates to the question of how individuals can achieve an extraordinary sense of selflessness to the extent that the coherence of the group becomes paramount over individual desires even to the extent of sacrificing their lives for it. In postmodern society where groups are oppressed by a system they consider to be illegitimate or meaningless, they may turn to a charismatic saviour who 'not only offers participation in an ecstatic communion, but also promises to lead a transformative crusade against the corrupt world' (Lindholm 1990: 175).

Notes

1. As Durkheim points out, these suicide types 'are not always found in actual experience in a state of purity and isolation. They are often combined with one another giving rise to composite varieties' (1897: 287). Egoistic suicide occurs as a result of excessive individualism when individuals become detached from the shared values and expectations of those around them. Durkheim explains the then higher suicide rates among Protestants over Catholics and Jews on account of the higher degrees of religiously driven individualism which characterizes Protestantism. Altruistic suicide occurs when the individual is so immersed in the social group that the individual in effect has no value: among observant Hindus, the past expectation was that the widow would throw herself on the funeral pyre of her dead husband – death became an obligation. Anomic suicide is associated with a lack of regulation in society: the individual is no longer located in a coherent social order. Fatalistic suicide occurs in societies dominated by inflexible rules against which there is no appeal by the individual. When a person's hopes and aspirations are blocked by oppressive

external forces, hopelessness ensues; this type of suicide is that committed by the despondent slave or that which occurred in concentration camps during the Second World War.
2. Though apocalyptic themes can be perceived in traditional Hindu and Japanese theology and among the Guarani, they do not have the centrality of the last days in Judaeo-Christianity, and hence Islam.
3. Job's Satan, for instance, is merely an instrument of the creator, not some independent ultimate principle.
4. Cohn argues that this occurred as Indo-Iranian culture became more militaristic with near perpetual warfare among the various Indo-Iranian societies (Cohn 1993: 94–95).

References

Adityanjee. 1994. 'Jauhar: Mass Suicide by Self Immolation in Waco, Texas', *Journal of Nervous and Mental Disease* 182: 727–28.
Augustine. 1945. *City of God*. London: Everyman.
Barkun, M. 1974. *Disaster and the Millennium*. New Haven, CT: Yale University Press.
Beckford, J.A. 1975. *The Trumpet of Prophecy: A Sociological Study of Jehovah's Witnesses*. Oxford: Blackwell.
Black, A. 1990. 'Jonestown – Two Faces of Suicide: A Durkheimian Analysis', *Suicide and Life-Threatening Behaviour* 20: 285–306.
Cohn, N. 1957. *The Pursuit of the Millennium*. London: Secker and Warburg.
_______. 1981. *Warrant for Genocide*. New York: Scholars Press.
_______. 1993. *Cosmos, Chaos and the World to Come: The Ancient Roots of Apocalyptic Faith*. New Haven, CT: Yale University Press.
Dein, S. 2001. 'What Really Happens When Prophecy Fails?', *Sociology of Religion* 62: 383–401.
Dein, S. and R. Littlewood. 2000. 'Apocalyptic Suicide', *Mental Health, Religion and Culture* 3: 109–14.
Devereux, G. 1955. 'Charismatic Leadership and Crisis', in G. Roheim (ed.), *Psychoanalysis and the Social Sciences: IV*. New York: International Universities Press.
Durkheim, E. 1951 [1897]. *Le Suicide*. New York: Free Press.
_______. 1965. *The Elementary Forms of the Religious Life*. New York: Free Press.
Erickson, E. 1965. *Childhood and Society*. Harmondsworth: Penguin.
Galanter, M. 1999. *Cults: Faith Healing and Coercion*. New York: Oxford University Press.
Girard, R. 1977. *Violence and the Sacred*. Baltimore, MD: Johns Hopkins University Press.
Grottanelli, C. 1985. 'Archaic Forms of Rebellion and Their Religious Background', in B. Lincoln (ed.), *Religion, Rebellion, Revolution*. Houndmills: The Macmillan Press.
Hall, J.R. 1987. *Gone from the Promised Land: Jonestown in American Cultural History*. New Jersey: Transaction.
Hall, J. and P. Schyler. 2000. *Apocalypse Observed: Religious Movements and Violence in North America, Europe and Japan*. London: Routledge.
Harlan, L. 1992. *Religion and Rajput Women: The Ethic of Protection in Contemporary Narratives*. Berkeley, CA: University of California Press.
Introvigne, M. 1995. 'Ordeal by Fire: The Tragedy of the Solar Temple', *Religion* 25: 267–83.
Juergensmeyer, M. 2000. *Terror in the Mind of God*. Berkeley, CA: University of California Press.
Kermani, D. 2002. 'A Dynamite of the Spirit: Why Nietzsche Not the Koran Is the Key to Understanding the Suicide Bombers', *Times Literary Supplement*, 29 March.
La Barre, W. 1970. *The Ghost Dance*. London: Allen and Unwin.

Lamberg, L. 1997. 'A Psychiatrist Explores Apocalyptic Violence in Heaven's Gate and Aum Shinrikyo Cults', *Journal of the American Medical Association* 278: 191–93.
Lanternari, V. 1963. *The Religions of the Oppressed: A Study of Modern Messianic Cults*. London: MacGibbon and Kee.
Lewis, J. 1994. *From the Ashes: Making Sense of Waco*. Lanham, MD: Rowman and Littlefield.
Lienhardt, G. 1964. *Social Anthropology*. Oxford: Oxford University Press.
Lifton, R. 1974. *Explorations in Psychohistory*. New York: Simon and Schuster.
Lindholm, C. 1990. *Charisma*. Oxford: Basil Blackwell.
Littlewood, R. 1993. *Pathology and Identity: The Work of Mother Earth in Trinidad*. Cambridge: Cambridge University Press.
Makiya, K. and H. Mneimneh. 2002. 'Manual for a "Raid"', *New York Review of Books*, 17 January.
McCoy, A. 1988. *The Guyana Murders*. San Francisco: Highland House.
Neiman, S. 2003. *Evil in Modern Thought: An Alternative History of Philosophy*. Princeton, NJ: Princeton University Press.
Robson, R. 1995. *Old Believers in Modern Russia*. De Kalb, IL: North Illinois University Press.
Roheim, G. 1940. 'The Garden of Eden', *Psychoanalytical Review* 27: 1–26.
Salib, E. 2003. 'Suicide Terrorism: A Case of Folie à Plusieurs', *British Journal of Psychiatry* 142: 475–76.
Storr, A. 1996. *Feet of Clay: A Study of Gurus*. Glasgow: Harper Collins.
Tabor, J. and E. Gallagher. 1995. *Why Waco? Cults and the Battle for Religious Freedom in America*. Berkeley, CA: University of California Press.
Takahashi, Y. 1989. 'Mass Suicide by Japanese Friends of the Truth Church', *Suicide and Life-Threatening Behaviour* 19: 289–96.
Toch, H. 1971. *The Social Psychology of Social Movements*. London: Methuen.
Weber, M. 1946. *From Max Weber: Essays in Sociology*, eds. H. Gerth and C. Wright Mills. New York: Oxford University Press.
Wolman, B. 1973. 'Sense and Nonsense in History', in B. Wolman (ed.), *The Psychoanalytic Interpretation of History*. New York: Harper.
Woodcock, G. and I. Avakumovic. 1968. *The Doukhobors*. London: Faber.
Worsley, P. 1973. *The Trumpet Shall Sound*. London: Paladin.
Wright, S. 1999. *Armageddon in Waco*. Chicago: University of Chicago Press.
Zee, H. 1980. 'The Guyana Incident: Some Psychoanalytic Considerations', *Bulletin of the Menninger Clinic* 44: 340–63.

Chapter 10

The Advent of the Adversary

If I cannot move the Higher Powers, I will move the Infernal Regions.
—Freud's epigraph for *The Interpretation of Dreams*, 1899 – quoting Juno in the *Aeneid*

The argument of this chapter is fairly straightforward. Any novel system of Euro-American healing or salvation which presumes a wider cosmological framework starts by offering a relatively straightforward psychological therapy, which is in harmony with understandings of health, life and generation, and which is aimed at the amelioration of a characteristic dilemma. This core dilemma, whether sickness or sin, has its own fundamental and logical solution which is advocated as the basic practice of the movement and which, with its own redemptive narrative, is incorporated as a primary principle into a standardized procedure and personnel, such as a healing session, medical practice, prayer group, or congregation. However, over time, challenges start to appear: (1) dissident members leave the group whether their dissent was occasioned by a personal quarrel, or by theoretical or practical disagreements; (2) there is external criticism and sometimes public action against the group for its disturbing novelty; (3) members experience disappointments and failures of prediction with doubts about the efficacy of their healing in particular instances; (4) they themselves are affected by sickness, age and debility.

The primary principle by itself now seems inadequate to explain these challenges: a more complex system is called for. The movement responds by elaborating a second principle, which explains all four challenges as related to another power, one which is opposed to health, life, and generation; this is of the same general nature as the primary principle – the original core healing process – but now of countervailing polarity. Opposition and interaction between the original principle and its new negative may proceed by a continued conflict which is considered to exemplify the current crisis, or by complementarity, balance, and incorporation, and by embodiment in certain persons and situations which reference the group's general principles and powers. The negative itself may become reified as a malevolent force, possibly personified, against which members must struggle. Whether personified or not, the opposition between the two serves to contain them as discrete and antagonistic counterparts.

Malicious Animal Magnetism

The Church of Jesus Christ, Scientist (generally known as Christian Science) has endured extensive prosecution and lawsuits concerning the failure of its members to obtain conventional medical treatment for their own families and for their patients – although its founder, Mary Baker Eddy (1821–1901), did finally accept morphine at the end of her own life. And the church's history has been synonymous with internal disputes, quarrels, and schisms since its foundation in 1879. The central religious teaching, partly veiled in the language of nineteenth-century popular science, is that Man is a perfect manifestation of a perfect God. Consequently, Man cannot truly be sick, suffer, sin or die. Through understanding the nature of God, we can obtain control over our body and mind.

Mrs Eddy's idealist position equated spirit with mind and counterposed them to the material: 'There is no life, truth, intelligence, nor substance in matter. All is infinite Mind. . . Spirit is immortal Truth; matter is mortal error.' And 'illness' and physiological events can thus refer only to a belief or suggestion.[1] Adherents of Christian Science prayed to understand that they lived in a world without sin, sickness, and death. Its founder predicted that in the future she would be able not only to alleviate pain but to spiritually influence the actual physical process which apparently caused pain (Gill 1998: 630). Humans would become less sexual, just like angels, and one key follower announced that her own child was parthenogenically conceived, Mrs Eddy having acted as the Holy Spirit: this announcement caused yet another quarrel and subsequent schism and external derision.

The church grew up in a New England milieu of Unitarian Universalism and Transcendentalism, Emersonian self-reliance and pragmatism; it was characteristically American in its emphasis on self-actualization and perfection. In childhood, Mary Baker, the daughter of a small farmer, had experienced various ill-defined ailments which continued into adulthood despite recourse to hydrotherapy, phrenology, homeopathy, mesmerism, and spiritualism. She was cured intermittently by 'Dr' Phineas Quimby, a watchmaker and mesmerist (hypnotist), who proposed that diseases were only a product of the mind, and a cure could be obtained by the patient achieving the correct view. He played down the fears of illness which he said were typically encouraged by the local doctors (Fraser 1996: 56). Quimby argued that the effective mesmerist took on himself the patient's illness (which he could then later dissipate) and that he did not have to be actually physically present at the healing session. In partial remission from her troubles, Mrs Eddy enthusiastically took up his ideas and began to practise herself.

In the third edition (1881) of her book, *Science and Health,* which went through multiple revisions in her own life and after, Mrs Eddy included a chapter on 'Demonology' in which she denounced two early followers with whom she had quarrelled. As Christian Science grew, a series of such favourites were taken up by her, promoted and then discarded, with continuing internal disagreements, splits, and secessions, as it faced a critical popular press as well as denunciations from competing local churches. Eddy herself was undoubtedly a difficult personality.[2] She began to play down the original significance of Phineas Quimby as her own group grew, and a continuing theme within Christian Science studies remains the actual significance of Quimby for Eddy's teaching. His mesmerism was no longer considered a healing practice, and indeed was now regarded as the quite unhealthy influence of the mesmerist on other people. Recognized as the force opposing the purely spiritual healing of Christian Science, this was now termed Malicious Animal Magnetism (MAM). By the 1860s Eddy, having started on her own healing mission, realized she was more successful in educating the students in her Metaphysical College than in actual healing. And Christian Science, like the Jehovah's Witnesses, is didactic in its rituals: early on the church similarly banned extempore prayer and indeed any vocal prayer. Church meetings and treatment consist of reassertions and paraphrases of the Bible and Mrs Eddy's *Science and Health* (first published in 1875). Unlike the Witnesses, Christian Science is what Brian Wilson (1970) calls a 'manipulationist' group in which the means to salvation remain religious if textual, with the goals really being secular – education, health, and happiness.

If disease is simply intellectual error, then prayer alone is insufficient to cure it. A serious Christian Scientist must perform daily mental work in repeated assertions that error is powerless, and that truth and goodness are all pervasive. Unless this work is done, error might seem to have power, so afflicting people through their worries with real sickness and death (Wilson 1970). Some of its themes of mind/body interaction appear again in forms of later secular psychotherapy: thus the bodily experience of soreness might be attributed to the recognition that somebody somewhere 'is sore' with you (Wilson 1970: 164), recalling the ideas of the psychoanalytically-influenced Psychosomatic Medicine of the 1940s in which a lump in the throat – a physical sensation – is caused by one not being able to 'swallow' something mentally. Pierre Janet (1925) argued that Christian Science was the predecessor to modern psychotherapy in its emphasis on the mental, yet MAM, here following Quimby's teaching, can act at a distance, thus recalling our idea of witchcraft – but a witchcraft which can only affect the mind not physical nature itself.[3]

MAM operated, like healing, through the inculcation of a 'belief': 'a belief in homesickness tried to tempt Mrs. Eddy' (Gill 1998: 523): i.e. in conventional terminology she was almost homesick. Her third husband's death through MAM, she argued, was through the sending to him of a belief in arsenic poisoning: 'the theory of arsenical poisoning [through MAM] allowed her to reconcile her Christian Science doctrine with the fact of [her husband's] death', says her biographer (Gill 1998: 291). She maintained that truth was always manifest in practical experience – what she termed a 'demonstration'.

To counter the seditious effects of MAM – endless schisms, law suits, accusations of conspiracy to murder and so on – groups of students were encouraged to mentally resist it together, and in her later years Mrs Eddy, now known as 'Mother', organized special shifts of her household staff, called the 'watchers', to guard against it by prayer in such cases of malicious press attacks, household accidents and lost articles, the common cold and even bad weather. Each watcher specialized in averting one particular form of MAM. As the explanation for misfortune, sickness and the deaths of patients and family, MAM became increasingly salient in Mrs Eddy's teaching: some students complained that the majority of her classes now focused on it rather than on healing (Gill 1998: 651). Fear of MAM, along with the Christian Science doctrine of the unreality of disease, could proceed to the neglect of conventional medical and obstetric procedures, thus often leading to a death, and so to the confirmation of the actions of MAM itself (Gill 1998: 331): MAM occasionally killed members of her staff who were then brought back to life by Mrs Eddy. Interpersonal accusations were followed by counter-accusations as favourites were dropped, and the students and staff quarrelled and feuded: Mary Baker Eddy's generally sympathetic biographer, Gillian Gill, concedes that paranoia was 'endemic' in the movement from the beginning (Gill 1998: 433).

Negative Orgone Energy

In modern physics, energy is the capacity of a physical system to perform work, a conserved extensive property of a system which cannot be observed directly. Conserved, neither created nor destroyed, it can be changed into different forms. The concept emerged historically out of the idea of a living force (Aristotle's ἐνεργεια: activity or operation) and has been used in the modern sense since Thomas Young in the early nineteenth century amidst continuing arguments as to whether energy was actually a discrete substance or only a physical quality. In 1847 Helmholtz proposed in his law of the conservation of energy that all types of energy (mechanical, electrical, chemical, and so on) are forms of a single universal energy (Kraft). 'Energy' then became a popular and powerful trope, both in the mechanical world (Rabinbach 1990) and also in literary culture (Gold 2012).

Brücke, a physiologist who taught Sigmund Freud in Vienna, argued that all living systems are energy systems and coined the term 'psychodynamic' to emphasize that the brain-mind system operates along the principles of physics. He reduced psychology to neurology and 'described mental processes indifferently in physical and psychological terms' (Ellenberger 1970: 479). The neurologist Beard likened the human being to an electrical battery, and the term 'psychic energy' was used to refer to the number of (newly discovered) brain cells: a limited number of neurons led to a weak nervous constitution (or neurasthenia) and thus to a weak will – as exemplified by women in comparison with men (Littlewood 1996). This rather material idea of psychic energy harked back to Mesmer's eighteenth-century notion of a magnetic fluid which pervaded the universe, and which was the basis for all matter, an idea which maintained a certain wayward existence in the continuing practice of hypnotism; experiments on transferring personalities by means of electromagnets continued to be carried out into the twentieth century. Freud, a neurologist, abandoned his early attempt to place psychic energy on such a distinct physical platform, but his disciple Jung developed that possibility in assuming that psychic energy was somehow related to physical energy; even if that could not be demonstrated, or psychic energy measured, its principles paralleled those of the physical, notably in its properties of conservation and transformation (Ellenberger 1970).

Freud's follower and later critic, the Austrian psychoanalyst Wilhelm Reich (1897–1957), took Freud and Jung's early and concrete reading of mental energy to its most developed form. Rebelling against Freud's apparent downplaying of libido (psychic energy), in the 1920s he considered his own ideas on energy, love, disease, and the cosmos to be purely natural science (Rycroft 1971). By the 1930s Reich argued he could isolate 'life energy' ('bioenergy', 'primordial cosmic energy') in the form of vesicles (bions) and store it in accumulators (the famous healing orgone boxes, for marketing which he was later imprisoned in the United States). Bions could be seen under a microscope or be recorded by a Geiger counter, electroscope or thermometer as Reich carried out numerous experiments in his laboratory: 'the discovery of libido in vitro' as he put it (Reich 1973: 9). Once stored, bions could be used to control the weather, cure cancer or be condensed into new life forms. Reich equated this orgone energy with love: blue in colour as exemplified by the hue of sexually excited frogs, it had the power to move the planets and reconcile all polarities.

Reich left Austria to escape the Nazis, and then was forced out of Norway by the medical establishment there, and settled uneasily in America with a few followers, becoming increasingly conspiracy minded as he grew older (Reich 1969). Orgone energy was, he now argued, opposed by its converse, negative (destructive) orgone energy, such as nuclear energy, and which was manifest in clouds and in the stillness of the landscape, and in the silence of birds as leaves lost their turgidity. Negative orgone energy was bioenergy that had become stale and blocked. It had become 'sequestered' (Rycroft 1968) from orgone energy and turned against it. When thus damned up, it caused serious personality disturbances (character armour) and neuroses, cancer, and fascism. Reich located the opposition between the two in the autonomic nervous system, with the parasympathetic subserving pleasure and the sympathetic anxiety (Rycroft 1968).

Freud had argued that in the face of the conflict between the instinctual sexual drive (libido) and group conformity, characteristic defences were developed by the ego which led to an individual's character. Reich argued that these defences were a pathological armour, just like psychological symptoms but represented in the body's posture and musculature. He proposed the healthy genital character which was motivated purely internally and naturally, and was not subject to the 'compulsive morality' of an authoritarian culture (itself formed on the basis of similar individual repressions). Such mature genitality was demonstrated by Jesus Christ, the archetypal genital character, who was in close communication with the world's organic forces. Eventually, Reich identified himself with Christ as a similar martyr of genitality. Therapy consisted initially of bodily exercises, often whilst naked, and on occasion sex with Reich. Sexual energy, if not regularly discharged, said Reich, would be converted into anxiety (this had been an early idea in Freud's preliminary psychobiological schema which he then discarded in the 1920s) and thence into sadism. 'Psychic health depends on orgastic potency. . . the capacity for surrender to the flow of biological energy, without any inhibition, the capacity for complete discharge of all damned-up sexual excitation', said Reich, for God 'represents nothing but the personification of the natural laws which govern men and make him part of the universal natural process. . . One day science will succeed in handling biological energy, as today it masters electrical energy. Not until then will the psychic plague [the generation of negative orgone energy] find its master' (Reich 1968: 39, 114, 340). As his pupils built machines to shoot down UFOs (Turner 2011), eventually humans would evolve into a healthy spherical form. This materialized life force, later to be negatively personified in the form of Modju, the grotesque dictator, led to his expulsion from the International Psychoanalytical Association and the German Communist Party[4] in the same year. It is still maintained by Reichian groups in the United States under the name of Bioenergetics.

Thanatos

Sigmund Freud's introduction in the 1920s (in his book *Beyond the Pleasure Principle*) of a second biological instinct, the death instinct (Thanatos), which was opposed to libido, has been variably attributed to his own diagnosis of cancer in 1922 and to his consequent debility, but also to the deaths of a daughter and grandchild, to doubts in his circle about the very efficacy of psychoanalytical treatment (Robinson 1969: 20), and to increasing disputes over succession in the 'Byzantine politics' (Roazen 1979: 363) of the psychoanalytic movement. Certainly, Freud had quarrelled with and split from a large number of colleagues,[5] but looking at the chronology of the introduction of his new idea suggests that it marginally predated the formal diagnosis of his own sickness (Sulloway 1980). Freud's initial positioning of instinctual libido against social conformity was, after the First World War (in which three of Freud's sons had risked their lives), replaced by an interest in our evident ability to destroy and self-destroy. In war-ravaged Vienna, a miserable and starving remnant of the once extensive empire (with Freud losing all his savings in the post-war inflation), both Freud and Reich turned to elaborating new bipolarities in which each of the pair had a similar nature rather than the old opposition between the quite distinct biological and social. Reich protested that the new theory of the death instinct meant that the primacy of Freud's original genital libido was betrayed, and he complained that all interest in sexual libido had now been lost (Reich 1973), but it is debateable how many of Freud's orthodox followers have fully accepted the death instinct. Freud acerbically commented that Reich explained the new death instinct, not as biology but as capitalism (Robinson 1969: 37).[6]

There had been earlier precedents for the new idea of Thanatos: Jung's patient and lover, Spielrein, had suggested a death instinct in 1912, and Freud's colleague Adler, as far back as 1908, had proposed a primary aggressive drive which Freud had then denied. In 1915 during the First World War, Freud had published an essay, 'Thoughts for the Times on War and Death', in which he argued that aggressive instincts seemed evidently stronger than was previously believed, and our main problem was how to channel aggression. He no longer attributed hatred to transformations of the libido alone but to some separate, and at first vague, non-libidinous instinct (Ellenberger 1970; Sulloway 1980). At the same time, he was also concerned with explaining the compulsion to repeat found in hysteria and in children's play and which was also found in shell shocked soldiers' morbid and self-punishing dreams of extreme violence. The 1920s reformulation of these concerns into Thanatos now 'sought to restore the intellectual unity that had been undermined by certain conceptual inconsistencies that emerged in the previous decade', comments Sulloway (1980: 395).

Together with dealing with the 'negative therapeutic reaction' (i.e. the not uncommon finding of the patient becoming clinically worse as the psychoanalytic treatment proceeded), Freud's 'death instinct' (he himself seldom used the actual term 'Thanatos')[7] was less a drive to death than an explanation of the compulsion to repeat traumas[8] and to return to an earlier, simpler, state, an explanation which harked back to his thoughts in the 1890s on a psychological entropy of tension reduction. (Perhaps a more appropriate term for the death instinct would have been Freud's preferred label, the Nirvana instinct.) If the death instinct of Thanatos and the life-affirming libidinal instinct of Eros are opposed, they always go together and are necessary in life, effectively shaping and complementing each other. Life is a dialectic between the two until Thanatos eventually prevails at our death, with dissolution of the organism and our return to inanimate matter, the state before birth. In this sense, said Freud, 'the aim of all life is death', Eros (libido) being the postponement of death through flight forward. Whilst libido is psychic energy and increases tension, Thanatos is the converse. And aggression is simply Thanatos directed outwards in the service of Eros.

Reich is more monist in his schema in that for him libido should always seek expression and ideally triumph. Freud, at least, had a preference for dualist positions and he was generally opposed to monistic schemata (Wolheim 1971: 180; Roazen 1979: 274, 338).[9]

Satan

The postulation of our second, 'negative' complement to the primary principle, as found in Eddy, Reich, and Freud, seems to owe something to the personification of evil as an opposing but subordinate principle in the Judeo-Christian tradition. Paul Ricoeur (1967) has argued that there has been an historical development from early ideas of human impurity to a more internalized and individualized sense of sin in a strong sense, and that existing small-scale enclosed communities, such as those typically studied by social anthropologists, seldom have an idea of a strong absolute Evil which is opposed to a strong absolute Good. Neither, we might presume, did the earliest civilizations of the ancient Mediterranean and Middle East: the closest the ancient Hebrews came to metaphysical evil was evil in a weak sense, as impurity, defilement, blasphemy or the breaking of a contract. The Hebrews revered only their own god, and he eventually became their idea of the one and only God. Like other early absolute Gods, he seemed to have manifest characteristics of what we would now characterize as a coincidence of opposites, good and evil: 'I am the Lord and there is none else. I form the light and create darkness: I make peace and I create evil: I the Lord do all these things' (Isaiah 45: 6–7).

The idea of evil in a 'strong' unregenerate form seems to have developed in settled agricultural communities (Parkin 1983), and Iranian religion dichotomized the two emerging principles into separate deities, with one good god of light and one evil god of darkness who endlessly contend but with some indication that the good one will eventually triumph. Humanity is the battleground. Where, as with the Hebrew Yahweh, there was strictly only one single God, his evil aspect became split off into a separate but still subordinate being. Lesser malign spirits had been personified as angelic tempters or obstacles (satans) sent or permitted licence by the high God – as happens in the Book of Job. In the post-exilic literature of the Hebrew Apocalyptics, these and various other doubtful characters came together with the evil aspect of divinity to yield eventually something approaching a single negative principle (Russell 1977: ch.5): the 'children of God' (who were certain angels),[10] along with various named[11] adversaries, accusers, obstacles, tempters, rebels, angelic watchers, the spirits of the giants and other reprehensible figures. Satan then is a coalescence of what were once distinct characters such as these fallen Hebrew angels and who also become identified with various Hellenistic nature spirits and demons and with the pagan gods.[12] Satan appears now as a unitary figure in the Christian New Testament but is named variously – as Diabolus, Belial, or Beelzeboul, the enemy, the tempter, the accuser, the evil one, the ruler of this world, the prince of demons, and he becomes associated with the serpent of Genesis. St Paul equates this Satan with absolute metaphysical evil.

It became evident that the coming of Christ had not resulted in the final abolishment of sin, which was put off till his second coming; as the Christians awaited this, the idea of a contemporaneous Hell, which barely features in the New Testament, was elaborated (Russell 1977). The earlier rather nebulous Middle Eastern and Mediterranean afterworlds, such as the Greek Hades, now became transformed into a counterpart to Paradise as the site of eternal torment for sinners (a notion perhaps encouraged by the clearly demonic afterworld proposed by Zoroastrianism – a religion which impinged on Christianity not only through its earlier influence on the Hebrews in their Babylonian exile but through the contemporary Mithraism and Manicheaism).

Another important dualism entered Christianity through Greek philosophy (and perhaps through the 'mystery cults' of the eastern Mediterranean) and was partially equated with the divine/satanic: that between spirit and matter which had important resonances in early Christian asceticism (Brown 1988; Littlewood and Dein 2012).[13] In the form of man versus nature (or as mind versus brain), it is still with us as vulgar 'Cartesianism'.

All of this of course introduced a problem: if God was supreme and good, then how could he permit a satan to do evil? Later Jewish and Christian thinking attempted to resolve the question through different solutions – that ultimately apparent evil is only a higher good, or it is the creation of human free will, or else evil has no real existence but is the inevitable product of a good world, or even that the whole thing is a mystery which only God can comprehend (Russell 1977). Whatever the solution, Satan remains subordinate to God and can still act on his behalf as a tempter, but his new enhanced form has greater autonomy than in the past; he increasingly acts as though he were somehow independent of his divine creator, a process which continued throughout Christianity (Russell 1977: 259). The Christian figure of Satan thus preserved the semi-dualism of the Hebrew Apocalyptics; although created by and remaining subservient to God, he has considerable autonomy in leading humanity astray, encouraged by his own pride and jealousy and his wish to supplant God (Luke 10:15). So Evil always threatens to become a separate, equal, but of course contrary, principle: 'the God of this world' (2 Corinth. 4:4). Semi-dualism allowed Satan to be the agent of natural evil – earthquakes, floods, epidemics – as well as of moral evil which depended on humanity's free will although of course influenced by Satan, God's original tempter: even in the early modern period Satan could still punish us as a divine warning to repent (Maxwell-Stuart 2011).

By the end of the second century of the Christian era, we have then something resembling the definitive Satan. God created the world and mankind and angels, but a number of angels led by Satan rebelled against God through their own pride and were thrown out of heaven. Satan, now identified with the serpent in the garden of Eden (or having entered him), promotes the Fall of Man who, knowing sin, is expelled from the garden. Man is currently alienated from God, but all will be resolved by God's victory at the end of time, and Satan will be bound forever.[14]

The parallelism between the kingdom of God and the kingdom of Satan is shown well by the figure of the Antichrist (McGinn 1994). A general word for a false prophet in the Epistles of John, in the Book of Revelation the Antichrist becomes *the* false prophet. A human figure, in whom some said Satan was incarnated, he was the leader of Satan's mundane deceivers, and the term was used by Athanasius and others to refer to various heretical leaders within Christianity, such as Arius: Protestants and other critics used the term to refer to certain popes. The Antichrist closely imitated Jesus, but as inversion: thus, he had the power to make trees grow upside down (Almond 2014: 174).[15] If Satan was lord of this earth, then some heretics (Gnostic Christians, Cathars) argued for a fuller dualistic system in which Satan had actually created the world. The late medieval equation of the satanic with folk magic and witchcraft envisaged a whole counter-church in which rituals, prayers, gestures, objects, vestments were all turned upside down in a demonic parody.[16] And some critics commented that this symbolic inversion equated to a belief in two antithetical Gods (Almond 2014: 213).

If Christianity postulated a metaphysical universe of two principles, then the New Testament had already been packed with this-worldly healing stories. The Christian promise is therapeutic, not only spiritually but also physically: the blind shall see, the deaf hear, the crippled walk, and so on. And there was some sense that in an imperfect world, Satan was the ultimate cause of sickness. And certain missionary orders and congregations (Adventists, Salvation Army, Christian Science) have taken on bodily healing as being virtually on a par with spiritual healing.

Negative Power and/or Complementary Power?

Cultural psychiatrists and anthropologists have typically described non-Western nosologies and therapies as more dispersed than in biomedicine, typically extending out into the social and political world less contained. Parkin (1995) has argued that there is something particularly Western (Christian) about the epistemologies of biomedicine in that the disease (or spirit) is ideally totally eradicated rather than accommodated. So, there is a therapeutic preference for the total elimination (or exorcism) of the undesirable rather than an accommodation with it, as in the way an intruding disease or spirit may be supplicated and bargained with in most non-Western therapies (e.g. Crapanzano 1991; Boddy 1990). If my thesis is correct, we can expect an affinity between Christianity and biomedicine in their severe sequestration of the undesirable (disease eradication, surgery, 'exorcism') as opposed to the affinity between the more dispersed (latticed) notions of pathology (and psychopathology) found in the non-Christianized small-scale communities traditionally studied by social anthropologists. The clinical implications are beyond the scope of this present chapter but follow the bipolarity of contained versus extended.

One can of course perceive binaries anywhere, but is the dualism or near dualism suggested by our examples aetiological (and thus to be overcome – as with Jung), or a frank bipolarity, or an ambivalence, or what? Whatever the theoretical elaboration, it seems likely that for the sick person or the sinner, the appearance of the second force is overwhelmingly powerful. It is as a concrete personage. The sick person and the sinner are not especially interested in the analytics of the system. They just want to be rid of this sickness, of sin. And whether analytically we regard the second principle as a simple negation of the first's emphasis on life and health, or as its complement, is fairly arbitrary, depending on whether we take the system under consideration as being the original principle alone or whether as manifest in the byplay between the first and the second in a wider set-up.

If I have argued a similar nature (but opposed polarity) for the two principles, then how distinctive is the second, 'negative', principle? Satan, for instance, always threatens to become an independent, autonomous power but (heresies aside) he does not. He still has a role as God's tempter of Man. Although assimilated to the material world, he remains, like God, a spiritual power, distinct from God but created by God. Mary Baker Eddy is practically concerned with combatting Malicious Animal Magnetism among her congregation and is not deeply metaphysical, relying on the moral schema already afforded by local Christianity. Freud is the most dualist in maintaining two quite separate biological principles (instincts), Eros and Thanatos, but they can interact to produce other patterns such as aggression. Reich starts from Freud's psychoanalysis but his second principle, negative orgone energy, develops out a transformation of his first principle, orgone libido, after which orgone and negative orgone seem mutually exclusive.

Malicious Animal Magnetism (although Christian Scientists of course must have known that mesmerism had preceded Christian Science) is regarded as a jealous and vindictive antithetical power like Satan, attacking Mrs Eddy's congregation. Negative orgone energy, also like Satan, seems – as blocked or sequestered primary energy – similarly gone astray, as having experienced a 'fall' from grace. And Freud? Although originating independently but in a similar way to the vital energy of Eros, Thanatos maintains a fairly complete autonomy as a sort of negative vital energy.

In all three, each of the pair of principles acts against the other, but in this 'complementary opposition' (Needham 1973) they generate the dynamic texture of life as lived: in retrospect, the initial power alone now seems inadequate, one-dimensional, absurdly simplistic, and pathetically optimistic. If, as Bateson (1972) argues, a single unlimited unilateral power is unbalanced, making no sense in a relational epistemology, then the second principle is necessary. The immediate dialectical symbiosis, each shaping the other,[17] (never a synthesis) of the two appears most evident in Freud: one imagines that Eddy and Reich would have been appalled by the possibility of concerted action by Christian Science and Magnetism acting together, of orgone and negative orgone, although the Christian idea of an eventual resolution lies behind both, given their generally optimistic metaphysics. Eddy and Reich, like mainstream Christianity, talk of a final bliss at the end of time with humans becoming angels, the negative power neutralized, overcome in struggle with the primary principle, whilst Freud's more dualistic (and pessimistic) schema envisages the two, Eros and Thanatos, in an eternal play. Until our death.

Acknowledgements

I am grateful to participants at two UCL research seminars (Medical Anthropology, History of Psychology) and to the 2015 World Association of Cultural Psychiatry Conference in Mexico, where this chapter was first presented.

Notes

1. Thus 'there had recently been a belief of a birth in the house' (Gill 1998: 286), i.e. a baby had been born.
2. 'Shallow, egotistic, mad, ambitious, mercenary, tyrannical, man eater, drug addict, mesmerist, illiterate, illogical, uncultured plagiarist' were some of the attributes then given to her (Gill 1998: xvii).
3. Certain contemporary African Christian interpretations of witchcraft would maintain the same: that it only works through affecting the mind. As referred to below in the text, in the causation of bad weather MAM seems to be able to bypass the receiving mind to directly affect the physical world itself, a teaching which was implicit but not really elaborated in Christian Science. On the whole MAM was deemed to work on a mind-to-mind basis.
4. In his earlier, more conventional thinking, Reich had argued that psychoanalysis could understand the Marxist dilemma of why the working class did not always act in their own class interests.
5. Breuer, Fleiss, Adler, Jung, Stekel, Kahane, Rank, Rado and arguably Ferenczi. After quarrelling he dropped his academic references to them when reprinting his papers. According to Helene Deutsch, Freud described one erstwhile associate as a 'bum' and as senile (cited in Roazen 1979: 490), Adler was 'loathsome' and 'trash', a 'pernicious creature', whilst Stekel had ideas the size of a pea, and Jung was 'crafty' (ibid.: 201, 268, 23l, 270). Another ex-colleague was 'a case of moral insanity' (ibid.: 232). Freud engineered the expulsion of Reich from the movement, and three close disciples committed suicide when in dispute with Freud – Tausk, Silberer and Federn: Roazen (1979) lists at least thirteen suicides among Freud's close associates. Like Mrs Eddy, he had to 'protect myself against people who have called themselves my pupils. . . Now I must accuse them and reject them' (ibid.: 272). As with Eddy, he had moved away from purely therapeutic

endeavours to concentrate on producing a new generation of loyal followers (in his case through training analyses).

6. '(T)his wish to die was somehow [Freud's] own. He was sick. He was miserable. He was alone', countered Reich (1973: 73). But Reich also attributed Freud's new teaching to the analytical movement's turn against his (Reich's) faithful emphasis on libido and towards what became ego psychology: away from the biology of instinct towards a psychology of consciousness.
7. 'Thanatos' had been popular in nineteenth-century Romantic literature as the urge to destruction and self-destruction, death being likened to orgasm (*la petite mort*), and was used by the psychoanalyst, Stekel. A popular book of short stories had been published under that name in 1906.
8. Previously noted among criminals by Gustave Tarde in 1890.
9. Whether we take the tendency to antithetical dualisms as a universal human proclivity, as do the followers of Lévi-Strauss, is beyond the scope of this chapter.
10. Who descended to earth to teach women agriculture and have sex with them to produce a race of giants (Genesis 6: 2 and the Apochryphal books of Enoch and Jubilees), and who introduced vanity, violence and sorcery into human society, and were punished by God. St Clement unusually attributed the eventual fall of these demonic angels to Man.
11. Originally as common nouns which then became proper nouns as the names of identified personages, as a satan becomes Satan.
12. Such as phallic Pan, winged Hermes and trident wielding Poseidon.
13. And, of course, a number of other dualisms were polythetically linked to God : Satan, such as Male : Female :: Spirit : Body :: Light : Darkness :: Knowledge : Ignorance, etc.
14. Origen's suggestion that even Satan would finally be redeemed did not catch on.
15. As Origen said, the Antichrist was the simulation and negative of Christ, of the same character but opposite moral potency (Almond 2014). I am indebted to my student Dr Athar Yawar for pointing out to me that the Antichrist (Dajjāl) also features considerably in Islam: a human deceiver, he will eventually be defeated by Jesus (Kabbani 2003).
16. Black candles, prayers backwards, kissing Satan's anus, etc. This had become possible at the end of the millennium (1000 CE) on some interpretations of the Book of Revelation 20:1–10.
17. Bateson's schismogenesis.

References

Almond, P.C. 2014. *The Devil: A New Biography*. London: Tauris.

Bateson, G. 1972. *Steps to an Ecology of Mind*. St. Albans: Paladin.

Boddy, J. 1990. *Wombs and Alien Spirits: Women, Men and the Zar Cult in Northern Sudan*. Madison, WC: University of Wisconsin Press.

Brown, P. 1988. *The Body and Society: Men, Women and Sexual Reincarnation in Early Christianity*. New York: Columbia University Press.

Crapanzano, V. 1981. *The Hamadsha: A Study in Moroccan Ethnopsychiatry*. Berkeley, CA: University of California Press.

Ellenberger, H. 1970. *The Discovery of the Unconscious: The History and Evolution of Dynamic Psychiatry*. London: Allen Lane.

Fraser, C. 1996. 'Mrs. Eddy Builds Her Empire', *New York Review of Books*, 11 July: 53–59.

Gill, G. 1998. *Mary Baker Eddy*. Reading, MA: Perseus Books.

Gold, B.J. 2012. *Thermopoetics: Energy in Victorian Literature and Science*. Boston, MA: MIT Press.
Janet, P. 1925. *Psychological Healing*. London: Allen and Unwin.
Kabbani, S.M.H. 2003. *The Approach of Armageddon: An Islamic Perspective*. Washington, DC: ISCA.
Littlewood, R. 1996. *Reason and Necessity in the Specification of the Multiple Self.* Occasional Paper No. 43. London: Royal Anthropological Institute.
Littlewood, R. and S. Dein. 2012. 'Did Christianity Lead to Schizophrenia?', *Transcultural Psychiatry* 50: 397–430.
Maxwell-Stuart, P.G. 2011. *Satan: A Biography*. Stroud: Amberley.
McGinn, B. 1994. *Antichrist*. New York: Harper Collins.
Needham, R. 1973. 'Introduction', in R. Needham (ed.), *Right and Left: Essays on Dual Symbolic Classification*. Chicago, IL: University of Chicago Press.
Oldridge, D. 2012. *The Devil*. Oxford: Oxford University Press.
Parkin, D. (ed.). 1983. *The Anthropology of Evil*. Oxford: Blackwell.
______. 1995. 'Latticed Knowledge: Eradication and Dispersal of the Unpalatable in Islam, Medicine, and Anthropological Theory', in R. Fardon (ed.), *Counterworks: Managing the Diversity of Knowledge*. London: Routledge.
Rabinbach, A. 1990. *The Human Motor: Energy, Fatigue, and the Origins of Modernity*. New York: Basic Books.
Reich, I.O. 1969. *Wilhelm Reich: A Personal Biography*. London: Elek.
Reich, V. 1973. *Reich Speaks of Freud*. Harmondsworth: Penguin.
Reich, W. 1968. *The Function of the Orgasm*. London: Panther.
Ricoeur, P. 1967. *The Symbolism of Evil*. New York: Harper and Row.
Roazen, P. 1979. *Freud and His Followers*. Harmondsworth: Penguin.
Robinson, P.A. 1969. *The Sexual Radicals*. London: Temple Smith.
Russell, J.B. 1977. *The Devil: Perceptions of Evil from Antiquity to Primitive Christianity*. Ithaca, NY: Cornell University Press.
Rycroft, C. 1968. *Reich*. London: Fontana.
Sulloway, F.J. 1980. *Freud, Biologist of the Mind: Beyond the Psychoanalytic Legend*. London: Fontana.
Turner, C. 2011. *Adventures in the Orgasmatron: The Invention of Sex*. London: Fourth Estate.
Wilson, B. 1970. *Religious Sects*. London: Weidenfeld and Nicolson.
Wolheim, R. 1971. *Freud*. London: Fontana.

Chapter 11

Religion and Psychosis

> O Lord, you have searched me and you know me. You know when I sit and when I rise; you perceive my thoughts from afar, you discern my going out and my lying down, you are familiar with all my ways.
>
> —Psalm 139:1–3 NIV

That religious experiences and psychosis (more particularly schizophrenia) share similar, or indeed identical, psychological characteristics has often been maintained since suggestions in classical Greece (Simon 1978). In both popular and medical perceptions, religious enthusiasm and experience have often been equated with madness. From the eighteenth century onwards, scholars have often argued that the founders of new religious dispensations might be conspicuously unusual or even frankly insane (Littlewood 1993).

The debate on the mental health of the shaman in particular has long continued among social anthropologists, some of whom have even ventured that all religious cognition is psychotic (e.g. La Barre 1970). In terms of empirical study, the evidence for this hypothesis has of course been problematic, given the difficulty of providing a conventional psychiatric assessment of the religious leader as they develop a new (or modified) religious dispensation. One exception is the founder of a new religion in the Caribbean, described by Littlewood (1993). It has generally proved easier, if less reliable, to offer a retrospective assessment of religious leadership based upon existing biographical sources (e.g. Littlewood 1996). Anthropological accounts of religious experience and certain aspects of psychopathology in contemporary Euro-Americans have argued that, from the phenomenological perspective, they may be identical (Dein and Littlewood 2007; Jackson and Fulford 1997). Any differentiation depends on the social consequences: in William James' reframing of Jesus, 'By their fruits you shall know them' (James 1902: 36).

To develop an argument on the convergence of religion and psychosis, we need to: (1) use coherent definitions of both, and to restrict 'religion' here to some Neo-Tylorean mentation, ignoring for the moment the social institutions and doctrines which insubstantiate this; (2) argue that they are essentially the same process, or that one is primary and the other is inherently piggy-backed onto it, or that both follow closely on some other third phenomenon in a way that other patterns, social or psychological, do not; (3) offer appropriate evolutionary explanations, either social or biological selection (or both), if we are arguing a long-term convergence.[1]

Several suggestions have been proposed to explain why schizophrenia (taken as cross-culturally found) persists and why, with its lower fertility, it has not disappeared through natural selection. One possibility argues that schizophrenia has an evolutionary advantage either for the individual's immediate kin or the larger group in terms of reproductive success or survival: Erlenmeyer-Kimling and Paradowski (1968) found, surprisingly, that female infants of parents with schizophrenia enjoy increased survival compared to other children. Karlsson (1984) argues that the evolutionary advantage of schizophrenia in Western societies lies in the enhanced creativity (and hence survival) of relatives. Crow (2000), arguing that the evolution of schizophrenia and language are intimately related, suggests a possible lack of cerebral asymmetry observed in schizophrenia along with its characteristic alterations in language use: as language per se confers selective advantage, then schizophrenia is dragged along too.

Stevens and Price (2000) propose a functionalist model of religion in which an expanding small-scale ancestral community must eventually split to conserve population size optimal for its ecological niche: charismatic leaders with schizotypal traits use 'paranoia,' 'delusions,' 'religious scenes' and neologisms to control and fractionate groups by seeking new social dispensations and settings. For Polimeni and Reiss (2002), schizophrenia, or something allied to it, could enhance the leader's ability to initiate and conduct religiously based rituals: such rituals are universally observed in all cultures and thus are likely both to be genetically rooted and perhaps critical for survival, presumably in terms of group cohesion and mobilization.[2] They argue that until the past few thousand years humans have always lived in hunter-gatherer societies with some form of 'shamanic' leadership. Psychosis might be advantageous for these individuals in generating novel and persisting religious rituals from an 'altered state of consciousness.' Due to a lack of contemporary empirical evidence and their extremely conjectural speculation, both these theories, like other social evolutionist scenarios, must remain extremely problematic.

One may ask whether what one terms 'religion' is an adequate general category for comparison. For religion is generally regarded as a shared cultural institution whereas schizophrenia is fundamentally an individual experience. Religious experience may take numerous forms, including feelings that all things are one, a sense of transcending time and space, a feeling of the holy, sacred, divine; and that such events and situations cannot be described in words (Beit-Hallahmi and Argyle 1997). Here we adopt the view that religion primarily involves recognition of the agency of ultrahuman agents, agreeing with Boyer (1994: 9) that the notion of ultrahuman entities who possess something like human agency seems to be the only evident universal found in religious cosmologies. Actual religious practice of the sort studied by social anthropologists is always organized around such agents and it is upon these that seem to be erected systematized reflection (doctrine), prescribed behaviours (rituals and so on) and communal structure (social organization). The acceptance of such agents may be the most commonly offered definition of religion in the social sciences (Sosis and Alcora 2003). For religious adherents themselves, gods do not just exist, they matter to those who believe in them, and they render everyday events significant through their association with a divine cosmology. We propose, along with Boyer (2001), that religious cognition is a specific form of cognition characterized by a focus on ultrahuman agents; it is counterintuitive, and it is costly in terms of time and emotional involvement.

That this sort of cognition might be related to schizophrenia is suggested by various findings. First, in schizophrenia, there is a substantial occurrence of religiously oriented delusions in all societies examined (Brewerton 1994; Moslowski et al. 1998; Siddle et al. 2002). Second, religious ideas and assertions of the 'paranormal' are especially common among those individuals in the West with schizotypal traits (Thalbourne and Delin 1994). Third, there are phenomenological parallels between schizophrenic and normative religious hallucinations (Dein and Littlewood 2007). Finally, there is emerging evidence for a continuum between religious normality and psychosis: members of new Euro-American religious movements have been found to have similar scores on various 'delusion scales' as those who have been diagnosed clinically with psychotic illnesses (Peters et al. 1999).

Shared Modules?

Can such a postulated link between 'religion' and 'schizophrenia' be regarded as intrinsic? There seems to be some evidence that religious thinking in schizophrenia is a strategy to cope with extreme experience (Mohr et al. 2006). The usual explanation is that religious beliefs and practice may provide a source of fundamental meaning, solace and stable purpose in a radically confusing world. Here we propose a rather different theory in which 'religion' and schizophrenia both represent applications or by-products of certain mental modules, which once had some adaptive advantage. Such modules include (1) human agency – our sense of personally owning, controlling or identifying with an experience or action, and (2) what psychologists term theory of mind (ToM) – our ability to attribute mental states such as cognition, intention and agency to other people, thus allowing the social individual to explain, predict and manipulate the behaviour of others. The two modules are related, for other recognized agents are presumed to act via intentions, motivations and desires just like ourselves. Both religious cognition and schizophrenia, compared with everyday cognitions, involve agency over detection and overextended ToM. In everyday religious cognition, agency detection and ToM modules function fairly normally; in schizophrenia, as we shall discuss below, both modules are impaired.

While religious cognition is based upon an intact ToM and agency detection mechanism, under certain circumstances (e.g. rituals, dancing, music) the ToM functions in a way that results in a breakdown of the boundary between the self and outside world. Schizophrenia and 'extreme' religious experiences[3] both involve breaches in our (Western) boundaries between self and 'other.' In both there is a subjective breach of a perceived psychological border to the self, conventionally termed the 'ego-boundary,' a breach which in psychosis is experienced fairly concretely (Jaspers 1926). In some way the subjective self becomes more permeable, and patterns of influence and agency may pass 'into' or 'out from' the self depending on the symptom type: '[The] patient knows that his thoughts and actions have an excessive effect on the world around him, and he experiences activity, which is not directly related to him, having a definite effect on him' (Fish 1967). In a similar way to this 'magical thinking' (as it was once called), in many religious experiences the boundary between self and divine is breached. This occurs in the extreme during mystical states where the self seems to be completely absorbed into the divine.

Although we suggest a cognitive mechanism shared between religion and schizophrenia, we are not arguing for a shared identity or that religion is a form of mass delusion, as has been suggested by some (Dawkins 2008; La Barre 1970; Schumaker 1995).

Agency and Religion

Religion in an extended sense is virtually universal and hence perhaps 'natural' (Boyer 1994). Following Stephen Jay Gould (1997), the evolutionary biologist who popularized the notion of a spandrel (an associated by-product of evolution itself not immediately adaptive), Boyer (1994), Barrett (2000) and Atran (2002) have offered a set of arguments, now termed the 'cognitive science of religion,' which attempts to describe the primary mental procedures upon which religious ideas are 'parasitic.' Religious cognition is seen as dependent upon psychological faculties, which have evolved for other purposes, and is not immediately adaptive in itself. Religion is thus an extraordinary use of everyday cognitive processes which cannot exist apart from the individual minds and in environments which can employ them. What gets newly transmitted in social life must fit well with existing patterns of cognition. Religious representations, especially those of deities with something like a mind, seem easily represented by the brain for they rest upon the cognitive processes which have developed for more immediate advantages. They have properties which fit with existing natural ontological categories such as personhood. They do differ from these categories in some respects but only slightly and are thus described by Boyer (1994) as minimally counterintuitive. For instance, the gods have wishes and emotions just like humans but they also possess novel qualities extended from everyday life like omnipotence and omniscience – or, in the case of ancient Egyptian religion, a falcon's head. Shades have a form yet they pass through walls. It is these counter-intuitive properties, argues Boyer, which renders them salient and hence memorable and persisting.

Agent Detection and Religious Representations

Atran (2002) is typical of this position: he regards religion as a spandrel on the cognitive mechanism responsible for agent detection, which, he argues, developed in evolution for inferring the presence of dangerous predators. A large psychological literature suggests that to attribute agency at times to non-humans and to inanimate objects is universal (Heider and Simmel 1944; Michotte 1963). Agency overgeneralization may be an innate feature of human cognition; even infants may see inanimate movement as purposive behaviour (Gergely and Csibra 2003). According to Atran our brains are primed to identify the presence of agents, even when such presence is unlikely. Barrett (2000), like Boyer (2001), argues that we have a hyperactive agent detection template which seeks out the presence and intentions of other beings around us. Boyer argues this is represented in children's imaginary companions which provide representations for the social mind. Similarly, Atran and Norenzayan (2004: 714) argue that 'widespread counterfactual and counter intuitive belief in supernatural agents could be explained by the fact that they trigger a naturally selective agency detection system, which is trip wired to respond to fragmentary information, inciting perception of figures, lurking shadows and emotions of dread and awe.' A by-product then is the susceptibility to infer ultrahuman beings. Ultranatural agents are readily conjured up because natural selection has resulted in a cognitive mechanism for privileging agency detection in the face of uncertainty: it is clearly more adaptive to mistakenly identify a shadow as a predator than the reverse. And the identified agency of another will be elaborated as akin to our own experience of personal agency: in other words, we take our own experiences and perceive them in others ('projection').

These ideas accord with Guthrie's (1993) ideas of the origins of 'animism' in anthropomorphism, which he then uses as an explanation for established religion. He too postulates that in the 'environment of evolutionary adaptation' it would have been beneficial for humans to be able to quickly and easily signal out the presence of other people and animals who might present danger. His examples of the everyday overextension of this include hearing voices in the wind or seeing faces in the clouds (Guthrie 1993).

If postulation of the existence of supernatural beings might relate to the misattribution of agency at certain times, it does not immediately explain the persistence of religion. Once suggested and organized, the gods then have social advantages for us in maintaining group cohesion and mobilization as the ultimate underpinnings of a culture in terms of norms and sanctions, and indeed in the very possibility of meaning open to a society.

Theory of Mind, Metarepresentation and Religion

Theory of mind allows us to anticipate the actions of others by imagining ourselves in another's place: what would X do if X was like me? Boyer (2001) argues that by developing a hypertrophied theory of mind we are able to predict the behaviour of others and thus facilitate cooperation and social interaction. Sociality is dependent upon predicting and anticipating the behaviour of others with a fair degree of accuracy. The essence of ToM, its central adaptive importance, and the reason why it has evolved, is that this adaptation is primarily concerned with making inferences concerning the dispositions, motivations and intentions of others.

Ultrahuman agents too are intimately involved in interactions with people: as in human interactions they employ the processes involved in social cognition (Bering and Johnson 2005). Supernatural agents do not just act; they are represented as having knowledge of humankind and as thus themselves possessing a theory of mind in attributing mental states such as belief and intention to people. As Bloom (2004) has argued, if one accepts the idea of minds (which cannot be empirically verified), it is a short step to postulate minds which do not have to be anchored in bodies, and thence another short step to both an immaterial soul and a transcendent deity.

Gods and spirits are not represented as having human features in general, but as having minds: they are held to have thoughts, memories and emotions and perceive events. Although corporeal features, such as having bodies, eating food or aging, may also be attributed to them, the only feature of humans that is invariably projected onto supernatural beings is mind (Boyer 1994).

Ultrahuman agents do not merely possess minds; they deploy these minds in interacting with human agents. Boyer argues that the special properties of supernatural agents that mean they matter to people are those that directly activate 'mental systems geared to describing and managing social interaction with other human agents' (2002: 77). In normal social interactions people make moves, the consequences of which then depends on the moves of others. Unlike humans who have limited access to the intentions of others, supernatural agents have full access to strategic information – the various sources of input that the social mind uses to evaluate a particular individual or situation and to influence ongoing social interaction.

Tremlin (2006: 115) argues 'in every culture the gods that matter know the truth, keep watch, witness what is done in private, divine the causes of events and see inside people's minds.' In Judaeo-Christian sacred texts several passages attest to the fact that God can read our mind. Psalm 139:4 (NIV) argues that 'Before a word is on my tongue you know it completely, O Lord.' Jesus, as the incarnation of a supernatural agent, is held to know people's thoughts (Mark 2:6–8). According to Ezekiel (11:5, NIV) 'Then the Spirit of the Lord came upon me, and he told me to say: "This is what the Lord says: That is what you are saying, O house of Israel, but I know what is going through your mind."' St Mark (13:11, NIV) describes the reverse, an external control over our thought and speech: 'Whenever you are arrested and brought to trial, do not worry beforehand about what to say. Just say whatever is given you at the time, for it is not you speaking, but the Holy Spirit.' Pettazzoni (1955: 20) argues for such divine omniscience being ubiquitous religious systems:

> Divine omniscience has another field of activity; besides the deeds and besides the words of mankind, it examines even their inmost thoughts and secret intents. In the prophecies of Jeremiah we are told that the Lord tries 'thereins and the heart' (Jer. XI, 20). The same thought is found among many other

> peoples, savage and civilized. Karai Kasang, the Kachin Supreme Being, 'sees' even what men think. The Haida say that everything we think is known to Sins Sganagwa. The Great Manitu of the Ankara knows everything, including the most secret thoughts. Tezcatlipoca knows men's hearts; Temaukel, the Supreme Being of the Ona-Selknam, knows even our thoughts and most private intentions. In Babylonia, the god Enlil knows the hearts of gods and men, and Shamash sees to the bottom of the human heart. Zeus likewise knows every man's thought and soul.

The idea that ToM may be a prerequisite for religious belief has been forcefully argued by Dunbar (2005). The notion of a God who is just, who watches over us, who punishes us but who can admit us to Paradise depends on the understanding that other beings – in this case a supernatural one – can have human-like thoughts and emotions. Dunbar proposes that several levels of metarepresentation may be required, since religion is a social activity, which depends on shared beliefs.

The Earth People of Trinidad revere a notion of the divine as sensate Nature, but this is a Nature who has a memory of Her own and of human experiences, who has suffered and who is seeking, through cataclysm, to return the whole universe into a more just and orderly state (Littlewood 1993). As divinity, She knows what humans are thinking and planning, and will respond to them: She is now impatient. (Whilst its immediate origin was in a personal psychotic identification, the idea of a divine Nature here recalls a Caribbean Christianity creolized with contemporary ecological ideas.)

We would argue that the application of ToM is not limited to living beings, whether real or imaginary, but rather it can extend thus to the natural world as well. Although agency may at times be attributed to inanimate objects, this is rare in the universalist religions. But the universe is imbued with purpose and intention. Are we cognitively predisposed, like the Earth People, to view the physical world teleologically? As Pascal Boyer (2001) puts it, 'Physical events around us are not just one damn thing after another; there often appear to be causes and effects. But you cannot claim a cause, at least literally. What you see are events and your brain interprets their succession as cause plus effect.' As Hume argues, we cannot see cause or purpose, all we actually see is 'one damn thing after another,' but our brain takes these observations and infers that the things and events around us are purposeful. Religious people are predisposed to infer purpose when observing the natural world and this same process renders events as intended and as personally significant.

Among the Earth People, as among others, events like thunderstorms or the passage of strangers are immediately given meaning as a divine incident which is a message to the group of ultimate significance: one always dependent, observes the ethnographer, on certain current debates, preoccupations and tensions among the group themselves (Littlewood 1993).

Alienation of Personal Agency in Religion and Schizophrenia

This distinction between self and other has been emphasized by the modern Western phenomenologists of religion. Otto (1958) describes the 'numinous' in religious experience as the ineffable core of religion: a dependence on something greater than ourselves. Durkheim describes 'the man who lives according to religion. . . as above all a man who feels within himself a power of which he is not usually conscious, a power which is absent when he is not in a religious state' (Pickering 1994: 192). Similarly in the nineteenth century, Feuerbach (1967) had talked of this self/ other dimension rather more psychologically when he claimed 'the ultimate secret of religion is the relationship between the conscious and unconscious, the voluntary and involuntary. The I and the not I in one and the same individual.' In a similar way James proposed surrender of the self as the essence of religion (1902: 403–404): 'At the same time the theologian's contention that the religious man is moved by an external power is vindicated, for it is one of those peculiarities of invasion from the sub-conscious region to take on objective appearances, and to suggest to the subject an external control.'

James (1902) describes here the loss of personal agency during mystical experiences: something he refers to as 'passivity' (as do contemporary psychiatrists). The oncoming of mystical states may be facilitated by preliminary voluntary operations, such as by fixing the attention, or going through certain bodily performances, or in other ways which manuals of mysticism prescribe; yet when the characteristic sort of consciousness has once set in, the mystic feels as if his own will were in abeyance, and indeed sometimes as if he were grasped and held by (or absorbed into) a superior power. While few religious experiences attain the degree of unification associated with the mystical state, we would contend that all religious experience involves an alteration in the sense of agency to varying degrees.

The founder and leader of the Earth People is understood as a partial incarnation of the divine Nature in one human: like (the plausible example of) Jesus, she alternates between her mundane being with habitual everyday memories and actions, and the identification with supreme divinity – omniscient, powerful and frequently irascible (Littlewood 1993).

Beyond recent interest in their putative biological correlatives (Bartocci and Dein 2005), there have been few empirical attempts to look at the mechanisms involved in such religious experience. Luhrmann (2005) appeals to a psychological phenomenon of 'absorption' to account for both spiritual experience and dissociative disorders: related both to dissociation and hypnotic states, this is the capacity to become absorbed in inner sensory stimuli and to lose a degree of external awareness. There is evidence from ethnography (anthropological accounts of spirit possession), psychology (experimental work on hypnosis and meditation) and religious history (accounts and manuals of Christian mysticism) that the practice of 'absorption' can go along with the development of hallucinations; as the state of absorption deepens there is also a shift in the sense of agency so that individual mental events come to happen to a person from the outside (similar to the earlier views of James and G.H. Mead), or indeed, at a less intense level, the indigenous psychologies and daily life of communities such as the Dinka (Lienhardt 1962).

Hyper-vigilance to perceived threat has been frequently cited as an explanation of paranoia. Individuals with paranoid delusions are especially sensitive to possible threats. Compared to non-deluded psychiatric patients or other people, those with persecutory delusions preferentially attend to threat-related stimuli and preferentially recall threatening episodes and attribute failures to the malevolent actions of others (Bentall and Kaney 1989; Ullman and Krasner 1969).

There is some evidence that schizophrenia is a phenomenon primarily of the misattribution of agency. Patients with schizophrenia often report the immediate experience of someone else controlling their thoughts and actions. Alternatively, they may feel that they are in control of external events or are convinced they know what other people think. Things or events are related to them in a special way or have a personal significance. Symptoms which suggest misattribution of agency include thought insertion and withdrawal experiences, passivity and certain auditory hallucinations (Fish 1967). In thought insertion the patient experiences thoughts that do not have the quality of being his own. In thought withdrawal the patient describes his thoughts being taken from his mind by an external force. Thought broadcasting is the experience that an individual's thoughts are not contained within his own mind: the thoughts escape from the confines of the self and may be experienced by those around. This may form the basis of the delusion that 'thoughts are being read.'

Among the wide range of manifestations in schizophrenia, these so-called 'first rank symptoms' are traditionally considered critical for its diagnosis. They are often seen to be primary. Schneider (1955) argues that these refer to a situation where patients interpret their own thoughts or actions as made by alien forces or other people. These symptoms reflect disruption of a mechanism which normally generates consciousness of one's actions and thoughts and allows direct attribution to their author alone. In schizophrenia patients may attribute to others rather than to themselves their own actions or thoughts; or in contrast attribute to themselves the actions or thoughts of others. Pierre Janet (1937) argued that the false attribution reflected personal representations of others' actions and thoughts in addition to the usual representation of one's own thoughts and actions. False attributions were due to the imbalance of the two representations. Those experiencing hallucinations thus misattribute their own intentions or actions to external agents.

Frith (1992) suggests that an internal monitoring deficit causes delusions of alien control: these abnormal experiences arise through a lack of awareness of intended actions. Such impairment might cause thoughts or actions to become isolated from the sense of will normally associated with them. Internally generated voices or thoughts might be interpreted as external voices (auditory hallucinations and thought insertion) and one's actions and speech might be construed as externally caused (passivity or delusion of control).

The presumed phenomenological parallels between religious experience and schizophrenia may be particularly apparent in Western cultures. Fabrega (1982: 56–57) discusses how Schneider's first rank symptoms depend on a 'Western' notion of self:

> These [first rank] symptoms imply to a large extent persons are independent beings whose bodies and minds are separated from each other and function autonomously. In particular, they imply that under ordinary conditions external influences do not operate on and influence an individual: that thoughts, are recurring inner happenings that the self 'has'; that thoughts, feelings, and actions are separable sorts of things which together account for self-identity; that thoughts and feelings are silent and exquisitely private; that one's body is independent of what one feels or thinks; and finally that one's body, feelings and impulses have a purely naturalistic basis and cannot be modified by outside 'supernatural' agents . . . and it is based on this psychology (i.e. a Western cultural perspective) that schizophrenic symptoms have been articulated.

Barrett (2004) emphasizes the fact that a comparative cultural phenomenology requires ethnographic underpinnings. He describes the difficulties of studying these first rank symptoms cross-culturally. Using data from the Iban of Borneo, he suggests that questions concerning auditory hallucinations translate with ease from English to Iban. In contrast, problems with thinking (thought withdrawal, insertion and broadcasting) make little sense in this group: unlike Western notions of thought as 'interior' and 'privatized,' among the Iban thinking is partly a bodily process and partly an interactional process. A cultural phenomenology of 'unusual' experiences must take account of indigenous conceptualizations of mind and self.

Within Western cultures there are a number of counter-suggestions to the ideals of mental autonomy and privacy. Such instances include telepathy and hypnosis, but more pervasive is the Christian belief in an omniscient God who knows inner thoughts. In the Christian tradition individuals can be punished, feel guilty or ashamed of these thoughts even if they are not verbalized. The experience of God's omniscience might act as a cultural model for articulating disorders of the privacy of thinking. Theology and the phenomenology of the self are dialectically related. We might speculate that the Reformation, with its interiorization and privatization of religion, might have facilitated the emergence of a bounded self and subsequently set the cultural grounds for the experience of schizophrenic thought disorder as we know it, especially those delusions and hallucinations which relate to loss of self–other boundaries.

Theory of Mind and Metarepresentation in Schizophrenia

Patients with schizophrenia have specific difficulties in inferring what others intend, think, or pretend, and this ToM impairment probably influences the way in which they use language and interpret speech (Brune 2005). For instance, delusions of alien control and persecution, the presence of thought and language disorganization, and other behavioural symptoms may be understood in light of a disturbed prior capacity to relate personal intentions to executing behaviour, and to monitor others' intentions. A common symptom in schizophrenia is the delusion of reference: the phenomenon that external events are experienced as personally meaningful and specifically related to the patient. Mundane events may be held to be personally significant and to be 'set up' specifically for that person. Frith (1992) explains this as a dysfunction of ToM. According to him the mechanism for enabling metarepresentation fails and the primary representation becomes detached from the patient's knowledge of others.

There is still much debate as to how an impaired ToM in schizophrenia is associated with other aspects of cognition and, indeed, whether theory of mind is impaired or exaggerated in some types of schizophrenia. Frith (1992) has argued that a compromised theory of one's own and others' minds in schizophrenia may account for (1) disorders of 'willed action' (e.g. negative and disorganized symptoms); (2) disorders of self-monitoring (e.g. delusions of alien control and hallucinations commenting on one's thoughts or other 'passivity' symptoms); and (3) disorders of monitoring other people's thoughts and intentions, including delusions of reference and persecution.

In relation to theory of mind, a substantial number of studies have been carried out to test the theoretical model put forward by Frith (1992). Paranoid patients have an intact ToM in the sense that they know that other people have mental states. They are, however, impaired in using contextual information, which leads them to make incorrect 'online' inferences about what these mental states are. The false beliefs found in delusional disorder are social and involve mistaken mental state inferences such as misjudging the motivations and intentions of other people. Such mistakes are inevitable, given the nature of the theory of mind mechanism: beliefs concerning the mental state of others cannot always be true because beliefs cannot be checked against objective criteria – there is no direct access to other minds.

There is some evidence that patients with schizophrenia have difficulty applying strategic social rules and tactics because of their impaired ToM (Sullivan and Allen 1999). More recently, Mazza and colleagues (2003) confirmed that ToM deficits in schizophrenia may be associated with impaired strategic social thinking: patients with predominantly 'positive symptoms' (hallucinations, etc.) who performed better on the ToM tasks than patients with negative symptoms (apathy, withdrawal) also had a more 'cynical' and pragmatic view of the world as measured using the Mach-IV scale, whereas patients with negative symptoms obtained lower scores in 'Machiavellianism.' Thus, impaired strategic social reasoning might reflect a deficit in appreciation of second order mental states (Mazza et al. 2003).

Conclusion: Schizophrenia, Religion and Creativity

We have compared religious thinking with cognition in schizophrenia and outlined some similarities and differences.[4] Specifically there are parallels in the ways in which boundaries between the self and outside world are breached. This is not to suggest that phenomenologically they are the 'same' experience or that they are associated with the same affective response, just that they depend on similar cognitive strategies involving agency and ToM. In religious cognition ToM is intact whereas in extreme religious experience there is a breakdown in the boundary between the self and outside world. In schizophrenia ToM is disordered – not only are there problems understanding other minds but there may be breaches of the self-other boundaries. And in schizophrenia, delusions of reference may be similar to the ideas held by religious believers that mundane experiences have personal significance and purpose. Both involve over attributions of intentions onto the outside world.

An interesting question is whether both originate in the same evolutionary trajectory. Although, like some evolutionary explanations, we lack empirical data to establish this position, we speculate here that everyday cognition, religion and schizophrenia are on a continuum; both 'religion' and schizophrenia perhaps derive from an over-attribution of agency and an overextension of ToM. There is some suggestion that schizophrenia and religion may have evolved together. Schizophrenia and schizotypy have been associated with creativity throughout recorded history (Claridge et al. 1990; Nettle 2001). Psychological experiments, biographical survey studies and neurophysiology support the hypothesis that schizotypal cognition is associated with creativity and divergent thinking (Barrantes-Vidal 2004; Claridge et al. 1990; Nettle 2006). Schizotypy is thought to be a disposition for schizophrenia (Claridge 1985), and schizotypic traits consist of tendencies to have abnormal perceptual or cognitive experiences.

Family studies and adoption studies indicate that schizophrenia in a family member is associated with an increased risk of schizotypy. On the other hand, it is also an indication of an increased likelihood of high creativity, leadership qualities, high musical skills and an intense interest in religion (Horrobin 1998). Horrobin proposes that schizophrenia was probably present in the earliest stages of human development, about 150,000–100,000 years ago, around the time that there was a cultural explosion of art and religion. Furthermore, schizophrenia and 'human genius' began to manifest themselves as a result of evolutionary pressures that ultimately triggered genetic changes in our brain cells, allowing us to make unexpected links with different events, an ability that significantly enhanced our intellectual abilities. Early manifestations of this creative change, according to him, include the 30,000-year-old cave paintings found in France and Spain. Thus, schizophrenia was the price paid for these cultural developments.[5]

A prediction of this hypothesis is that schizophrenia has evolved, and is maintained, in part as a by-product of recent positive selection and adaptive evolution in humans (Crow,1997; Horrobin 1998): creativity may be one type of 'compensatory advantage' for those carrying the genes for psychosis. Such creativity may have been associated with the potential for symbolic cognition including the possibility for the attribution of agency and ToM onto ultrahuman entities.

Notes

1. While the origins of religion can only be dated with some confidence back to the practice of burial with grave goods (50,000 BCE), we would argue here that its cognitive antecedents can probably be traced from the period of hominid evolutionary adaptive functioning (late Pleistocene). Archaeologists trace religion back to our earliest Sapiens progenitors (Dickson 1990; Mithen 1999). In the absence of written records or distinctive pathoanatomical features, we clearly cannot attempt to date the origin of schizophrenia or other psychoses to before the earliest medical texts (c. 1000 BCE), but we are proposing that it is the antecedents of both religion and schizophrenia that are significant in terms of natural selection (whilst allowing for later selection from biological advantages or disadvantages of institutions stemming from religion or schizophrenia: see Note 2).

2. Once established, religious systems are, we argue, likely to be biologically advantageous (through group cohesion and mobilization) and thus persist. In other words, a social pattern is biologically advantageous, as in Fox's (1980) theory of culturally mandated incest avoidance having biological advantages through its social consequences (exchange of sisters and hence the formation of alliances). The origin of social formations among humans is still poorly understood. Various theories have been proposed including kin-selection in which cooperation is genetically rewarded by favouring kin (Hamilton 1964), reciprocal altruism in which reciprocal acts are returned later (Trivers 1971), indirect reciprocity in which one's reputation for cooperation is rewarded indirectly through the favour of third-party observers (Nowak and Sigmund 1998), and costly signalling in which generosity signifies high fitness to mates or allies (Zahavi 1995). While these theories may explain cooperation among non-humans, among humans cooperation still occurs even when kin-selection, reciprocal altruism, indirect reciprocity and costly signalling are not immediately apparent (Gintis 2003). Punishment may function to ensure cohesion and cooperation (Andreoni et al. 2003). Recently, Johnson and Kruger (2004) have argued that ancestral cooperation was promoted because norm violations were deterred by the threat of supernatural punishment. There is ethnographic data to support this contention: religious believers alter their behaviours to avoid supernatural retribution (Boyer 2001). Gods, dead ancestors, and other ultrahuman entities are commonly held to bring about misfortune. In contemporary evangelical Christianity and Islam misfortune is attributed to sin; those who act contrary to God's will are punished. In many traditional societies the emphasis is upon other-worldly punishment for the violation of religious norms. The question however is why gods would not want us to engage in such behaviours. When we posit that gods have minds and know the thoughts of humankind, this is generally in the context of moral behaviour: gods appear to have little interest in other aspects of our life. According to the work on just-world beliefs, we operate under the assumption that others will 'get what they deserve', especially when they have little control over negative events (Lerner 1980). Johnson and Bering (2009) argue that it is easy to understand how some behaviour in the moral domain is connected to an uncontrollable and unrelated life event; our innate cognitive tendency to search for reason and intention in life events predisposes us to see gods as agents who are deeply involved in our life events. Thus, negative events are easily attributed to divine agency.
3. While the cognitive science of religion approach convincingly accounts for religious cognition, we would argue that this approach to date has not developed a coherent theory of religious emotion and religious experience – a composite whole involving cognitive, affective and behavioural components. Some recent research is promising in this respect (Boyer and Lienard 2006; Whitehouse 2004).
4. In this chapter, we have restricted ourselves to considering schizophrenia rather than psychosis in general, but similar arguments could be applied to manic-depressive illness, though here alienation of agency is likely to be less profound.
5. These mutations involved changes in lipid metabolism. Initially, they predisposed proto-hominids to schizotypy. It was only later (around 100,000 years ago) that mutations to the phospholipase A2 cycle gave us the potential for schizophrenia, bipolar disorder and psychopathy. Frank psychosis was avoided by the ingestion of a fatty acid rich water diet.

References

Andreoni, J., W. Harbaugh and L. Vesterlund. 2003. 'The Carrot or the Stick: Rewards, Punishments, and Cooperation', *American Economic Review* 93: 893–902.

Atran, S. 2002. *In Gods We Trust: The Evolutionary Landscape of Religion*. Oxford: Oxford University Press.

Atran, S. amd A. Norenzayan. 2004. 'Religion's Evolutionary Landscape: Counterintuition, Commitment, Compassion, Communion', *Behavioral and Brain Sciences* 27: 713–30.

Barrantes-Vidal, N. 2004. 'Creativity and Madness Revisited from Current Psychological Perspectives', *Journal of Consciousness Studies* 11: 58–78.

Barrett, J. 2000. 'Exploring the Natural Foundations of Religion', *Trends in Cognitive Sciences* 4: 29–34.

Barrett, R. 2004. 'Kurt Schneider in Borneo: Do First Rank Symptoms Apply to the Iban?', in J. Jenkins and R. Barrett (eds.), *Schizophrenia, Culture and Subjectivity: The Edge of Experience*. Cambridge: Cambridge University Press.

Bartocci, G. and S. Dein. 2005. 'Detachment: Gateway to the World of Spirituality', *Transcultural Psychiatry* 42(4): 545–69.

Beit-Hallahmi, B. and M. Argyle. 1997. *The Psychology of Religious Behaviour, Belief and Experience*. London: Routledge.

Bentall, R. and S. Kaney. 1989. 'Contents for Specific Processing and Persecutory Delusions: An Investigation Using the Emotional Stroop Test', *British Journal of Medical Psychology*, 62: 355–64.

Bering, J. M. and D.D.P. Johnson. 2005. '"O Lord. . . You Perceive My Thoughts from Afar": Recursiveness and the Evolution of Supernatural Agency', *Journal of Cognition and Culture* 5: 118–42.

Bloom, P. 2004. *Descartes' Baby*. New York: Basic Books.

Boyer, P. 1994. *The Naturalness of Religious Ideas: A Cognitive Theory of Religion*. Berkeley, CA: University of California Press.

______. 2001. *Religion Explained*. London: Heinemann.

______. 2002. *Religion Explained: The Evolutionary Origins of Religious Thought*. New York: Basic Books.

Boyer, P. and P. Lienard. 2006. 'Why Ritualized Behavior? Precaution Systems and Action-Parsing in Developmental, Pathological, and Cultural Rituals', *Brain and Behavioral Sciences* 29: 595–613.

Brewerton, T. 1994. 'Hyper-Religiosity in Psychotic Disorders', *Journal of Nervous and Mental Diseases* 182: 302–304.

Brune, M. 2005. 'Theory of Mind in Schizophrenia: Review of the Literature', *Schizophrenia Bulletin* 31: 21–42.

Claridge, G.S. 1985. *Origins of Mental Illness*. Oxford: Blackwell.

Claridge, G., R. Pryor and G. Watkins. 1990. *Sounds from the Bell Jar: Ten Psychotic Authors*. London: The Macmillan Press Ltd.

Crow, T.J. 1997. 'Is Schizophrenia the Price That Homo Sapiens Pays for Language?', *Schizophrenia Research* 28: 127–41.

______. 2000. 'Schizophrenia as the Price That Homo Sapiens Pays for Language: A Resolution of the Central Paradox in the Origin of the Species', *Brain Research Reviews* 31: 118–29.

Dawkins, R. 2008. *The God Delusion*. Boston, MA: Houghton Mifflin.

Dein, S. and R. Littlewood. 2007. 'The Voice of God', *Anthropology and Medicine* 14: 213–28.

Dickson, D.B. 1990. *The Dawn of Belief: Religion in the Upper Paleolithic of Southwestern Europe*. Tucson, AR: University of Arizona Press.

Dunbar, R. 2005. *The Human Story*. London: Faber and Faber.

Erlenmeyer-Kimling, L. and W. Paradowski. 1968. 'Selection of Schizophrenia', *American Naturalist* 100: 651–65.

Fabrega, H. 1982. 'Culture and Psychiatric Illness: Biomedical and Ethnomedical Aspects', in A. Marsella and G. White (eds), *Cultural Conceptions of Mental Health and Therapy*. Dordrecht, Netherlands: Reidel, pp. 39–68.

Feuerbach, L. 1967 cf1841. *Lectures on the Essence of Religion*. New York: Harper and Row.

Fish, F. 1967. *Clinical Psychopathology*. London: Wright.

Fox, R. 1980. *The Red Lamp of Incest*. New York: Dutton.

Frith, C. 1992. *The Cognitive Neuropsychology of Schizophrenia*. Hove, UK: Lawrence Erlbaum.

Gergely, G. and G. Csibra. 2003. 'Teleological Reasoning in Infancy: The Naive Theory of Rational Action', *Trends in Cognitive Sciences* 7: 287–92.

Gintis, H. 2003. 'Solving the Puzzle of Prosociality', *Rationality and Society* 15: 155–87.

Gould, S. 1997. 'The Exaptive Excellence of Spandrels as a Term and Prototype', *Proceedings of the National Academy of Sciences USA* 94: 10750–55.

Guthrie, S. 1993. *Faces in the Clouds: A New Theory of Religion*. Oxford: Oxford University Press.

Hamilton, W.D. 1964. 'The Genetical Evolution of Social Behaviour. 1 & 2', *Journal of Theoretical Biology* 7: 1–52.

Heider, F. and M. Simmel. 1944. 'An Experimental Study of Apparent Behaviour', *American Journal of Psychology* 57: 243–59.

Horrobin, D.F. 1998. 'Schizophrenia: The Illness That Made Us Human', *Medical Hypotheses* 50: 269–88.

Jackson, M.C. and K.W.M. Fulford. 1997. 'Spiritual Experience and Psychopathology', *Philosophy, Psychiatry and Psychology* 4: 41–65.

James, W. 1902, 1958. *The Varieties of Religious Experience*. New York: Simon & Schuster.

Janet, P. 1937. 'Les Troubles de la Personnalité Sociale', *Annales Medico-Psychologiques* 11: 149–200.

Jaspers, K. 1926. *General Psychopathology*. Reprinted (1963), trans. J. Hoenig and M.W. Hamilton). Manchester, UK: Manchester University Press.

Johnson, D.D.P. and J.M. Bering. 2009. 'Hand of God, Mind of Man: Punishment and Cognition in the Evolution of Cooperation', in J. Schloss and A. Platinga (eds), *The Nature of Belief: Scientific and Philosophical Perspectives on the Evolution of Religion*. New York: Oxford University Press, pp. 26–43.

Johnson, D.D.P. and O. Kruger. 2004. 'The God of Wrath: Supernatural Punishment and the Evolution of Cooperation', *Political Theology* 5(2): 159–76.

Karlsson, J. 1984. 'Creative Intelligence in Relatives of Mental Patients', *Hereditas* 100: 83–86.

La Barre, W. 1970. *The Ghost Dance*. London: Allen and Unwin.

Lerner, M. 1980. *The Belief in a Just World*. New York: Plenum.

Lienhardt, G. 1962. *Divinity and Experience: The Religion of the Dinka*. Oxford: Clarendon Press.

Littlewood, R. 1993. *Pathology and Identity: The Work of Mother Earth in Trinidad*. Cambridge: Cambridge University Press.

______. 1996. 'Psychopathology, Embodiment and Religious Innovation: An Historical Instance', in D. Bhugra (ed.), *Religion and Psychiatry*. London: Routledge, pp. 178–97.

Luhrmann, T.M. 2005. 'The Art of Hearing God: Absorption, Dissociation and Contemporary American Spirituality', *Spiritus: A Journal of Christian Spirituality* 5: 133–57.

Mazza, M., A. De Risio, L. Surian, R. Roncone and M. Casacchia. 2001. 'Selective Impairments of Theory of Mind in People with Schizophrenia', *Schizophrenia Research* 47: 299–308.

Mazza, M., A. De Risio, C. Tozzini, R. Roncone and M. Casacchia. 2003. 'Machiavellianism and Theory of Mind in People Affected by Schizophrenia', *Brain and Cognition* 51(3): 262–69.

Michotte, A. 1963. *The Perception of Causality* [T.R. Miles and E. Miles, trans.]. New York: Basic Books.

Mithen, S. 1999. 'Symbolism and the Supernatural', in R.I. Dunbar, C. Knight and C. Power (eds), *The Evolution of Culture*. New Brunswick, NJ: Rutgers University Press, pp. 147–69.

Mohr, S., P. Brandt, L. Borat, C. Gillieron and P. Huguelet. 2006. 'Towards the Integration of Spirituality and Religiousness into the Psychosocial Dimension of Schizophrenia', *American Journal of Psychiatry* 163: 1952–59.

Moslowski, J., D. Jansenvanrensberg and N. Mthoko. 1998. 'A Poly-Diagnostic Approach to the Differences in Symptoms of Schizophrenia in Different Cultural and Ethnic Populations', *Acta Psychiatrica Scandinavia* 98: 41–46.

Nettle, D. 2001. *Strong Imagination: Madness, Creativity and Human Nature*. Oxford: Oxford University Press.

______. 2006. 'Schizotypy and Mental Health Amongst Poets, Visual Artists, and Mathematicians', *Journal of Research in Personality* 40(6): 876–90.

Nowak, M.A. and K. Sigmund. 1998. 'Evolution of Indirect Reciprocity by Image Scoring', *Nature* 393: 573–77.

Otto, R. 1958. *The Idea of the Holy*. New York: Oxford University Press.

Peters, E., S. Day, J. McKenna and G. Albach. 1999. 'Delusional Ideation in Religious and Psychotic Populations', *British Journal of Clinical Psychology* 38: 83–96.

Pettazzoni, R. 1955. 'On the Attributes of God', *Numen* 2: 1–27.

Pickering, W. 1994. *Durkheim on Religion*. Atlanta, GA: Scholars Press.

Polimeni, J. and J. Reiss. 2002. 'How Shamanism and Group Selection May Reveal the Origins of Schizophrenia', *Medical Hypothesis* 58: 244–48.

Polimeni, J. and J. Reiss. 2003. 'Evolutionary Approaches on Schizophrenia', *Canadian Journal of Psychiatry* 48: 34–39.

Schneider, K. 1955. *Klinische Psychopathologie*. Stuttgart: Thieme Verlag.

Schumaker, J. 1995. *The Corruption of Reality: A Unified Theory of Religion, Hypnosis and Psychopathology*. New York: Prometheus Books.

Siddle, R., G. Haddock, N. Tarrier and E.B. Faragher. 2002. 'Religious Delusions in Patients Admitted to Hospital with Schizophrenia', *Social Psychiatry and Psychiatric Epidemiology* 37(3): 130–38.

Simon, B. 1978. *Mind and Madness in Ancient Greece*. Ithaca, NY: Cornell University Press.

Sosis, R. and C. Alcora. 2003. 'Signalling, Solidarity and the Sacred: The Evolution of Religious Behaviour', *Evolutionary Anthropology* 12: 264–74.

Stevens, A. and J. Price. 2000. *Evolutionary Psychiatry: A New Beginning*. London: Routledge.

Sullivan, R.J. and J.S. Allen. 'Social Deficits Associated with Schizophrenia in Terms of Interpersonal Machiavellianism', *Acta Psychiatrica Scandinavica* 99: 148–54.

Thalbourne, M.A. and P.S. Delin. 1994. 'A Common Thread Underlying Belief in the Paranormal, Mystical Experience and Psychopathology', *Journal of Parapsychology* 58: 3–38.

Tremlin, T. 2006. *Minds and Gods: The Cognitive Foundations of Religion*. Oxford: Oxford University Press.

Trivers, R.L. 1971. 'The Evolution of Reciprocal Altruism', *Quarterly Review of Biology* 46: 35–57.

Ullman, L. and L. Krasner. 1969. *A Psychological Approach to Abnormal Behaviour*. Oxford: Prentice Hall.

Whitehouse, H. 2004. *Modes of Religiosity: A Cognitive Theory of Religious Transmission*. Walnut Creek, CA: AltaMira Press.

Zahavi, A. 1995. 'Altruism as a Handicap – The Limitations of Kin Selection and Reciprocity', *Journal of Avian Biology* 26: 1–3.

Chapter 12

NEGLECT AS PROJECT

How Two Societies Forget

A new dispensation demands that details, indeed memories, of the old ways be forgotten as fresh ideals and modes of action become paramount. This chapter proposes that an initial step in forgetting involves neglect – more specifically the neglect of certain patterns of comportment or material evidence or practice that recall a past now considered undesirable. In a millennialist Caribbean community, past memories and technical practices are discouraged by 'ideological work' that constantly weighs the old order against a new world in the process of creation: 'directed forgetting'. For a post-communist Albanian village, by contrast, neglecting a technology appears to be a more transparently 'spontaneous' process. For both, memories are insubstantiated in an older material world, which must be avoided or destroyed.

Remembering has generally thought to be a more interesting question than forgetting. Memories, whether collective or personal, are seen as needing constant cueing – by insistent reminders of the centrality of that which is to be remembered, whether by internal recall or by ritualized and collective acts, modes of comportment and linguistic address, styles of bodily behaviour, or formal verbal consolidation (Connerton 1989; Rundus 1971). By contrast, forgetting has traditionally been regarded as a simple fading away or insidious neglect of the inessential (Nora 1989; Rivers 1921). Nearly a century ago, Rivers (1921) gave the example of there no longer being suitable game for bow and arrow, which now lie forgotten in a corner of the hut, soon to be lost altogether. But what of instances when a society seeks actively to dispense with some current set of technical acts and sentiments, as when Japanese Samurai agreed not to use firearms?[1]

For some groups, public remembrance may be actively discouraged for being too individually painful (Gay y Blasco 2001; Stewart 2004). Whole societies, particularly minorities and migrants, may engage in a continued process of selective editing of the past, choosing and discarding particular events and knowledge to deal with current dilemmas (Douglas 1995; e.g. 'structural amnesia' in Southeast Asia: Carsten 1995; Spanish Gitanos: Gay y Blasco 2001; Albanian migrants: Kretsi 2002; Roma: Stewart 2004), as do new national governments in Werbner's (1998) 'antimemory'. Cole (2001) and Shaw (2002) look at how the past may continue implicitly to intrude in the present as 'memories' in Betsimaraka (Madagascar) sacrifice and in Temne divination; but neither author considers how collective or individual forgetting first occurs at the time, even if the present determines what memories persist in a 'two-way temporality' (Shaw 2002) as memories embody and rework the past. They work forwards and back.

This intrusion of the past is perhaps less of a problem for successive generations in the absence of written texts, where the death of the physiological individual means there can be no prompting. A is preferred to B, and so it is encouraged and performed; B becomes neglected and eventually becomes impossible because it is forgotten both individually and collectively. Connerton (1989) emphasizes this collective social memory, as does Bloch (1998) after Halbwachs' classic *Les cadres sociaux de la mémoire*. Halbwachs (1994 [1925]) argued that collective memory is actually primary – you cannot remember outside a society's politics. Ricoeur (2004), like Cole (2001) and Shaw (2002), goes some way to reconciling the positions. Memory exists intersubjectively, 'stretched across individuals' (Cole 2001: 29). Yet, individual and collective memory mutually construct each other (Cole 2001). Halbwachs emphasized the localization of memory in commemorative practice and sites, and the way in which memory supports and sustains a group's identity.

The problem of forgetting when a memory is profound and powerful has recently been addressed in Western society in the case of the individual forgetting, or apparent forgetting, of traumatic memories that unconsciously or otherwise influence current functioning (Antze and Lambek 1996; Kirmeyer 1996; Littlewood 1996; Ricoeur 2004; Schacter 2003).[2] The therapeutic procedures for retrieving 'hidden memories' or for assisting obsessed individuals to 'forget' their troubling thoughts have alerted us to the paradox of motivated forgetting: that the more we try actively to dismiss from our thoughts some undesirable memories, the more we are recalling them to mind (Forty and Küchler 1999). Ricoeur (2004) terms this the presence of absence.

How does the generation that seeks to change actually commence the process of committing the customary to oblivion? This has not generally been a concern for social anthropologists, seen perhaps as too psychological a question (Rausing 2004); Cole (2001: 322) simply refers us back to the work of psychologists. The reverse has indeed sometimes been a concern for national authorities when, as in South Africa, the recovery of the events of a recent malign period has been seen as essential to any future reconciliation; but often, as with the case of fascist Spain (Espinosa 2003) or the communist Baltic states (Rausing 2004), the recent traumatizing past has been promptly lost to view. As Espinosa (2003) notes of the post-Franco period, memory can be seen as synonymous with rancour, forgetting with reconciliation. Often a local community can retain no knowledge of painful national events whilst retaining and commemorating local happenings. Levi (1963 [1945]) recounts how a southern Italian village in the 1930s had apparently no knowledge of the First World War yet had detailed accounts of the past exploits of local brigands against the central government. Cole (2001) cites the apparent forgetting of the traumatic 1947 revolt in Madagascar against the French.

Clearly, the separation from the past is easier if there is a geographical separation from the older but still persisting social order. Thus, many utopian and millennialist communities have sought a new physical site for their new activities away from the metropoles (Holloway 1966; Nordhoff 1966 [1875]; Woodcock and Avakumovic 1968). The past is truly 'away', another country. Missionaries, colonial officials, or national governments can prohibit certain practices, which might well have a continuing underground existence, but societies that decide to achieve radical change use techniques of forgetting and change through which they organize and reform themselves (Burridge 1969), a procedure referred to by sociologists of chiliastic movements as ideological work, in which implicit and explicit steps back towards the old have to be constantly called to mind and policed (Berger 1981). These steps come particularly to use in crises of inadequate forgetting.

Evidently there is a problem in that the more the former and now forbidden are called to mind, whether reproved or not, the more they continue as some sort of mental or physical potential. Newly constituted societies thus often find that a successful solution is to move one step away, so to speak, and, by direct emphasis on some other more easily achieved practical habitus (in Bourdieu's sense), make the forbidden ideology inaccessible: 'social practices that enable or disable certain kinds of memories' (Cole 2001: 11). Thus the millennialist sect of the Earth People, by explicitly stipulating nudity and intensive labour on the land, render unnecessary more specific prohibitions concerned with embodied practice, past costume, urban comportment, and commerce; and these do not have to be selected out for remark (thus presenting the danger of remembrance), so the forbidden past is thus steadily forgotten.[3] It was evident that for the children born into the community, certain urban forms of activity and thinking had become effectively impossible because they had not been publicly enacted or verbalized by anybody for some years: conscious accumulative practice (Connerton 1989: 34) had become habit (cf. Bourdieu 1977; Ricoeur 2004).

The two communities discussed here, an Africanist commune in the Caribbean and a post-communist village in Albania, both seem to have agreed to forget aspects of the past and to forge a new future. The Earth People are concerned to neglect and thus abandon almost the whole of modern technology and urban civilization as they perceive it; the villagers of Derret i Vogël are more specifically occupied with neglecting practices of the period of Albanian communism (1944–1992). The disengagement of the Earth People is more severe but perhaps easier to achieve because of their geographical isolation and nakedness, whilst the members of the Albanian village constantly have to avoid those technical and social achievements of communism that remain in their vicinity. The Derret villagers seek a rapprochement with Western European society more generally, and, rather than neglecting whole technologies as such, seem to neglect a particular social practice for its political origin and its potential for village conflict. The two communities are similar in that the new social order is perceived by both as a return to an idealized past: to a pre-European Africa in the case of the Earth People; to a pre-communist tribal (*fis)* society in the case of the Albanian village. What has to be forgotten is perceived by both as an unnatural distortion of some primordial way of life: hence a negation of the negation, such as is commonly found in millennial groups (Littlewood 1993). For the Earth People the new way is inevitably a severely re-created 'past'; for the Albanians it is a return to an idealized family life of the older generation before 1944. In the case of the Earth People, 'forgetting' is actively prescribed by teaching rooted in the daily exhortations of their leader: 'manipulated' or 'commanded', as Ricoeur (2004: 46) puts it; Cole's (2001: 22) 'directed forgetting'. In Albania, forgetting appears more 'spontaneous' and individual, a general reluctance to confront and thus relive a period seen as oppressive and conflictual. Trinidad is 'modern' if we follow Connerton (1989) in arguing that modernity is characterized by a deliberate erasure of the past to facilitate a new start, ironically dependent on memories of the past. Gupta (2005) meanwhile argues that the intersubjectivity espoused by the modernist project inevitably involves a high degree of communal forgetting.

Paraphrasing Dennett (1991: 117), we might term the Trinidadian case Orwellian forgetting (rewriting the past), and the Albanian case Stalinist forgetting (forgoing the past). Both necessitate practical neglect as the necessary first stage to forget devalued practice and thought.

The Earth People

The Earth People are an antinomian 'Africanist' community on the north coast of the Caribbean Island of Trinidad, which originated in the visions of their leader, Mother Earth (Jeanette MacDonald). From 1975 until 1976, she experienced a series of revelations and came to understand that the Christian teaching of God the Father as creator was false and that the world was the work of a primordial Mother, whom she identified with Nature and with the Earth. Nature gave birth to a race of Black people, but her rebellious Son (the Christians' God) re-entered his mother's womb to steal Her power of generation and created Europeans. The Whites, the Race of the Son/Sun, then enslaved the Blacks and have continued to exploit them. The Way of the Son is the way of Science – of cities, clothes, schools, factories, and wage labour. The Way of the Mother is the Way of Nature – a return to the simplicity of the Beginning, a simplicity of nakedness, cultivation of the land by hand and with respect, and of gentle and non-exploiting human relationships.

Jeanette herself is a partial manifestation of the Mother who will fully enter into her only at the End. Her task at the time of the initial fieldwork was to facilitate the return to Nature by organizing the community known as Hell Valley, to prepare for the return to the Beginning and to teach her people, the Mother's Children. She has to combat the false doctrines of existing religions, which place the Son over the Mother, and to correct the distorted teaching of the Bible, where she is represented as the Devil. She stands for Life and Nature in opposition to Science and Death. As the Devil, she is opposed to churches and prisons, education and money, contemporary morals and fashionable opinions. The exact timing of the End is uncertain but expected in Jeanette's physical lifetime. Then Time will end, Sickness be healed, and the Nation speak one language. Mother Earth's revelations ceased in 1976 after she burned all her young family's possessions in an episode called The Miracle, through which she brought the sun closer to the earth. At this time her family were still living with her in an abandoned village some fifteen miles from Pinnacle, the nearest settlement, and they were joined by an assortment of young men, mostly old friends and neighbours from Port-of-Spain. Her ideas were now consolidated in reflection and debate. She continued to have visions in her dreams, but these were similar to those of other members: premonitions and answers to immediate organizational problems (Littlewood 2004). The origins of expected behaviour in the group reflect the original visions, chance events, and the subsequent organization of the community. (Some remain uncertain to me: for instance, the obligation to enter the same doorway by which one departed. My supposition is that this may refer to the divine incest.) For the Earth People, every 'gesture of social life points away from details that would provoke memory and recollection'

(Kirmeyer 1996: 188). While around sixty individuals have been active Earth People at different times, in October 1981 twenty-two were resident in the Valley, with perhaps twenty sympathizers and occasional members in town. There were annual naked marches into Port-of-Spain which sometimes ended in arrests, together with raids on the settlement by police and social workers, who placed the younger children in an orphanage.

In opposition to the material world, the group all went naked, sleeping out on the bare ground, and maintained themselves through fishing and cultivation of the land using only cutlasses. The centre of the community was an old wooden house in the deserted village, together with some added 'African' huts. For about half a mile in each direction, the secondary bush and scrub of the seasonal rainforest had been cleaned and a variety of trees and perennial cultigens were grown: medicine bushes; trees and plants for cordage and wrapping and for basketry and calabashes; timber for building; plantain and banana; roots like cassava, sweet potatoes, dasheen, yam, tannia; aubergine, pineapple, tomato, pigeon peas, callaloo, okra; Indian corn, pumpkin, ginger, sugar cane, christophene; trees bearing oranges, grapefruit, guava, nuts, mango, avocado, pawpaw, pomerac, tamarind and breadfruit; garlic and bushes with pepper, shadobenny, and other herbs. Above the settlement, reaching into the lower reaches of the mountains of the northern range, were cocoa and coffee, cannabis and tobacco. In the nearby bush were cress and watermelon, mauby bark, mammy apple, passion fruit, star apple, nutmeg, and soursap, whilst along the coast grew coconut and almond. The variety of their crops, virtually every Trinidad food plant, justified the boast of the Earth People that they were living in the original Eden.

Although all members accepted Mother Earth's role as some sort of primordial maternal figure, the group were 'this worldly' in their emphasis on present cultivation of the land and on the preparation and consumption of food. Daily agricultural labour ended with a swim in the sea and Mother Earth ritually dealing out cooked vegetable food. Each new member took a 'fruit name' – like Breadfruit, Coconut, Cassava, or Pumpkin. Relations between members were fairly egalitarian, and not especially 'religious', generally recalling those of the average Trinidad working-class family. Supposedly the group were living in the Beginning of the End, a run-up to the imminent, very physical, end of the world, but little time was spent on millennial speculation. Painted words on the main house proclaimed 'Fock [sic] God' – a sentiment in accord with the group's opposition to Christianity and Islam.

Obscenity and Nudity: 'Ideological Work' among the Earth People

Because God is 'right', Mother Earth teaches the Left, and the Earth People interchange various conventional oppositions: 'left' for 'right'; 'evil' or 'bad' for 'good'. Seeming obscenities are only Natural words for She Herself is the Cunt, the origin of all life. The Earth People are encouraged by their leader to exchange the words when referring to people and ideas – 'You all left now?' – but only rarely when giving spatial directions. Like the others, Mother Earth herself may slip into conventional usage. Among newer members of the community such slippage is a source of amusement whilst also recognized as 'humbling you'self', that is, induction into the group.

As our current education is upside-down, the real meanings of many words can be found only by a fresh inversion restoring the original state: '"God" is "dog" backward an' they say he is a man's best friend and so he God'. As with so much of Life in the Valley, slippage between inside and outside meanings is the source of continued hilarity, particularly when it involves children or new members. Contradictions, puns, and 'nonsense' are joyfully seized upon. Like obscenities, calypsos, and village humour, they champion the wordplay and fragmentary subversions of an African-American English.

The Life is not really to be understood through words anyway; these are an imperfect reflection of Nature, suited to the double-talk of the Scientific world:

> Words is just a confusion. The power is in you. Is the book I'm speaking about when you really think about it because is the book the children are learning from, not really from their true self – the senses. So, then they become a slave to the book. The book becomes the main part of slavery now.

The limits of Trinidadian tolerance are breached by what the Earth People term the culture of the body. Although the community are sometimes referred to by others as the Naked People, we may argue that they are 'nude' rather than 'naked', for they defiantly engaged in a social activity motivated by a recognition that they are contravening a fundamental value. The Western notion of 'nudity', on which the Earth People draw, entails a way of seeing which is conventionalized and idealized: a deliberate shedding of clothes on behalf of other meanings of the act, whether sexual display or antinomian revolt. McCauley and Lawson (2003) argue that because nudity is 'emotionally provocative' and hence newly memorable, it is more easily transmitted as a new ritual practice.

In Trinidad a naked plantain is one eaten without any sauce, undressed and signalling poverty. One important measure of a woman's respectability is her struggle to send her children to school in clean and ironed clothes. Even to go bareback (shirtless) is hardly for respectable men, and no woman would publicly bare her breast to feed her baby. When they venture into the bush, village women are clothed in hat, boots, and kerchiefs wrapped about; at other times (Carnival always excepted) even trousers are hardly acceptable for rural women and, like shorts, indicate the dubious morals of the promiscuous *jagomet*. No adult in the West Indies has gone naked in public since slavery, and probably rarely then (Braithwaite 1971). At Mother Earth's prompting I gave a talk about the Earth People at the psychiatric hospital in which she had been once interned. Incredulity at my own going naked in the Valley prompted the usual criticisms of nudity: it led to promiscuity and laziness, to squatting in filth and excrement, and the abuse of children.

When someone comes to join the group, they are encouraged immediately to relinquish their clothes, which are burned or used for toilet purposes. The year before I first arrived in the Valley, the Earth People had decided to wear bag (sacking) kilts when outside the community. Public provocation was played down in favour of the idea that Natural life was only really possible in the bush, and nudity in town was restricted to particular demonstrations of protest in the central square. Mother Earth's own argument for nudity recalls that of the semiologist: clothes are just a means of social distinction increasing rather than diminishing sexual interest. As Mother Earth puts it, 'Everything has its meaning, its sign. Everything has its spirit. Clothes now, they build it in signs to always get it sell'. It is the religion of the Europeans which has persuaded African people that they cannot live together among the elements, and resilience is valued in the Valley. My own experience suggests it is comparatively easy to work in the sun with no clothes on; the test is in the night when one lies naked on the cold ground above the cliff with no covering. The frequent cuts, thorns, and scorpion stings consequent on going without shoes are shrugged off, and the Valley member with a poisoned foot who seeks an extended period away from his labours is accused of still being under the influence of the Son: 'Without clothes, baby skin develop toughness quicker . . . that is how we put ourselves down to Nature to regain our spirit' (Mother Earth).

Members of this celibate community obtain a good deal of amusement from the idea that everybody believes them to be engaged in an endless orgy. But nakedness does involve us in a raw physical intimacy, an unveiling of bodily activities other than sex. The male Earth People freely urinate outside the men's hut while continuing general conversation (not a local Trinidad practice), but they have built two earth latrines which are enclosed by wooden planks and remain relatively private, although the sounds sometimes emanating from them are a subject for ribald merriment: 'Free up you'self now!' During her menstrual periods Mother Earth keeps a rag between her legs, changing this at intervals. She may call attention to it, and the newer male recruits complain rather queasily.

Public renunciation closely follows the mode of discipline and control within the group. The Earth People recall themselves as having been 'searching' when they met Mother Earth. While a decision to join coming from one's spirit is preferable to calculation, none of the group describe anything that could be called a sudden conversion. Adherence is simply taking off one's clothes and living in the Valley. A slow understanding dawning on the potential member is preferred. The community is experienced as a logical extension of the experiential world, a broadening and validation of it; there can be no shame or guilt attached to one's earlier life, merely a need to forget it.

Compared with other new religious movements in the West, the Earth People are 'open' – prosaic and flexible – with relatively free movement to and from the group. Membership is signalled by immediate participation in most group activities alongside established members. Any sudden protestations of full conviction in Mother's teachings would be rather suspect; what is assumed is an immediate readiness to join in the way of life, principally by taking off one's clothes and labouring in the Valley; the boundaries of the group are physical above all. The only initial commitment required is an acknowledgement of the undesirability of urban and middle-class goals, and of the centrality of Nature as manifest in the person of Mother Earth. Even for established members, a readiness to work hard and to subordinate personal interests to those of the group – 'humbling you' self' or 'sacrificing you' self' – is valued above ideological rectitude. The enthusiastic participant is allowed greater latitude in disagreeing with theoretical questions than the one who is less hard-working. Commitment is in taking off one's clothes; while recruits have little personal property beyond clothes to renounce, the difficulty of returning to town without them (or money) reinforces the group's cohesion.

It is the physical work without modern tools which Mother Earth recognizes as the principal way of neglecting the urban past. As she told me:

> Some of them that come comes with a spirit of seeing themselves and working the land. Some come they want to play. They not really thinking of what they're doing so then they usually leave because working they find that is too hard to do. So, they don't stay, they leave. But those who stay they go through little cutses, biteses, you know, and fight up with it.

Everyday life in the Valley offers no continuing revelations, no prayers or possession states, no supplications of a divinity, no contact with any external power, but rather engagement with Nature in an immediate sense. Ultimate reality is present in the authority of Mother Earth and through her in daily tasks. No one moment seems more central than another, but if any activity could be said to be 'sacramental', it is the production and consumption of food. Food must be provided for those who will come at the End, and the land has to be prepared now. In fact, more food is harvested than is immediately required: baskets are overflowing, piles of yams rot in the out-houses. Agricultural techniques are those traditionally used in the coastal villages. Many of these have now been discarded by the remaining country people, less for reasons of economic maximization than because they are just 'primitive' (Littlewood 2007). While the Earth People do not employ fertilizers or machines, they still use cutlasses, axes, and small scythes, the implements which remained intact around the house after the Burning in 1976 and also those still found most commonly in the villages. The materials employed are wood, bark, and creepers, which are strung, knotted, matted, twisted, plaited, and lashed. Water transport comprises a dug-out canoe and two rafts. Hessian is used for sails, bags, and the short kilts now worn on the way to town.

Decisions as to land use are agreed collectively (there are no private plots), but usually only after suggestions by Mother Earth. All adult male members work on the land during the majority of the daylight hours, cutting, burning, planting, weeding, and gathering. The food collected is brought back to the storage area to be cooked under the supervision of Mother Earth. The main meals, usually twice a day, are communal; Mother Earth calls each member by name and his calabash is filled with food, which is eaten sitting on the ground in the same place where he sleeps at night. The parallel rows of sleeping places recall an old British school dormitory and provide a personal space where individual tools may be stored together with small pieces of carving or other work in progress.

Members have a claim to use objects made by them, but to refuse to lend them on the basis that they are 'owned' would be *antisocial* and thus implying distinction. At the same time, there is considerable bickering over the borrowing of tools, incidents which Mother Earth uses to reinforce notions of personal responsibility for one's own tools and responsibility to the group as a whole.

While work involves clearing the land and removing unproductive bush, the ultimate aim is to allow Nature to blossom unhindered. Machines are quite unacceptable, but a limited degree of technical innovation – say a more efficient way of burning scrub – is often debated. The acceptance by members that they live in a 'compromised' pre-utopia does not in itself determine exactly where the line is to be drawn. There are continual and heated discussions. Crises in the group usually prompt a more natural line. When things are progressing smoothly, what we may call a 'technical' approach becomes accepted; conflicts herald a purist return to the central teaching. The point of general accommodation seems to be bounded by some conception of African life as portrayed in the cinema, together with the technology used on the coast up to the 1960s. On occasions the line is drawn depending on frank comfort: 'We suppose not to use light, but we still use flambeaux as we accustom to it from the city'. Points that are never for negotiation are nudity and the refusal to use animals for labour. The goats are tethered only lest they wander into the bush. When going to town – a dangerous site of memories (cf. Halbwachs 1994 [1925]; Nora 1989) – the group set off to walk the whole way but are not altogether reluctant to accept a lift in the back of a passing truck. They are quite happy to accept food from sympathizers when in town, and some of the younger members volunteer for errands away from the Valley just so that they can sample packaged foods again: 'To say to contradict the food outside, you can' do that because you eat it sometime an' before we come to our senses we was eating it . . .', as Cassava put it to me.

Debates as to the acceptability of hunting agouti or using nets to fish are of greater significance. A general discussion as to whether to grow rice was solved by sending me to the University Department of Agriculture to beg some hill rice, a generally acceptable compromise: 'That we own spirit talking to we!' (Breadfruit). Discussing one's own personal past life is *social* and discouraged, as is using one's original name. But Mother Earth's directed amnesia can hardly be totally successful at first. The gap between the ideal future-in-the-present and the compromised memory provides the texture of daily life inside the Valley, but it is especially salient in the physical separation between the Valley itself and Rome.[4] The outside world remains necessary as a source of new recruits, and the Valley maintains relations with it through the persistence of past sentiments and through some economic transactions. On occasions they beg or scrounge necessary articles, or purchase salt, rice, sacking, cutlasses, and even kerosene from the Pinnacle stores, or barter fish, copra, and fruit using cash equivalents.

Too close to Pinnacle Village to risk any confrontation and knowing that many of the villagers remain resentful of their squatting on Pinnacle land, the Earth People make no attempt on such occasions to gain new recruits, although they are prepared to 'put out' their views if challenged. In the village are families who were friends with Mother Earth before her visions, and they are the people most likely to trade with Hell Valley. Intrusions from the past, if modest, are not generally regarded as threatening. Sometimes a passer-by along the Turnpike, usually an itinerant preacher or hiking student, stops for a meal and discussion. He is welcomed and work stops as the Earth People gather round to teach him and show him their crops and offer gifts of their best produce to carry away. They welcome the occasional coverage in the media but complain of misrepresentation, particularly of being described as violent.

Post-communist Derret i Vogël

The Catholic village of Derret i Vogël lies two kilometres from Montenegro in mountainous northern Albania, west of the Accursed Mountains. It now has a population of around 700 (900 in 1990), representing thirteen different patrilineal *fis* (clans, lineages). The eighty-one households are grouped by *fis* in districts inside the village, many next to each other in joint male sibships (*vllazni*).[5] None are conspicuously wealthy, but very few are poor. Houses are now generally concrete, built with remittances from family members working abroad. They are widely dispersed, each on its own household land. The village is more or less self-sufficient in basic food – milk, pigs, chickens, sheep, maize, pumpkins, tomatoes, cabbage, onions, cucumbers, grapes, plums, figs, and trellis vines. Wheat and coffee are bought in the town of Shkodër two hours away by truck along an unmetalled road. Potatoes, maize, and young pigs are sold to the town, and also a mountain herb recalling thyme (*sherbil*) which is exported from Shkodër for medicines. There is no longer land telephone communication, but by 2003 most of the better-off families had mobiles. With no piped water in the village, the electricity supply is precariously maintained for six hours per day; cooking is carried out by the women generally on wood stoves or on open fires in the house yard. In addition to household work, women fetch water from the well, firewood from the forest, and do much of the heavy agricultural work. The men work as drivers or farmers, with cash also earned from smuggling, small pensions, and compensation in cashable coupons for periods of imprisonment in the communist period (for each *familje persekutesme*, persecuted family).[6] Two families have been able to buy a truck with remittances from sons abroad, and provide occasional transport to town or other villages.

Before 1944, the Catholic northern mountains were largely inhabited by a land-owing peasantry (Durham 1985 [1909]), for the terrain was not suitable for the accumulation of large estates. The mountains were the last area of resistance to the communist Hoxha regime, and the village land was fully collectivized only in the late 1960s. Until 1993, cars, fridges, television, beer, and wheat flour were unknown in the village, and rare in the town. The north was relatively neglected by the communists and there was little industrial investment, although the proximity of the village to the border meant more than the usual allocation of military bunkers,[7] and a subterranean army barracks and artillery station were built into the nearby mountains overlooking the village, where the forest was cut down for timber and for security. The village was controlled by a People's Council of its sixty or so communist (Party of Labour) members and the old system of *bayrak* (region, literally Banner or mobilizable force) and *fis* organization was abolished. The villagers now say publicly that 'everybody was a prisoner' in that forced levies and youth camps for building roads, railways, and electrical infrastructure were ubiquitous. The ex-communists do not disagree. The cemetery was bulldozed when religion was abolished in 1965, and all village produce was taken away for external distribution after private possession of animals was finally prohibited in the late 1960s; meals (still prepared by women) were served in a communal canteen as Hoxha tried to eradicate the power of the joint *vllazni* household and its organization through male kin and their wives. Nevertheless, villagers recall that the local communist party was essentially kin-based, and the People's Council organized heavier working days for the families of non-members. But health care and education in the primary school were regular and efficient, unlike now.

Enver Hoxha died in 1985, and the regime gradually lost its grip on the population. As news of student demonstrations in the nearby town of Shkodër reached the village in 1990, some men immediately set off there in their carts to join in; and later when the communist period was clearly over, many joined the new Democratic Party. The exact details of who did what, when, are already publicly obscure, although incidental memories (Cole 2001) may intrude. The events are not commemorated. A period of destruction of buildings of the communal era certainly set in: canteen and store, school, crèche, cultural centre, buildings for collectivized animals, the reservoir and the irrigation system were all triumphantly razed or severely damaged. Some materials were recycled for private building, and the collective's potato shed was converted into a makeshift church. Local communist members were thrown out of office but not harmed physically. Others such as the teachers left the village and their dormitory was burned. As Gjergj, the son of an old political prisoner, pointed out to me one day when we were fishing in the river with stolen dynamite: 'My father said, "What's the point, we all still have to live together". I protested, "But how can you now receive them [as guests in your house]?" My father replied, "All that is over. It is too painful to recall"'.[8]

Gjergj still does not visit the old Communist Party members who all still live in Derret,[9] although he talks politely enough with them when we meet in the three village bars. Collectivized animals and land were spontaneously redistributed within weeks[10] without major quarrels, back to the *fis* who had previously owned them, up to the slopes of the mountains which remain state land. Party members acquiesced and indeed participated. The low stone walls which divided the plots were rebuilt and are kept in perfect repair. Schwandner-Sievers (1999) has described the return to the old *fis* and Kanun (customary law) boundary markers and traditions as a 're-traditionalization' for the Kanun (Littlewood 2002) and the old lineages of the patriclan were again emphasized, although the administration of the regional *bayrak* of Hoti was not reintroduced, but replaced by a new elected regional council

(Saltmarshe 2001). A local village council with an elected *kryeplak* (mayor, originally senior elder) was established, and a literate inhabitant wrote an enthusiastic popular history of the area in the form of a genealogy of the predominant local *fis*, with a pronounced but hardly elaborated anti-communist bias (Smajlaj 2001), thus linking the present village to the past of tradition. Marriage custom in the mountains[11] had hardly been affected by communism (with local Party of Labour officials following it themselves),[12] but bride-price (Hasluck 1954) has never been reintroduced, being substituted by extensive formalized gift-giving from the bridegroom to the bride and the bride's family at engagement and wedding. 'Re-traditionalization' has occurred particularly at the local and family level rather than that of wider political institutions.

In the early 1990s, immediately after the end of communism, the village entered a brief economic boom as petroleum and other goods were smuggled over the nearby border into Montenegro in defiance of the economic embargo placed on Yugoslavia during the Bosnian war. Women recall that the village was temporarily so wealthy that 'the men were drunk every day'. Contraband is now limited to leading horses over the mountains or the purchase of consumer goods in Montenegro for resale in Albania, carried on the back or with bribing of the border guards. The central government has never established secure control over the country, certainly not in the north, where banditry and armed robbery remain common (Schwandner-Sievers 1999), with the police being regarded by villagers as easily bribeable or as simply inept. They told me that they regard their country now, ten years after communism, as dangerous, corrupt, and chaotic.[13] But none miss the order and security of the Hoxha period. All the men complain of being abandoned by Western Europe ('Are we Africans?') and encourage their own sons to emigrate, legally or illegally, to Greece or Italy, and send back support for their families (Kretsi 2002). Most households have one member abroad in this way, and in the village televisions and indoor toilets are becoming more common. Expatriate money has provided a new church and school, a health centre, and a pump for the village well.

'Capitalism' with its foreign NGOs is described as modern, as a bountiful source of wealth, as open and generous, and as more naturally rooted than communism in the local kin structures; few villagers would perceive any problems with a business economy, which is regarded as an ideological rather than an economic set of affairs. Rausing (2004) notes of post-communist Estonia that the 'temporary amnesia' for the Soviet period inevitably still includes certain communist ways of comportment and thinking. And the 'return to tradition' in northern Albania has not involved a resurgence of moral explanations couched in the form of the evil eye or witchcraft (cf. de Waal 2005), which, as in the communist period, are seen as folkloric.

Townspeople in Shkodër still lament the loss of the free public services (which are seen as a right) and asked me with incredulity, as did the villagers, if it was really true that, in Britain, if one did not pay for electricity or water supplies, these were cut off.[14] It is recognized that all officials, at the town and regional councils, doctors, and police have to be bribed to carry out their duties; rubbish, unknown in the communist period, now lies along all the roads and beaches of Albania. At the same time, there remains strong trust between the members of a *fis* lineage: they are the preferred people to borrow money from[15] or to work with, even if a *fis* member expects to be paid more in your enterprise than a non-member. Yet there is nevertheless a gradual shift away from the *fis* and the brother-based household to nuclear families and smaller households (Doja 1998).[16]

Amnesia and Autonomy: Derret's Moral Economy

If local and national aspirations are orientated to Western Europe and to something like a market economy as it is locally understood, there are still continuities with the communist period: a lack of clear distinction between the particular political party in power and the state, a dependency on both, the politicization of the police and civil services, and a preference for illicit bribes and personal favours. The local zero-sum economics of the pre-communist peasantry passed through a short-lived period of perceived infinite abundance for all (late communism and immediate post-communism), to return back to a situation where no one can advance materially except through a loss gained by others, or by bribery, emigration, or foreign aid. There are few voluntary civil associations, and those largely of ex-political prisoners or of local NGOs in some towns who agitate for overseas development funding. Foreign NGOs have not moved beyond the town, and the incursion of foreign missionaries in the 1990s did not touch Derret. Though the public services of the communist period are mourned, they are seldom commented on; all is focused on future individual opportunities and the current thwarting of them by the post-communist Socialist Party. To advance is to possess the secret language of the NGOs (Sampson 1996).[17] The widespread destruction in the towns which followed the collapse of the Democratic Party's 'pyramid savings schemes' in 1997 did not significantly affect the villagers, who had few savings to invest, and they remain committed to the Democrats, who form the current 2008 central government, rather than to the Socialists. All is present-centred. The burning in the 1990s of the town archives has meant that the communist period (and earlier) is at one historical level irretrievable.

Derret is still scattered with the remains of buildings of the Hoxha period – the burned canteen, dairy, and culture centre, the abandoned school, and the less destructible and ubiquitous concrete bunkers. All these, though apparent to the view of anybody, are 'seen through' as if they are not there.[18] No one comments publicly on them, the younger children are not sure what the burned buildings were, and adults answer my (and the local children's) questions about some remaining substantial structure with awkwardness: 'Oh what? Oh that's nothing – it's from the old days'. The bunkers and broken buildings are now covered with briars and weeds. The suggestion that the communist-era buildings could have remained economically useful elicits official incomprehension: in 1991 they were justly destroyed as representative of the old regime. No one bothers to go and visit the extensive subterranean barracks in the nearby mountains, which are by-passed by the villagers in their annual movement of animals to the higher pastures. Indeed, some are not sure exactly where they are. The return to the old has meant that each dispersed household is again self-sufficient, with its one or two cows, its pig, its flock of sheep or goats, and its single horse. Unless the returned communist building was on a clearly identified piece of *fis* land, the central area of the village has been abandoned. No collective enterprise was converted into individual production. The man to whom the dairy land was returned simply sold off the milk churns for distilling household raki and encouraged the building to fall down. The People's Council had built a small reservoir on the edge of the village, from which a series of concrete channels alongside each lane conducted irrigation water to every patch of arable land; these are now all blocked with rubbish or broken (cf. de Waal 2005). No one suggests restoring them. The reservoir itself was claimed by a man whose *fis* originally owned the land: he planned to turn it into a fish farm, but nothing happened. Its paved lining is now holed and peeling, no longer waterproof but with a small dirty pool in the bottom.

But like the dairy, dining halls, old school, and cultural centre, barracks and bunkers, no one ever comments on it – at least in public discussion. The reservoir is there, and it is not there. Outside the village and beyond the town, disused and burned factories similarly line the bigger roads. The nitrate mine to the east is effectively abandoned. The communist-era railway to Montenegro barely functions and then only for occasional goods traffic. No one complains about these. Nor are they mentioned very much in conversation between villagers, although individuals are prepared to talk privately about them and about their own experiences in the communist period. As Saltmarshe remarks (on the exploitation of Albanian women under communism):

> Much remains unsaid on this subject; however, I doubt that it will ever be publicly remembered . . . It was almost as though there exists a pact of forgetting concerning this and other matters such as those who worked for or

informed the *sigurimi* [security police]. The willingness and capacity to forget is an important component in any transformation. (2001: 92)

Conclusions

Rather different from the Earth People, for whom memories of past pleasures threaten the collective future and have to be suppressed by the leader, in Derret i Vogël the local past just seems too painful and dangerous for the community to consciously bear in mind, and thus to recall 'publicly'.[19] Criticisms of the Hoxha period in public are made very generally and referred away from the village. My drinking encounters there with an old communist, once an educated party cadre and now an aimless and rather pathetic old man always begging a drink in a household or bar,[20] often ended after too much raki with our both exchanging communist salutes, Cuban slogans, and singing the Internationale. We were observed by those around us with silent pity but completely without rancour or complaint. Objections were just directed to my indulging his drinking, not to any breach of the new democratic principles or to any questionable retrieval of a forbidden past. The end of communism in the village was exciting but relatively untraumatic – and thus perhaps less memorable (Sturken 1997); to discuss it now publicly would entail personal disagreements between victims and party members, recovering the real traumas of the past, and possibly resurrecting disputes over land ownership. By contrast, graves and sites of sudden death by accident in both the communist and post-communist eras are freely borne in mind, and neighbours and kin are invited to visit and lay flowers.

As the bodily comportment of the Earth People is now seen as more 'free', so in the Albanian village, individuals are now seen as more liberated: newly married women again wear heavy make-up if they can afford it and some men beards (both banned by Hoxha), fights break out easily at village feasts, and life is seen as generally more chaotic. The Church has not established its precedence, and few households possess a Bible or catechism. Both societies signal liberation from the past and also a future abundance with food. If excess production of food is characteristic of the Trinidad commune, so in Albania hospitality has reverted back to a celebration of the household guest:[21] food is offered in abundance, the feet of male visitors are again washed by the women[22] and they are expected to eat to excess. But beyond the attempt to 'return' to the past, there is a sense of something missing that cannot be publicly stated or even considered (cf. the old German Democratic Republic post-unification: Eng and Kazanjian 2003). There is an empty space with no attempt to 'wash it' by reconfiguring it as a traditional narrative (to use Cole's [2001] Betsimaraka idiom on colonialism).

The two modes of technological neglect are clearly each rather different. Both may be said to be projected – to be intentional. Both the Albanian village and the Earth People are barely literate and exist in the margins of the global capitalist system, but Derret village, just like the wider West Indian society, aspires to a Western and urban way of life. The Earth People's rejection of this is collective, formal, didactic, and hierarchical, embedded in a distinctive and novel ideology of neglect, and consciously directed. (Similarly Meyer 1998 and van Dijk 1998.) By contrast, in Derret i Vogël there is no formal or public expectation of what is to be discarded; based in autobiographical memories and intersubjective sentiments, and not centrally mandated, it is, however, none the less ideological in demonstrating concurrence between everyday practice and the explicit and shared social order (cf. Bloch 1998). It appears part of a wider loss of embodied practices – a loss of collective provision, school education, forced labour, and revolutionary festivals.

In terms of immediate production, both groups 'suffer' economically through conscious neglect, not ignorance. By using only slightly more effective techniques, the Earth People could easily net fish or gather coconuts from the now abandoned groves along the coast (Littlewood 1993) and then market the copra. An Albanian agreement to continue to use the once efficient communal irrigation system would avoid women and horses spending hours carrying barrels of water from the well some considerable distance to the houses and fields. And the village has had to build the school and the clinic all over again. Communal enterprises such as the bakery, even when passing back into individual *fis* ownership, could have continued as a private business, but each family prefers subsistence agriculture – to be grimly self-sufficient, baking their own bread, and milking their own cows and goats, preparing their cheese and buttermilk, loading the horse with hay, fetching water and gathering fuel. Whilst 'capitalism' is seen as a bountiful (but foreign and barely intelligible) system, the individual ownership of a large-scale enterprise locally would give rise to accusation of corruption and crime (Littlewood 2002). When I pointed to examples of modestly successful enterprises in town, such as small shops or garages, the villagers always retorted that that was only possible by continued bribery of the old nomenklatura, still the local bureaucracy (cf. Frisby 1998). Instead, the village as a whole looks for material advancement either to outside remittances or to future European Union funding.

In neither case, Earth People or Derret i Vogël, is economic efficiency paramount. Both still know it is possible. The Earth People neglect a more effective technical past as corrupt and oppressive, as does the Albanian village. Whilst both attempt to increase production within the limits they have deliberately set themselves, for neither is material maximization per se an obvious goal. For both, neglect of the practically possible is the first stage to forgetting a compromised past.

Notes

Fieldwork with the Earth People in Trinidad was conducted first on a Social Science Research Council Post-Doctoral Fellowship in 1980–1982, and again in 1987 and 1992. I have generally used here the present tense for 1981 and used material from Littlewood (1993). I stayed in Derret i Vogël, Albania, twice between 2001 and 2003, conducting fieldwork in basic Albanian.

1. Or the Edict of Nantes which proscribed remembrance.
2. I am concerned here not with the vexed question of whether powerful memories can indeed be suppressed but retrieved through particular psychological techniques, but with the apparently easier question of how practices and ideas, once taken for granted on a daily basis, can be gradually forgotten as a motivated act.
3. Ricoeur's (2004) methodological forgetting.
4. Western urban society, similar to the Rasta Babylon (Chevannes 1995).
5. If two married brothers move out of the patrimonial household, they build adjoining houses which retain a variable amount of shared resources.
6. The *armiq të popullit* (enemies of the people) of the communist period. The major sources of communist support were the Islamic and Orthodox population in the south, where the party originated. To an extent, the neglect of communism now is a continuation of the old northern neglect of the centre, the south, and the government. The north retains a strong sense of marginality.
7. Enver Hoxha is supposed to have built one concrete bunker for every two inhabitants in Albania. When prompted, the villagers recall that there were frequent military alerts in the communist period when villagers took their places in their allotted bunkers. No external threat ever materialized.
8. Similar remarks are made by all in private conversation as if the recent past cannot be contained. Ricoeur (2004) suggests that forgiveness and forgetting are closely allied.
9. The communist leader of the old People's Council is now restricted to his house by a disabling stroke. This is attributed to his heavy drinking and to his own disappointments: for poverty is seen to lead to madness (*çmenduri*). There has been nothing like a 'Truth Commission' in Albania; trials of ex-communist officials were abandoned in the 1990s, and Hoxha's widow, imprisoned after his death for corruption, has been released.
10. Contrast Hahn's (1994) Hungarian village, where the locals were reluctant to abandon collectivization after the end of communism. In Albania, redistribution of communal land elsewhere has been a major cause of family quarrels and blood feuds (de Waal 2005; Schwandner-Sievers 1999).
11. Exogamy outside the *fis* arranged by the elders with virilocal residence (Doja 1999). But 'love marriages' have become more common and accepted as modern.
12. Marriage within the clan, indeed within the village, is equated with family incest (incest). A local joke is that in the pre-war Zog era, a woman in public walked seven paces behind her husband; under Hoxha this was reduced to three (probably referring to the communist reduction of the limits of prohibited consanguinity from seven generations to three). Clearly there is another incident of forgetting here which I do not consider: the

communist era's own forgetting of its pre-communist past (Misha 2002) (whose centrally directed mode recalls that of the Earth People).

13. Derret itself seems to have remained fairly peaceful as, owing to the late collectivization (1960s), there were few subsequent disagreements about where the original boundaries lay.
14. The local town abandoned attempts to cut off water and electricity to non-payers after near violent protests, recalling Durham's 1908 quote from northern Albania: 'We won't have a poor Government. We want a rich one. If this constitution is not rich enough to give us these things it can go to the devil' (Durham 2001: 15).
15. Indeed, it is almost impossible to borrow money elsewhere, except project grants from the district council (which require a bribe).
16. This had been encouraged by the communists distributing rations by the household, rather than by its members. The fewer in the household, the more food each individual received. Doja (1998) argues that a gradual turn to the nuclear family and a decline of the community role of the *zoti i shtepisë* (household head) continued throughout the twentieth century.
17. Schwandner-Sievers (2002: 25) describes local expectations of the West as 'almost [like] a "cargo-cult" in their visions'.
18. When looking through my photographs on preparing this chapter, I was amused to see that I too had neglected to photograph these bunkers and abandoned buildings, though I took plenty of the new church and of farm production.
19. As 'passive' rather than 'commanded amnesia' (Ricoeur 2004). When prompted privately by me, individuals, of course, had personal memories of the past events – episodes of heroism and of suffering. But these are publicly inaccessible, unavailable. Even the village and regional events when communism was overthrown are not celebrated or marked. The small antique/junk shop in Shkodër contains old bits of costumes and objects from the countryside but virtually no items from the relatively recent communist era, nor are these retained at home.
20. As one villager complained to me, 'If we say "Sorry, we are just about to eat", he will say "Good, I'll stay"'.
21. 'The house of the Albanian belongs to God and the guest' (Gjeçov 1989 [1933]: 132). Women again serve food to their men and guests and retire to eat afterwards, often from plates on the floor.
22. It might be expected that young women, brought up under communism, would now regret the loss of educational opportunities and the return to a highly constrained female role. This is true for some. But like further south (de Waal 2005), women again generally centre their aspirations on marriage and traditional values.

References

Antze, P. and M. Lambek. 1996. *Tense Past: Cultural Essays in Trauma and Memory.* London: Routledge.

Berger, B. 1981. *The Survival of a Counter-Culture: Ideological Work and Everyday Life Among Rural Communards.* Berkeley: University of California Press.

Bloch, M. 1998. *How We Think They Think.* Boulder, CO: Westview Press.

Bourdieu, P. 1977. *Outline of a Theory of Practice* (trans. R. Nice). Cambridge: Cambridge University Press.

Braithwaite, E. 1971. *The Development of Creole Society in Jamaica 1770–1820*. Oxford: Clarendon Press.
Burridge, K. 1969. *New Heaven, New Earth: A Study of Millenarian Activities*. Oxford: Blackwell.
Carsten, J. 1995. 'The Politics of Forgetting: Migration, Kinship and Memory on the Periphery of the Southeast Asian State', *Journal of the Royal Anthropological Institute* (N.S.) 1: 317–35.
Chevannes, B. 1995. *Rastafari and Other African-Caribbean Worldviews*. London: Macmillan.
Cole, J. 2001. *Forget Colonialism? Sacrifice and the Art of Memory in Madagascar*. Berkeley: University of California Press.
Connerten, P. 1989. *How Societies Remember*. Cambridge: Cambridge University Press.
de Waal, C. 2005. *Albania Today: A Portrait of Post-Communist Turbulence*. London: Tauris.
Dennett, D. 1991. *Consciousness Explained*. London: Allen Lane.
Doja, A. 1998. 'L'évolution et la folklorisation des traditions culturelles', *East European Quarterly* 32: 95–123.
______. 1999. 'Morphologie traditionnelle de la société albanaise', *Social Anthropology* 7: 37–55.
Douglas, M. 1995. 'Forgotten Knowledge', in M. Strathern (ed.), *Shifting Contexts: Transformations in Anthropological Knowledge*. London: Routledge, pp. 13–30.
Durham, E. 1985. *High Albania*. London: Virago.
______. 2001. *Albania and the Albanians: Selected Articles and Letters 1903–1944*. London: Centre for Albanian Studies.
Eng, D.L. and D. Kazanjian (eds). 2003. *Loss: The Politics of Mourning*. Berkeley: University of California Press.
Espinosa, F. 2003. *La Columna de la Muerte: El Avance del Ejército Franquista de Seville a Bandujoz*. Barcelona: Crítica.
Forty, A. and S. Kuchler (eds). 1999. *The Art of Forgetting*. Oxford: Berg.
Frisby, T. 1998. 'The Rise of Organised Crime in Russia: Its Roots and Significance', *Europe-Asia Studies* 50: 27–49.
Gay y Blasco, P. 2001. '"We Don't Know Our Descent": How the Gitanos of Jarana Manage the Past', *Journal of the Royal Anthropological Institute* (N.S.) 7: 631–47.
Gjecov, S. 1989. *Kanuni i Lekë Dukagjini* (The Code of Lekë Dukagjini) (trans. L. Fox). New York: Gjonlekaj.
Gupta, D. 2005. *Learning to Forget: The Anti-Memoirs of Modernity*. Delhi: Oxford University Press.
Hahn, C. 1994. 'After Communism: Reflections on East European Anthropology and the "Transition"', *Social Anthropology* 2: 229–49.
Halbwachs, M. 1994. *Les Cadres Sociaux de la Mémoire*. Paris: Albin Michel.
Hasluck, M. 1954. *The Unwritten Law in Albania*. Cambridge: Cambridge University Press.
Holloway, M. 1966. *Heavens on Earth: Utopian Communities in America 1680–1880*. New York: Dover.
Kirmeyer, L. 1996. 'Landscapes of Memory: Trauma, Narrative and Dissociation', in P. Antze and M. Lambek (eds), *Tense Past: Cultural Essays in Trauma and Memory*. London: Routledge, pp. 173–98.
Kretsi, G. 2002. '"Shkelquen" oder "Giannis"? Namenwechsel und Identitätsstrategien zwischen Heilmatkultur und Migration', in K. Kaser, R. Pichler and S. Schwandner-Sievers (eds), *Die weite Welt und das Dorf: Albanische Emigration am Ende des 20. Jahrhunderts*. Vienna: Boehlau.
Levi, C. 1963. *Christ Stopped at Eboli* (trans. F. Frenaye). London: Readers' Union.

Littlewood, R. 1993. *Pathology and Identity: The Work of Mother Earth in Trinidad.* Cambridge: Cambridge University Press.

______. 1996. 'Reason and Necessity in the Specification of the Multiple Self', (RAI Occasional Paper 43). London: Royal Anthropological Institute.

______. 2002. 'Trauma and the Kanun: Two Responses to Loss in Albania and Kosova', *International Journal of Social Psychiatry* 48: 86–96.

______. 2004. 'From Elsewhere: Prophetic Visions and Dreams Among the People of the Earth', *Dreaming* 14: 94–106.

______. 2007. 'Coconuts and Syphilis: An Essay in Over-Interpretation', in R. Littlewood (ed.), *On Knowing and Not-Knowing in the Anthropologies of Medicine.* Walnut Creek, CA: Left Coast Press, pp. 18–27.

McCauley, R.N. and E.T. Lawson. 2003. *Bringing Ritual to Mind.* Cambridge: Cambridge University Press.

Meyer, B. 1998. '"Make a Complete Break with the Past": Memory and Postcolonial Modernity in Ghanaian Pentecostal Discourse', in R. Werbner (ed.), *Memory and the Postcolony.* London: Zed, pp. 182–208.

Misha, P. 2002. 'Invention of a Rationalism: Myth and Amnesia', in S. Schwandner-Sievers and B.J. Fischer (ed.), *Albanian Identities: Myth and History* London: Hurst, pp. 33–48.

Nora, P. 1989. 'Between Memory and History: Les Lieux de Mémoire', *Representations* 26: 7–25.

Nordhoff, C. 1966 [1875]. *The Communistic Societies of the United States from Personal Observations.* New York: Dover.

Rausing, S. 2004. *History, Memory and Identity in Post-Soviet Estonia: The End of a Collective Farm.* Oxford: Oxford University Press.

Ricoeur, P. 2004. *Memory, History, Forgetting* (trans. K. Blamey and D. Pellauer). Chicago: Chicago University Press.

Rivers, W.H.R. 1978 [1912]. *The Disappearance of Useful Arts.* Cambridge: Cambridge University Press.

Rundus, D. 1971. 'Analysis of Rehearsal Processes in Free Recall', *Journal of Experimental Psychology* 89: 63–77.

Saltmarshe, D. 2001. *Identity in a Post-Communist Balkan State: An Albanian Village Study.* Aldershot: Ashgate.

Sampson, S. 1996. 'The Social Life of Projects: Importing Civil Society to Albania', in C. Hann and E. Dunn (eds), *Civil Society.* London: Routledge, pp. 121–42.

Schacter, D. 2003. *How the Mind Forgets and Remembers.* New York: Souvenir Press.

Schwandner-Sievers, S. 1999. 'Humiliation and Reconciliation in Northern Albania: The Logics of Feuding in Symbolic and Diachronic Perspectives', in G. Elwert, S. Feuchtwang and D. Neubert (eds), *Dynamics of Violence: Processes of Escalation and De-Escalation in Violent Group Conflicts.* Berlin: Duncker und Humblot, pp. 133–52.

______. 2002. 'Narratives of Power: Capacities of Myths in Albania', in S. Schwandner-Sievers and B.J. Fischer (eds), *Albanian Identities: Myth and History.* London: Hurst, pp. 3–25.

Shaw, R. 2002. *Memories of the Slave Trade: Ritual and the Historical Imagination in Sierra Leone.* Chicago: Chicago University Press.

Smajlaj, L.P. 2001. *Kërkime mbi të vërtetën.* Shkodër: Camaj-Pipa.

Stewart, M. 2004. 'Remembering without Commemoration: The Mnemonics and Politics of Holocaust Memories Among European Roma', *Journal of the Royal Anthropological Institute* (N.S.) 10: 561–82.

Sturken, M. 1997. *Tangled Memories: The Vietnam War, the AIDS Epidemic, and the Politics of Remembering.* Berkeley: University of California Press.

van Dijk, R. 1998. 'Pentecostalism, Cultural Memory and the State: Contested Representations of Time in Postcolonial Malawi', in R. Werbner (ed.), *Memory and the Postcolony*. London: Zed, pp. 155–81.
Werbner, R. 1998. 'Smoke from the Barrel of a Gun: Postwars of the Dead, Memory and Reinscription in Zimbabwe', in R. Werbner (ed.), *Memory and the Postcolony*. London: Zed, pp. 71–104.
Woodcock, G. and I. Arakumovic. 1968. *The Doukhobors*. London: Faber.

Chapter 13

Against Belief

The Usefulness of Explanatory Model Research in Medical Anthropology

Introduction

Do our informants' statements reflect their underlying concepts about illness? How do people's statements about sickness relate to their subsequent behaviours? How valid are the models that the anthropologist formulates from his/her informant's statements? These are questions that anthropology has addressed and continues to attempt to answer. A major concern of medical anthropologists is to elicit their informants' understandings of sickness and healing variously labelled as 'explanatory models', 'health beliefs'[1] or just 'understandings'. Within medical anthropology, there is a central notion that what people say and do needs to be understood in terms of explanatory models they carry in their minds. In fact, the common perception of non-anthropologists is that medical anthropology is the study of beliefs and practices associated with illness in diverse cultural groups and the ways in which these can be used in applied settings. Here, we examine explanatory models of illness both in physical and mental disorder.

For many years, the medical behavioural sciences – medical psychology, the sociology of illness behaviour and public health studies – have relied on belief and behaviour models firmly rooted in a positivist or empiricist paradigm. From its inception, the notion of belief has been ubiquitous in medical anthropology, with some of its founders readily resorting to the term. Recent writings continue to emphasize health beliefs. For example, after a description of the 'belief system' of a Papuan New Guinea group, Lepowsky (1990:

1049) asks 'What happens when Western Medicine is introduced to people who believe virtually all serious illness and death are due to sorcery, witchcraft or taboo violation'. Good (1994) rightly points out how belief stands as an unexamined proxy for culture. Much of this emphasis on belief derives from the assumption (often implicit) that changing health-related beliefs will necessarily result in more rational adaptive health-related behaviour. Lack of knowledge and maladaptive behaviour were held to be sources of ill health. For example, Paul wrote in 1955, 'If you wish to help a community to improve its health, you must learn to think like the people of that community' (Paul 1955: 1). Belief is held to determine behaviour in some mechanical way. However, is this born out of anthropological experience?

The health belief model was developed in the 1950s (Becker 1974). Within this paradigm, individuals are educated to modify irrational behaviour and to seek care appropriately. Research using this model, however, has failed to cast light on cultural differences in illness behaviour and rates of morbidity and mortality. Subsequent researchers have developed a variety of models that link health beliefs to health and illness behaviour (Connor and Norman 1998). Examples include the Theory of Reasoned Action (Fishbein and Azjen 1975) and Social Learning Theory (Bandura 1986), both of which have been influential in public health programmes. These models hold a narrow empiricist theory of culture as belief and require a rational autonomous patient who can maximize perceived benefits of treatment and respond adaptively to disease. This is by no means a value-free or culture-free model. The explanatory model concept was developed initially as a clinical application of an anthropological concept (Good 1986). They are sets of beliefs or understandings that specify how an illness episode is caused, its mode of onset and symptoms, pathophysiology and its treatment. According to Kleinman (1980: 106), these are formed and employed to cope with specific health problems and consequently need to be analysed in that concrete setting. Kleinman makes it clear that explanatory models are attributes of individuals, drawing on general knowledge but remaining at least partially as idiosyncratic and situational. They are frequently fragmentary, not fully worked out. They often change and are influenced by individual experiences. They do not determine medical behaviour in a mechanical way (Kleinman 1980: 107, 109). However, they may provide patients with the information they need when choosing and evaluating medical strategies, communicating with other people about sickness and making their own distress recognizable to them (Kleinman 1980: 71, 72). As they are pragmatic, they are strongly orientated towards making statements about causality.

Explanatory Model Instruments

There is no doubt that the explanatory model concept has been highly influential in medical anthropology and is known among health professionals with little knowledge of anthropology. The concept has often been deployed to teach clinicians the 'native's point of view'. In fact, clinicians have recently taken an interest in eliciting patients' explanatory models with a view to changing health beliefs or improving satisfaction in the clinical encounter. A number of instruments have been developed recently by psychiatrists and psychologists to elicit patients' explanatory models both in psychiatry and general medicine. These include the EMIC, SEMI and IPQ. The EMIC (Weiss 1997) and the SEMI (Lloyd et al. 1998) deploy both qualitative and quantitative methods to elicit patients' explanatory models.

The EMIC (Explanatory Model Interview Catalogue) has been devised to measure the epidemiology of cultural beliefs. It is a collection of locally adapted explanatory model interviews examining patterns of distress (including symptoms, social, economic disruptions and stigma), perceived causes, preferences for health seeking and treatment, and general illness beliefs. It has process rules and a system of presenting data, but is lengthy and expensive to use. However, its focus on illness experience, particularly patterns of distress, has helped to clarify the nature of illness burden, providing 'a useful alternative to the traditional indicators used more commonly in public health such as mortality, morbidity, economic impact and disability, which may be inadequate for conveying the magnitude of suffering arising from some diseases' (Weiss 1997: 257; Chan et al. 1994). The SEMI (Short Explanatory Model Interview) uses vignettes to elicit explanatory models (EMs) and consists of a fixed range of predetermined questions from which patients can choose the ones closest to their own views.

There has been some work examining the Illness Perception Questionnaire (IPQ; Weinman et al. 1996), psychiatric patient's explanatory models of psychiatric illness. This has largely concentrated on severe mental illness. Omark's (1980) study of 'nervous breakdown' among people in Florida revealed that 'stress' and 'pressure' were regarded as the most likely causes of this folk illness. There have been a number of studies that examine health beliefs and explanatory models in people in Western societies suffering from mental health problems (Burrow 1993; Nunally 1961; Rippere 1981) using various methodologies ranging from closed questions in an interview to questionnaire or a quantitative experimental design.

Priest et al. (1996) found that 20% of people with depression and other minor mental health problems thought that their illness was biological in origin (genetic or chemical causes), whereas 80% understood it in terms of social factors (stress, bereavement or childhood experiences). Williams and Healy (2001) looked at first-time presenters to a mental health service and found that explanatory models did not consist of a coherent set of beliefs, but a variety of explanations held simultaneously or taken up and dismissed rapidly. These authors fail to examine whether these models have any predictive validity.

Problems with the Explanatory Model Approach

Of course, patients do have cultural understanding of and explanations for their illness, but this may not be very sophisticated and may not directly relate to decisions about treatments. Anthropological experience suggests that people who attribute magical or supernatural causes to misfortune are generally aware of the immediate mechanical or biological causes of these events as well, as illustrated by Evans Pritchard's study of witchcraft among the Azande. However, when people say a god or witch caused a specific illness, they imply not the precise powers of these supernatural agents but the reasons for acting as they do in moral terms: the 'why' rather than the 'how' (Boyer 2001). They rarely discuss how they do this. If the ancestors make someone ill, they have only the faintest notion of how they do it. In fact, this is not a relevant or interesting question for most people.

In many cases of sickness, pragmatic measures are adopted. There is little conceptualization of the practice in symbolic terms (Ohnuki-Tierney 1984; Lewis 1975). For example, Lewis (1975: 234, 235), in his work among the Gnau of Papua New Guinea, differentiated unexplained illness from explained illness. In the former, either 'they did not know why it had occurred, or in which knowledge of any cause was denied or illness was accounted for solely by an observable directly connected sequence of ordinary events' (such as accidentally pouring boiling water on the skin). Treatments for the unexplained illnesses were purely pragmatic (such as lancing a boil) and little further consideration was given to them. However, in 'explained' illness, recourse was made to ideas deriving from their cosmology (their conceptualizations were more elaborate). These included notions of spirits, magic, sorcery or breaking of a taboo. The treatment for these illnesses often involved long rituals. Lewis (1975) points out that explanation was more likely as the illness became more severe, but for an illness with an obvious cause or visible source, it was less likely.

There are several major criticisms of the explanatory model approach. They fail to specify in any detail the extent to which individual explanatory models are shaped by culture and the extent to which they are idiosyncratic formulations. Garro (1986) criticizes the explanatory models in that they do not take into account political and economical determinants. Since they are primarily concerned with beliefs and knowledge that individuals bring to the illness situation, they pay relative little attention to the objective social order as a critical determinant of medical behaviour. Similarly, Morsy (1990) criticizes those studies which privilege culture and perception above local and global power relations, both of which constrain many aspects of the care-seeking process.

Some medical anthropologists have adopted the tools of cognitive psychology (D'Andrade 1976; Young 1978; Young and Garro 1982; Garro 1986) to look at natural decision-making and have developed formal models for the nature of the information considered and how it is processed. Alan Young (1982) has written a cogent critique of the explanatory model approach using the 'rational man' paradigm, which utilizes ideas congruent with contemporary thought in cognitive psychology. According to him, medical anthropologists over-simplify the process of producing statements about sickness and reduce it to the statement and the cognitive structures (explanatory models, conceptual categories) that are supposed to generate the statements. They typically bracket out non-cognitive and non-rational determents of the statements they study. Emotional states and the ability to discourse about medical matters may influence what people say about illness. In the course of a sickness episode, a person is likely to produce several kinds of knowledge, including theoretical, empirical, rationalized knowledge, intersubjective knowledge, and the knowledge the person produced by negotiating the meaning of objects, events and experiences in interaction with other people. Therefore, it is incorrect to assume that every statement the patient makes about a set of medical events can be properly worked into a single account of these events.

One of the essential aims of ethnography is to produce representations of the knowledge of the people we study even if it can only be reached implicitly by observing practices and imagining their interpretations. Language may not accurately reflect underlying concepts. Bloch (1998: 23) argues that anthropological accounts work from an incorrect theory of cognition: 'As a result when they attempt to represent the way that the people studied conceptualise their society, they do so in terms which do not match the way *any* human beings conceptualise anything fundamental and familiar in *any* society or culture'.

It cannot be assumed that words used by a person can be a straightforward guide to their concepts. Underlying concepts about many domains of life are far more sophisticated than the language used to refer to them suggests. In fact, concepts may not be stored in a linguistic form. Recent research in cognitive psychology suggests that much knowledge, especially the knowledge involved in everyday practice, does not take a linear logic-sequential form (ideas are expressed as logical sentences) but is organized in highly complex and integrated networks or mental models, most elements of which are connected to each other in a number of ways (Churchland and Sejnowski 1989).

Concepts involve implicit networks of meanings formed through the experience of and practice in the external world. These models are only partly linguistic; they also integrate visual imagery, other sensory cognition, the cognitive aspects of learned practices, evaluations, memories of sensations, and memories of typical examples (Bloch 1998). Models are based as much in experience, practice, sight, and sensation as in language. These ideas are particularly pertinent to sickness, which is characterized by the experience of altered sensations in the body. The quality and experience of a pain cannot be easily described in words, but the patient will remember having the same pain before. Memory is both somatic and linguistic: 'this body becomes a phenomenological memoir that opens a new way of interpreting distress and suffering and illness' (Pandolfi 1990: 255).

We are arguing that anthropological experience suggests that people do not hold sophisticated or coherent explanations of illness. People generally do not hold well-systematized belief systems but bits of information that may often be conflicting. It is the expert who over-systematizes a society's way of life. As Evans Pritchard (1937: 540) argued in 1937, the Azande witchcraft beliefs 'are not invisible ideational structures but are loose associations of notions'. Bloch (1998) echoes these sentiments and notes that when ideas are brought together in an ethnography and presented as a conceptual system, their insufficiencies and contradictions become apparent. In real life they do not function as a whole but as bits.

Health-Seeking Behaviour

Ideas about treating illness and lay explanatory models are shaped by contingent circumstances and forms of practical 'reasoning in action'. They are not always expressed orally, especially in one-off interviews that tend to produce orthodox responses. Knowledge elicited from interview studies may not include elements relevant to the decision-making process of those questioned. Malinowski has pointed out that people may say one thing and do another. Beliefs may not reflect actions.

We are not denying that underlying concepts influence what the person does in practice, more the notion that people hold underlying beliefs which directly influence their actions. Models 'of' may not be models 'for' (Holy and Stuchlik 1983). Health-seeking behaviour may not relate to underlying explanatory models. There is a large amount of data from medical anthropological research that suggests that treatment choice is determined primarily by social and political factors rather than underlying explanatory models (Pelto and Pelto 1997). Objective social factors and structures of inequality may be more constraining than subjective beliefs. For example, in James Young's (1981) classic study on medical decision-making in a rural Mexican community, cultural beliefs such as the general categorizing of illnesses and treatments into 'hot' and 'cold' categories had little effect on specific treatment-seeking decisions. Similarly, studies using the EMIC (Weiss et al. 1992) among leprosy patients suggest that those who held theories of humoral imbalance rather than biomedical theories of infection, sanitation and hygiene had the best biomedical clinic attendance records for leprosy treatment.

Alan Young (1982: 270) writes: 'Social forces help to determine which people get which sickness; symbols of healing are simultaneously symbols of power and medical practices are simultaneously ideological practices'. The use of biomedical healing as opposed to traditional healing may be a symbol of privileged status. Myntti (1988), in a study of Yemenite healing, suggests that the Muslim ulama (learned religious figures), a group wielding economic power based on their role as wealthy urban entrepreneurs, have come to prefer biomedical healing to traditional Islamic healers as a symbol of their privileged status.

In terms of treatment outcomes, patients may not be interested in how a treatment works (Last 1981) as long as it works. The weight of empirical evidence suggests that people are keen to utilize biomedical treatments regardless of their cultural beliefs without giving up traditional explanations of illness. A study of the use of traditional healers among South Asian psychiatric patients in East London, using both quantitative and qualitative interviews (Dein 2001), revealed that 28% of the sample had resorted to a traditional healer during the course of their illness. Biomedical and traditional models of illness were held concurrently. The use of traditional healing did not appear to be directly related to the underlying model of illness nor to religious affiliation, with both Hindu and Muslim patients consulting both types of healer.

For instance, a sixty-six-year-old Hindu man, born in Sri Lanka but living in the UK since the age of eighteen years, had a diagnosis of schizophrenia. His underlying model of illness was based on Ayurvedic principles that emphasize imbalance of certain humours. To control his auditory hallucinations he used lime juice, a 'cold' food to treat excess bile (a 'hot' condition). However, whenever he became very unwell, he took Western medicine (neuroleptic drugs) that helped his voices. He held that biomedical treatments helped symptoms although they did not treat the underlying cause (in this case a humoral imbalance). Hence, underlying explanatory models did not directly predict health-related behaviour.

We would take issue with this sort of work, that attempts to elicit patients' explanatory models or beliefs about illness. How useful are these for clinical practice and do they relate to what people actually do? Is there any evidence that taking into account patients' explanatory models improves satisfaction with treatment? There are other problems with this type of qualitative research deploying semi-structured interviewing. Qualitative health research often fails to distinguish between normative statements (what people say they should do), narrative reconstructions (biographically specific interpretations of past events) and actual practices. Bourdieu (1980) points out the inherent normative bias of responses to questioning. Questionnaires raise special issues in anthropology on account of the difference in culture between questioner and respondent. Literacy, rules of speech, privacy and secrecy may affect the design administration and usefulness of these questionnaires. If an utterance is understood as reflecting a belief, it must be assumed to be made sincerely. Hahn (1973: 215) talks of the ethnography of sincerity; we are constantly in doubt about what natives really believe. All discourse is located in social relationships and assertions about illness experience are typically embedded in narratives concerning life and suffering.

The Need for Observation

It is not enough to elicit our informants' statements about illness. What we need is to observe what they actually do in practice. Beliefs and actions are not separate. They are embodied and derive from actions. Explanations are problematic in themselves. How do they relate to subsequent actions? Questionnaires cannot pick up our informants' concepts about illness. We need to discover knowledge in action rather than normative statements about what is appropriate or possible. Such knowledge cannot be obtained without extensive fieldwork.

Social anthropology has a distinctive approach to gathering and interpreting data deriving from the underlying assumptions of the nature of social reality and social action (Lambert and McKevitt 2002). Two key features of this approach are an emphasis on holism and participant observation. Holism is the assumption that for any particular outcome or phenomenon to be explained, there are a great many inter-related factors at work. A social institution cannot be understood in isolation from other social institutions. Medical anthropologists are likely to collect data about economic features, social relationships including kinship and marriage, religion and political systems. To this extent, anthropologists are often critical of other disciplines that adopt simple explanations for illness and health-care responses. On account of this holistic approach, medical anthropologists are expected to learn the language of their informants, to perform general descriptive research of their fieldwork location and to understand the social institutions and social structure before specifically focusing on illness. This is necessarily a time-consuming process as it can take many months to become familiar with all the relevant cultural features in a given community setting. The most characteristic research strategy deployed by social anthropologists is participant observation – direct observation while participating in a study community including interviewing and extensive observation of events and of naturally occurring discussions. This also includes elicitation of narratives of illness episodes that may reveal the logic linking specific events over time. In terms of methodology, medical anthropologists traditionally interview informants. They not only ask but also observe what is going on through participant observation. This may be time-consuming and expensive, but it is the only way to understand what our informants understand about sickness and how it informs their health-seeking actions. Knowledge cannot be obtained without extensive fieldwork. Medical anthropologists focus on specific pathologies and explore the explanatory models, taxonomies and a variety of other areas of cultural knowledge in relation to the topical focus.

So, can there be any compromise between using structured and semi-structured interviewing and full anthropological fieldwork involving participant observation in a community? In the last ten years, largely deriving from medical anthropology's involvement in public health programmes, there has been a move to Rapid Ethnographic Assessment Procedures. These aim to produce basic data for designing health-care intervention programmes for specific health problems such as diarrhoea within a few weeks, using a systematic set of questions and methods. Proponents of this approach argue that many health-care programmes have been initiated without any sort of 'culture-specific map' (Scrimshaw and Hurtado 1987). The extensive version of the holistic approach is rejected in favour of a more limited style of multifactor research. In this genre of research, it is assumed that some descriptive materials are already available so that researchers do not have to spend time obtaining it. There is an emphasis on specific questions and observations about the illness.

This approach has often been resisted by anthropologists who refer to it as 'quick and dirty' applied research that lacks the in-depth holistic contextual approach upon which anthropological research should be based. Of course, over a period of time, there would be more and better information. However, I would argue that these rapid assessment procedures or focused ethnographic studies can produce a lot of useful data quickly and are useful for applied research such as that involved in public health programmes. Rapid assessment techniques are not ideal in an academic sense but are a useful way of obtaining information quickly in a health-care setting.

Conclusion

This chapter has examined the limitations of the belief paradigm in medical anthropology. I would agree that the term is overused in medical anthropological writing. It is important to be aware that representing other cultures in terms of belief authorizes the position and knowledge of the anthropologist. The characterization of others' beliefs can be seen to play a validating role similar to that of missionaries who described native religious beliefs. The crisis of representation in anthropology has increasingly questioned the position of the anthropologist in relationship to the groups of people he/she studies and writes about. The use of the term 'belief' has become more self-conscious and ironic. The concentration on folk beliefs has excluded analytic attention to the role of socio-political factors in health care. Synchronic analyses of the cognitive, affective and behavioural dimensions of local health systems have often ignored the relationships between local and global power relations that produce and shape sickness. An attempt to redress this issue can be found in the writings of critical medical anthropologists (see Taussig 1980; Frankenberg 1988). As Keesing, a social anthropologist, points out: 'Cultures do not simply constitute webs of significance, systems of meaning that orient humans to one another and their world. They constitute ideologies, disguising human political and economic realitiesy Cultures are webs of mystification as well as significance' (Keesing 1987: 161).

For example, hunger may become medicalized as 'nerves', as has been described in Brazil (Scheper Hughes 1988), the concern of biomedicine rather than a political and social concern. Beliefs about illness may function as ideologies. This misrepresentation is in keeping with the interests of the hegemonic class, although the processes by which these misrepresentations occur often remain unexplored. Similarly, Gramsci points out how cultural forms render existing social relations 'natural'. However, the relation between ideology and praxis is problematic. Eagleton (1991)[2] discusses how ideologies are often seen as action-oriented sets of beliefs rather than speculative theoretical systems. In order to be successful, ideology must work both practically and theoretically. However, ideologies may distract from action rather than bring about practical activity.

The idea of belief gives primacy to the individual actor as the site of disease and the source of rational and irrational behaviour reproducing the epistemology of the biosciences. Perhaps Lupton (1994: 14) is correct in her assertion that medical anthropology has suffered from its close links with biomedicine and its need to appear institutionally useful, with medical anthropologists acting as cultural translators or public relations personnel in health-care settings. The focus has been on an understanding of the way in which patients construct illness and their experience of it, hence providing doctors with a tool for better diagnosis and enhanced understanding of the experience of illness. 'Folk' illness is considered an inferior version of real biomedical illness. We continue to use terms such as 'folk' and 'primitive' in relation to the beliefs of our patients, be it those who are well educated or less educated, as Stoeckle and Barsky (1981: 233) pointed out twenty years ago. They argue: 'In their avoidance of the social criticism, perspective for fear of losing access to the health arena, medical anthropologists have often supported hegemonic ideologies supporting medical assumptions and have neglected the macro, socio-economic perspective for a more politically neutral micro level of analysis.' However, the situation is slowly changing with the developments of critical medical anthropology.

Notes

1. The notion of belief is problematic for some social anthropologists. Some authors (e.g. Needham 1972) have criticized the notion of belief, arguing that the study of belief entails a number of problems: how do we know what people really believe? Is it relevant what they believe, or is it the statement of belief which is important to the anthropologist? Is belief an internal state inaccessible to the ethnographer? Asad (1983) argues that the emphasis on belief as an interior state was specific to a modern private religiosity. There is evidence that the term 'belief' may not have counterparts in the ethnopsychological language of many societies. Good (1994) points out how we have 'knowledge' whereas the cultures we study hold 'beliefs'. Recently, the term 'belief' has been replaced by the term 'cultural knowledge' by cognitive anthropologists. For the purposes of this chapter, I hold that beliefs are real phenomena held in the minds of informants.
2. Eagleton (1991) in his book *Ideology* discusses the various uses of the term 'ideology' in sociological thought and in my opinion successfully clarifies a very confusing topic. The term 'ideology' has various meanings, ranging from a body of ideas characteristic of a particular group or social class to false ideas that help to legitimate a dominant political power.

References

Asad, T. 1983. 'Anthropological Conceptions of Religion: Reflections on Geertz', *Man* 18: 237–59.

Bandura, A. 1986. *Social Foundations of Thought and Action: A Social Cognitive Theory*. Englewood Cliffs, NJ: Prentice-Hall.

Becker, M. 1974. 'The Health Belief Model and Personal Health Behaviour', *Health Education Monographs* 2: 324–508.

Bloch, M. 1998. *How We Think They Think: Anthropological Approaches to Cognition, Memory and Literacy*. Boulder, CO: Colorado Press.

Boyer, P. 2001. *Religion Explained: The Human Instincts That Fashion Gods, Spirits and Ancestors*. London: William Heinemann.

Burrow, S. 1993. 'The Treatment and Security Needs of Special Hospital Patients: A Nursing Perspective', *Journal of Advanced Nursing* 18: 1267–78.
Chan, L., A. Kleinman and N. Ware. 1994. *Health and Social Change in International Perspective.* Boston: Department of Population and International Health, Harvard School of Public Health.
Churchland, P. and T. Sejnowski. 1989. 'Neural Representation and Neural Computation', in L. Nadel and P. Cooper (eds), *Neural Connections, Mental Computations.* Cambridge, MA: MIT Press.
Connor, M. and P. Norman (eds). 1998. *Predicting Health Behaviour.* Buckingham: Open University Press.
D'Andrade, R. 1976. 'A Prepositional Analysis of US American Beliefs About Illness', in K.A. Baso and H. Selby (eds), *Meaning in Anthropology.* Albuquerque: University of New Mexico Press.
Dein, S. 2001. 'The Use of Traditional Healing in South Asian Psychiatric Patients in the UK: Interactions Between Professional and Folk Psychiatrists', *Transcultural Psychiatry* 38: 245–59.
Eagleton, T. 1991. *Ideology: An Introduction.* New York: Verso.
Evans-Pritchard, E.E. 1937. *Witchcraft, Oracles and Magic Among the Azande.* Oxford: Oxford University Press.
Fishbein, M. and I. Azjen. 1975. *Belief, Attitude, Intention and Behaviour: An Introduction to Theory and Research.* Boston: Addison-Wesley.
Frankenberg, R. 1988. 'Rejoinder', *Medical Anthropology Quarterly* 2: 454–59.
Garro, L. 1986. 'Decision Making Models of Treatment Choice', in S. McHugh and T.M. Vallis (eds), *Illness Behaviour: A Multidisciplinary Model.* New York: Plenum Press.
Good, B. 1986. 'Explanatory Models and Care Seeking: A Critical Account', in S. McHugh and T.M. Vallis (eds), *Illness Behaviour: A Multidisciplinary Model.* New York: Plenum Press.
______. 1994. *Medicine, Rationality and Experience: An Anthropological Perspective.* Cambridge: Cambridge University Press.
Hahn, R. 1973. 'Understanding Beliefs: An Essay on the Statement and Analysis of Belief Systems', *Current Anthropology* 14: 207–29.
Holy, L. and M. Stuchlik. 1983. *Actions, Norms and Representations: Foundations of Anthropological Enquiry.* Cambridge: Cambridge University Press.
Keesing, R. 1987. 'Models "Folk" and "Cultural": Paradigms Regained', in D. Holland and N. Quinn (eds), *Cultural Models in Language and Thought.* Cambridge: Cambridge University Press.
Kleinman, A. 1980. *Patients and Healers in the Context of Culture: An Exploration of the Borderland Between Anthropology, Medicine and Psychiatry.* Berkeley, CA: University of California Press.
Lambert, H. and C. McKevitt. 2002. 'Anthropology in Health Research: From Qualitative Methods to Multidisciplinary', *British Medical Journal* 325: 210–13.
Last, M. 1981. 'The Importance of Knowing About Not Knowing', *Social Science and Medicine* 15: 387–92.
Lepowsky, M. 1990. 'Sorcery and Penicillin: Treating Illness on a Papua New Guinea Island', *Social Science and Medicine* 30: 1049–63.
Lewis, G. 1975. *Knowledge of Illness in a Sepik Society.* London: Athlone Press.
Lloyd, K., K. Jacob and V. Patel. 1998. 'The Development of the Short Explanatory Model Interview (SEMI) and Its Use Among Primary-Care Attenders with Common Mental Disorders', *Psychological Medicine* 28: 1321–27.

Lupton, D. 1994. *Medicine as Culture: Illness, Disease and Body in Western Societies*. London: Sage.
Morsy, S. 1990. 'Political Economy in Medical Anthropology', in T. Johnson and C. Sargent (eds), *Medical Anthropology: A Handbook of Theory and Method*. New York: Greenwood Press.
Myntti, C. 1988. 'Hegemony and Healing in Rural North Yemen', *Social Science and Medicine* 27: 515–20.
Needham, R. 1972. *Belief, Language and Experience*. Oxford: Basil Blackwell.
Nunally, J. 1961. *Popular Conceptions of Mental Health*. New York: Holt, Rinehart & Winston.
Ohnuki-Tierney, E. 1984. *Illness and Culture in Contemporary Japan*. Cambridge: Cambridge University Press.
Omark, R. 1980. 'Nervous Breakdown as a Folk Illness', *Psychological Reports* 47: 862.
Paul, B. 1955. *Health, Culture and Community: Case Studies of Public Reactions to Health Programs*. New York: Russell Sage Foundation.
Pandolfi, M. 1990. 'Boundaries Inside the Body: Women's Sufferings in Southern Peasant Italy', *Culture, Medicine and Psychiatry* 14: 255–73.
Pelto, P.J. and G.H. Pelto. 1997. 'Studying Knowledge, Culture and Behaviour in Applied Medical Anthropology', *Medical Anthropology Quarterly* 11: 147–63.
Priest, R., C. Vize and A. Roberts. 1996. 'Lay People's Attitudes to Treatment of Depression: Results of Opinion Poll for Defeat Depression Campaign Just Before Its Launch', *British Medical Journal* 313: 858–59.
Rippere, V. 1981. 'How Depressing: Another Cognitive Dimension of Commonsense Knowledge', *Behaviour Research and Therapy* 19: 169–81.
Scheper-Hughes, N. 1988. 'The Madness of Hunger: Sickness, Delirium and Human Need', *Culture, Medicine and Psychiatry* 12: 429–58.
Scrimshaw, S. and E. Hurtado. 1987. *Rapid Assessment Procedures for Nutrition and Primary Health Care: Anthropological Approaches to Improving Programme Effectiveness*. Tokyo: United Nations University, UNICEF and UCLA.
Stoeckle, J. and A. Barsky. 1981. 'Attributions: Uses of Social Science Knowledge in the "Doctoring" of Primary Care', in L. Eisenberg and A. Kleinman (eds), *The Relevance of Social Science for Medicine*. Dordrecht: D. Reidel, pp. 223–30.
Taussig, M. 1980. *The Devil and Commodity Fetishism*. Chapel Hill, NC: University of North Carolina Press.
Weinman, J., K. Petrie, R. Moss-Morris et al. 1996. 'The Illness Perception Questionnaire: A New Method for Assessing the Cognitive Representation of Illness', *Psychology and Health* 11: 431–45.
Weiss, M. 1997. 'Explanatory Model Interview Catalogue (EMIC): Framework for Comparative Study of Illness', *Transcultural Psychiatry* 34: 235–63.
Weiss, M.G., D.R. Doongaji, S. Siddhartha et al. 1992. 'The Explanatory Model Interview Catalogue (EMIC): Contribution to Cross-Cultural Research Methods from a Study of Leprosy and Mental Health', *British Journal of Psychiatry* 160: 819–30.
Williams, B. and D. Healy. 2001. 'Perceptions of Illness Causation Among New Referrals to a Community Health Team: Explanatory Model or Explanatory Map?', *Social Science and Medicine* 53: 465–76.
Young, A. 1981. 'When Rational Men Fall Sick: An Enquiry into Some Assumptions Made by Medical Anthropologists', *Culture, Medicine and Psychiatry* 5: 317–35.
______. 1982. 'The Anthropologies of Illness and Sickness', *Annual Review of Anthropology* 11: 257–85.

Young, J. 1978. 'Illness Categories and Action Strategies in a Tarascan Town', *American Ethnologist* 5: 81–97.

______. 1981. *Medical Choice in a Mexican Village*, New Brunswick, NJ: Rutgers University Press.

Young, J. and L. Garro. 1982. 'Variation in the Choice of Treatment in Two Mexican Communities', *Social Science and Medicine* 16: 1453–66.

Conclusion

Paracletes, Pathologists

The invitation to reprint some papers, from a period extending over the last twenty years, inevitably presumes questions of contemporary relevance and context. Are our various themes and arguments significant today? New patterns of individual pathology have continued to emerge for which that link between private virtue and public order which social anthropology explores remain of central importance: in its studies of gender, society, cultural representation and symbolism, religion, and social and individual power. It will be evident here that we consider the ideas of earlier social scientists – Durkhein, Evans-Pritchard, Lévi-Strauss – to be still of interest.

Our current medical education involves little of the concerns of social anthropology. Much of the recent work in cultural psychiatry (comparative psychiatry, transcultural psychiatry – whatever you want to call it) comes from historians interested in how psychiatric categories have emerged, or else from social activists concerned with equity in treatment. With the decline of the Culture and Personality school in the United States in the 1950s, there has no longer been any central paradigm of society and mental illness. The successor interests, which have emerged from the Culture and Personality school include cognitive anthropology and the anthropology of emotions and of the self, both already topics for European social anthropology. More pragmatic and epidemiological concerns have resulted in 'global mental health' which downplays theory in favour of health economics, the necessary alleviation of distress, with cross-national qualitative studies and the examination of the individual experience of mental illness (e.g. Kirmayer and Minas 2000; Luhrmann and Morrow 2017). Questions of the universality of the patterns of distress and therapy identified in Western societies have been generally put aside. At times cultural psychiatry threatens to relapse into qualitative medical sociology or ethnographic journalism. The very notion of 'therapy' has been pursued through a historical and literary lens (e.g. Young 1995).

The more recent editions of the Diagnostic and Statistical Manual of Mental Disorders (DSM), the standard American nosology, themselves a reaction to its earlier attempts at classification through psychoanalytic theory, have been criticized for pursuing the old biomedical idea of discrete and bounded categories of disease. An interesting alternative is the idea of affective circulation pursued by our colleague Sushrut Jadhav in which we follow the ideas and consequences of a psychological state through the human and natural worlds (a little like the 'pigs for the ancestors' cybernetic anthropology of the 1950s) to sketch out a non-essentialized notion of psychopathology and thence to a future post-human anthropology: this would yield a field-based characterization of a pattern rather than one based on detailing attributes (although one could if one wishes then correlate one with the other).

Cultural psychiatry textbooks now largely rehearse earlier work and earlier conclusions (e.g. Tseng 2001). The neglect of variation in psychopathology has resulted in a return to the presumption that the pattern identified in Euro-American societies is the fundamental and universal prototype, so that the *dhat* syndrome of South Asia (Choudhury 2020) is generally regarded as a variant of anxiety disorder. The cultural underpinnings of disorders in the West are ignored in favour of individual and psychological variables.

Particularly in American medical anthropology, there has been a shift from seeing the specification of the identified syndrome as of central interest (as it is in DSM) to a concern with the ethical dilemmas and political constraints of medical provision and policy. The anthropological commentor has been ascribed a role as a moral critic of biomedicine, with the beliefs of local communities now understandable but remaining at variance with the goals of medicine, and the sympathetic physician still relying on their own current ethical concerns. This is perhaps reminiscent of the way in which colonial anthropology, at one level, served the interest of imperial governance. Medical anthropologists have been critically aware of this, whilst simultaneously carrying it out, leaving them in the position of a not very efficient advocate, advisor and guide to the oppressed. The parallels and continuity between the colonial order and 'international mental health' are, we believe, striking.

Interest in differences in cultural response to different types of therapy has resulted in the new provision of psychotherapy for refugees and migrant and minority communities in the West (Kareem and Littlewood 1992; Ababio and Littlewood 2019), using an eclectic psychotherapy that confronts racism. In France, there is still interest in the utility of pre-migration indigenous healing in the new context. What is the meaning and efficacy of local healing practice particularly among migrant groups? How do therapeutic practices themselves migrate (Martin 2024)? How does 'therapy' itself overlap with lifestyle and individual religious conversion? What does it mean to say religion 'heals'? And what is the role of self-help groups and single-issue therapy practices? How is their approach to biomedical or social aetiologies maintained?

The former interest in culture specific patterns – the 'culture-bound syndromes' (Simons and Hughes 1985) – is now seen as an exotic or trivial interest in what for West European was the striking characteristic of non-Western societies. But they were exotic in that they explored the strange boundaries between what appeared to be medical illness and the social order. They represented salient issues of a particular community's dilemmas or contradictions, as extreme if sometimes contentious representations of human distress in its distinctive milieu. To essentialize such social dramas as a medical disease independent of local meaning or other experience of distress is certainly to render them exotic curiosities. To ignore them altogether is to leave human adversity bland and familiar, to affirm that the European's experience alone is true, and thus to naturalize the patterns of our Western psychiatric illness, to affirm them as transcending our intentions, as necessary and immutable.

And if we avoid all salient considerations of the naturalistic and personalistic logics (Body: Soul?) of our central antinomy and merely ram them both together, we perhaps end in the ultrahuman and religious. Culture-bound syndromes are fundamental in that they are concerned with such questions as personhood, identity, consciousness, social order, distress and death. Recent confrontations by LGBTQ+ activists have stimulated interest in the old anthropological concerns with the question of sex/gender and, together with new developments in biomedical technologies, again with 'nature' versus 'culture'. Non-binary genders evoke new patterns of personal and family life, recalling past studies of two-spirit (berdache) societies with their 'third sex' (Littlewood 2002a). A greater acceptability of sperm donor tracing recalls concern with 'genetic sexual attraction' (post-adoption incest [Greenberg and Littlewood 1995] and through that back to nineteenth-century anthropology's fascination with incest. Considering the work on culture-specific patterns of psychopathology, we might examine how they pass, modified or not, from one individual to another, and from one milieu to another (Littlewood 1988; Lipsedge and Littlewood 1997), for example eating disorders, body image disorder and dysmorphophobia: their relationships to transgender issues, new ways of parenting and non-biological kinship.

And what, if any, are the links between self-adornment, tattooing, self-mutilation, self-harm, self-sacrifice and martyrdom? Emergent intentional communities, with their particular patterns of affiliation and control, demand revision of our existing models of social structure and support. With the onset of technological forms of modernity and increased globalization, communities previously isolated by geography, culture or religion demand new consideration of hybrid identities. The recent return to authoritarian politics in Europe and elsewhere prompts a reconsideration of the old Culture and Personality studies on charisma and leadership, of which the examination of medical conspiracy theories is just a part of the relationship between leader and follower, not to mention the social imagery of resentment, retribalization, nostalgia and the salient mistrust of representative government, in a turn to political violence and frank paranoia. And of course, there is the resurgence of religion itself, once condemned to oblivion by secular social scientists: the emergence of Evil as postulated by certain Protestant groups in combination with an enthusiasm for 'neoliberal' capitalism necessitating questions of personal agency and justice which link into the fights against abortion rights and women's ownership of their bodies. Did identity politics fuel neoliberalism? No single disciplinary approach by itself can provide an adequate analysis of any of these.

The current popularity of the idea of 'trauma' would argue for an interest in its history, epistemology and presumed explanation of political crises, let alone personal predicaments and academic notions of causality. How do particular disciplinary proceedings, such as forensic diagnostic interviews and parole board hearings, recall other patterns examined by anthropologists, such as witchcraft confessions? And warfare? How are restraints in war maintained with new technologies? Does the resolution of the blood feud (Chapter 7) offer any clues for negotiation in contemporary large-scale conflicts? And continuing unresolved issues such as the possible link between purity norms and individual obsessionality? And, more daringly, experience in new off-world environments such as space stations where conventional idioms of, say, privacy and pollution are being challenged (Parkhurst and Jeevendrampillai 2024).

How can we understand the increasing medicalization of 'normal' everyday distress (see for instance Pickersgill 2014 on DSM-5): ADHD, gambling, 'sex addiction' and so on? What impact will the rapprochements between culture and biology, recent advances in neuroscience and genetics, have on our understanding of the cultural basis of mental illness? (Kirmayer, Lemelson and Cummings [2017] have made an interesting contribution to this question.) There needs to be a move in cultural psychiatry away from the notion of 'culture' itself to examine how structural constraints, power and the resources and constraints on medical care impact individual illness experience: from cultural competency to structural competency (McGuinness and Lipsedge 2022; Kaiser and Kohrt 2019).

Finally, what of religion? What social frameworks have developed to help individuals make sense of adversity in secular society? Are there secular theodicies: the psychologist as the new priest? What are the secular forms of such religious notions as apocalypticism? Climate anxiety? Do religious frameworks really enable coping with suffering and how does this differ across societies (Dein 2013)?

If cultural psychiatry has recently restricted itself to issues of equity, to the fair and adequate provision of mental health services to disadvantaged and minority groups, medical anthropology has also concentrated on illness recognized by Western medicine and media, ignoring issues of social cognition, local epistemologies and nosologies (see Jenkins and Barrett 2004, for an exception).

Both trends are of course essential. They are of course likely to obtain government funding and provide teaching and career opportunities. But compared to some older, now neglected interests, they are perhaps less exciting.

References

Ababio, B. and R. Littlewood (eds). 2019. *Intercultural Therapy: Challenges, Insights and Development*. London: Karnac/Routledge.

Choudhury, A. 2020. *Koro: Clinical and Social Developments in the Culturally Defined Sexual Retraction Syndrome*. Cham: Palgrave Macmillan.

Dein, S.L. 2013. 'Religion and Mental Health: The Contribution of Anthropology', *World Psychiatry* 12: 34–35.

Folmer, S. and G.K. Palmes. 2009. 'Cross-Cultural Psychiatry in the Field: Collaboration with Anthropology', *Journal of the American Academy of Child and Adolescent Psychiatry* 48: 873–75.

Greenberg, M. and R. Littlewood. 1995. 'Post-Adoption Incest and Phenotypic Matching: Experience, Meanings and Biosocial Implications', *British Journal of Medical Psychology* 68: 45–62.

Jenkins, J.H. and R.J. Barrett. 2004. *Schizophrenia, Culture and Subjectivity*. Cambridge: Cambridge University Press.

Kaiser, B.N. and B.A. Kohrt. 2019. 'Why Psychiatry Needs the Anthropologist: A Reflection on 80 Years of Culture in Mental Health', *Psychiatry* 82: 205–15.

Kareem, J. and R. Littlewood (eds), 1992. *Intercultural Psychotherapy: Themes, Interpretations and Practice*. Oxford: Blackwell.

Kirmayer, L.T. and H. Minas. 2000. 'The Future of Cultural Psychiatry: An International Perspective', *Canadian Journal of Psychiatry* 45: 438–45.

Kirmayer, L.T., R. Lemelson and C.A. Cummings (eds). 2015. *Re-Visioning Psychiatry: Cultural Phenomenology, Critical Neurosciences and Global Mental Health*. Cambridge: Cambridge University Press.

Kleinman, A. 1998. *Rethinking Psychiatry: From Cultural Category to Personal Experience*. New York: Free Press.

Lipsedge, M. and R. Littlewood. 1997. 'Psychopathology and Its Public Sources: From a Provisional Typology to a Dramaturgy of Domestic Sieges', *Anthropology and Medicine* 4: 25–43.
Littlewood, R. 1988. 'La Migration des Syndromes Liés à la Culture', *Psychopathologie Africaine* 20: 5–16.
———. 2002a. 'Three into Two: The Third Sex in Northern Albania', *Anthropology and Medicine* 9: 37–50.
———. 2002b. 'Military Rape', in R. Littlewood, *Pathologies of the West: An Anthropology of Mental Illness in Europe and America*. Ithaca, NY: Cornell University Press.
Luhrmann, T. and J. Morrow. 2017. *Our Most Troubling Madness: Case Studies in Schizophrenia Across Cultures*. Berkeley: California University Press.
McGuiness, T. and M. Lipsedge. 2022. 'Excited Delirium, Acute Behavioural Disturbances, Death and Diagnosis', *Psychological Medicine* 52: 1601–11.
Martin, K. 2024. 'Culture and Class in Contemporary Chinese Psychotherapy', *Anthropology Today* 40: 7–9.
Parkhurst, A. and D. Jeevendrampillai. 2025. 'Yesterday's Coffee Is Tomorrow's Coffee', in R. Lynch, J. Calabrese and R. Littlewood (eds), *Matter Out of Place: Anthropological Explorations of Bodies, Dirt and Morality*. Oxford: Berghahn.
Pickersgill, M.D. 2014. 'Debating DSM-5: Diagnosis and the Sociology of Critique', *Journal of Medical Ethics* 40: 521–25.
Simons, R.C. and C.C. Hughes. 1981. *The Culture Bound Syndrome: Folk Illness of Psychiatric and Anthropological Interest*. Dordrecht: Reidel.
Skultans, V. and J. Cox. 2000. *Anthropological Approach to Psychological Medicine*. London: Jessica Kingsley.
Tseng, W. 2001. *Handbook of Cultural Psychiatry*. San Diego: Academic Press.
Young, A. 1995. *The Harmony of Illusions: Inventing Post-Traumatic Stress Disorder*. Princeton, NJ: Princeton University Press.

Index

www.ingramcontent.com/pod-product-compliance
Ingram Content Group UK Ltd.
Pitfield, Milton Keynes, MK11 3LW, UK
UKHW021825130926
8597IPUK00004B/16